The Prevention of Oral Disease

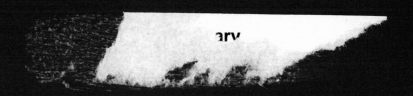

The Prevention of Oral Disease

Fourth Edition

Edited by

J. J. Murray CBE

Emeritus Professor of Child Dental Health and
Former Dean of Dentistry University of Newcastle upon Tyne

J. H. Nunn

Professor of Special Care Dentistry, Trinity College, Dublin

J. G. Steele

Senior Lecturer in Restorative Dentistry
University of Newcastle upon Tyne

OXFORD

UNIVERSITY PRESS

OXFORD
UNIVERSITY PRESS

Great Clarendon Street, Oxford OX2 6DP

Oxford University Press is a department of the University of Oxford.
It furthers the University's objective of excellence in research, scholarship,
and education by publishing worldwide in

Oxford   New York

Auckland Bangkok Buenos Aires Cape Town Chennai
Dar es Salaam Delhi Hong Kong Istanbul Karachi Kolkata
Kuala Lumpur Madrid Melbourne Mexico City Mumbai Nairobi
Sao Paulo Shanghai Taipei Tokyo Toronto

Oxford is a registered trade mark of Oxford University Press
in the UK and in certain other countries

Published in the United States
by Oxford University Press Inc., New York

First edition published 1985
Second edition published 1989
Third edition published 1996
This edition first published 2003
Reprinted 2004, 2007

A catalogue record for this title is available from the British Library

Library of Congress Cataloging in Publication Data
(Data available)

ISBN 978-0-19-263279-1

10 9 8 7 6 5 4

Typeset by Cepha Imaging Private Ltd, Bangalore, India
Printed in Great Britain
on acid-free paper by
Ashford Colour Press Ltd, Gosport, Hampshire

Preface to the Fourth Edition

This book was conceived almost twenty years ago. Its aim was to gather together the scientific evidence concerning the prevention of dental disease. Subsequent editions built on this aim and expanded the scope of the book. Now the primary importance of prevention in all aspects of disease is generally accepted and it is time for the book to take a different direction. I am delighted that two colleagues, June Nunn and Jimmy Steele, have agreed to join me in developing this fourth edition. They have been instrumental in developing the shape of the book. Many changes have been made; some authors of chapters in the first edition have agreed that others should be given the opportunity to present information in their chosen field of expertise. I am most grateful to them for enabling this book to develop over the twenty year period.

The manuscript of this book was edited, and the proofs corrected, at a time of personal difficulty and sadness. This edition is dedicated to the memory of Valerie Murray (28.04.1943-19.08.2002) and Professor Gerald Winter (24.11.1928-22.12.2002). Their love and support, friendship and guidance, sustained me for over thirty years.

Newcastle upon Tyne   J. J. M.
February 2003

Preface to the Third Edition

When the idea of this book was first suggested in the early 1980s its main aim was to concentrate on the prevention of dental caries and periodontal disease. One reviewer, although complimentary overall, suggested that the book would have been improved by including a chapter on the prevention of trauma. I rejected this idea immediately—as I felt the reviewer had not understood the main purpose of the book.

The second edition reflected developments in the field of prevention, chapters on dental health education, root caries, and other problems affecting the dentition in middle and old age, and the difficulties in preventing dental disease in handicapped persons were added.

In planning the third edition it became obvious that if more chapters were to be added, then considerable revision of existing material was required. Professor Crispian Scully kindly agreed to write a chapter on the prevention of diseases of the oral mucosa. A chapter by Dr Richard Welbury on the prevention of trauma has been included (the reviewer of the first edition, Professor Dennis Picton, obviously had a clearer idea of where the book should be developing than I did!), and Professor Aubrey Sheiham has contributed a chapter on the prevention of oral disease from an international perspective. Dr Jimmy Steele, who has recently completed a study of the elderly in Salisbury, Darlington, and Richmondshire, provided a chapter on ageing in perspective. Unfortunately, Professor Emeritus J.R.E Mills died in January 1995 after a long illness. He suggested to me some time ago that a new author should review the topic 'Preventive orthodontics'. Dr Peter Gordon kindly agreed to prepare a chapter on 'The prevention of malocclusion'.

A final section has been added, looking briefly at the oral health needs in the twenty-first century.

In order to accommodate these changes, my chapter on 'Dental caries—a genetic disease?' has been omitted from the new edition. The sections on diet and fluorides and their effect on dental caries have both been reduced, partly by editing the text and partly by eliminating some of the references. For a fuller consideration of these topics the reader is referred to Andrew Rugg-Gunn's book, *Nutrition and dental health* or to the third edition of our book, *Fluorides in caries prevention*.

The title of the book has been changed slightly to *The Prevention of Oral Disease* to reflect the wider remit of the third edition.

The first edition was essentially a 'Newcastle' book in that a majority of contributors were either working in, or had worked at, Newcastle Dental School and Hospital. The present list of authors covers eight dental schools. I hope that this edition will be accepted as a 'British' contribution to our knowledge about the prevention of oral disease.

Newcastle-upon-Tyne   J.J.M
March 1995

Preface to the Second Edition

In the five years since the first edition was prepared the impetus for the prevention of dental disease has increased. Reviews of the book have been generally favourable, but in some cases pointed out areas that might have been included in a text on the prevention of dental disease. Most reviewers appreciated that the aim was not to provide details of clinical techniques but rather to concentrate on documented evidence. This general aim has been maintained: chapters on dental health education, root caries and other problems affecting the dentition in middle and old age, and the difficulties involved in preventing dental disease in handicapped persons have been added. The chapter on fissure sealants has been expanded so that the question of cost-effectiveness of preventive techniques can be considered in greater detail. The downward trend in dental caries in developed countries has been reviewed, together with a consideration of changes in child and adult dental health over the last 20 years, as found by results from national surveys. The implications of providing a preventively oriented service to deal with rapidly changing levels of oral disease are considered against a back-ground of dental services that have developed from a curative base.

I am most grateful to Mr J.R. McCarthy, Chief Dental Adviser, Dental Estimates Board, for providing me with details from the Board's Annual Reports, to Ms Diana Scarrott, Under Secretary, British Dental Association, for information on the General Dental Services, and most especially to Miss Sally Baldwin, who has been responsible for the secretarial work involved in compiling this second edition.

Newcastle-upon-Tyne   J.J.M.
September 1988

Preface to the First Edition

The Survey of Children's Dental Health in England and Wales in 1973 showed that over 90 per cent of our children leave school with untreated dental disease and over 50 per cent have had at least one general anaesthetic for dental treatment. This high level of dental disease seems to have been accepted with equanimity by the public at large, as though it were inevitable. It means that in adult life, at best a large amount of repair is required to maintain teeth in the mouth, at worst, that decayed teeth must be extracted. The extent of the problem can be judged by the fact that 30 per cent of all adults aged 16 years and over in Britain have no natural teeth at all.

And yet, and yet. Are things changing?

Over the last ten years there has been an increasing emphasis on good dental health and a number of encouraging reports, not only from Britain, but also from America, Australia, Scandinavia, and other European Countries that dental caries is decreasing in children. The idea is gaining round that dental disease is not inevitable, but preventable and that the possibility of keeping one's teeth for life is not just for the lucky few but is possible for almost everyone.

I was delighted to be given the opportunity of trying to draw together some of the main factors involved in the prevention of dental disease and am most grateful to my colleagues for agreeing to contribute the various chapters which make up this book. We do not attempt to cover all dental disease but concentrate on the prevention of dental caries and periodontal disease in order to draw together the available clinical and epidemiological information. In many instances we have referred to previous publications and have reproduced diagrams from other workers: due acknowledgement is made in the text. We would also like to thank our publishers for their help and encouragement. If our present knowledge could be translated into practice the impact on dental health would be immense and the practice of dentistry would change considerably. We hope that this book will help in some small way to encourage the movement towards prevention.

Newcastle-upon-Tyne   J.J.M.
January 1983

Acknowledgements

I would like to thank Oxford University Press for encouraging me to develop the theme of the prevention of oral disease. This book has been produced in line with Oxford University Press' latest thinking on the production of books for both undergraduate and postgraduate students. The number of references for each chapter has been reduced markedly; instead key references are now included at the end of each chapter. A series of key words or bullet points have been built in to each chapter in order to direct the reader to the main issues.

Part of the material on fluoride dentifrices was first published in the third edition of *Fluorides in Caries Prevention* and I thank Butterworth-Heinemann for permission to reproduce this material. Diagrams from the national surveys of child and adult dental health have been reproduced by kind permission of Miss Jean Todd and the Government statistical services. Our thanks go to the editors of Archives of Oral Biology, British Dental Journal, Caries Research, and the World Health Organization for permission to reproduce illustrations. Thanks go also to Emma Tavender, Review Group Co-ordinator, Cochrane Oral Health Group, for permission to publish summaries of topical fluoride reviews. Figures 17, 18, and 19 in Chapter 3 are reproduced by kind permission of the NHS Centre for Reviews and Dissemination.

I am most grateful to Mrs Judy Preece, Audio-Visual Centre, Newcastle University for the way she has interpreted my incomprehensible squiggles over many years, particularly for drawing Figures 1.3 and 16.6 in this edition.

Finally, I thank all contributors and their secretaries for their help, and most especially Mrs Helen Cox, who has been responsible for most of the secretarial work involved in the compiling of this edition.

To provide the opportunity for everyone to retain a healthy functional dentition for life, by preventing what is preventable and by containing the remaining disease (or deformity) by the efficient use and distribution of treatment resources.

Aim of the Dental Strategy Review Group,
Towards Better Dental Health HMSO 1981

The retention throughout life of a functional, aesthetic natural dentition of not less that 20 teeth (shortened dental arch) and not requiring recourse to a prosthesis.

The Goal of Oral Health
WHO 1982

Oral Health is a standard of health of the oral and related tissues which enables an individual to eat, speak and socialize without active disease, discomfort and embarrassment and which contributors to general well being.

Oral Health Strategy Group 1994

The ethos of preventive dentistry should prevail in every clinical department.

The First Five Years,
General Dental Council 2002

Contents

List of Authors

Dr P H Gordon
Child Dental Health
School of Dental Sciences
University of Newcastle
Framlington Place
Newcastle upon Tyne NE2 4BW

Professor P A Heasman
Restorative Dentistry
School of Dental Sciences
University of Newcastle
Framlington Place
Newcastle upon Tyne NE2 4BW

Dr A Hegarty
Oral Medicine & Special Needs Dentistry
Eastman Dental Institute for Oral Health Care Sciences
University College London
256 Gray's Inn Road
London WC1X 8LD

Mr W M M Jenkins
Consultant in Periodontology
Glasgow Dental Hospital & School
378 Sauchiehall Street
Glasgow G2 3JZ

Professor E Kidd
Professor of Cariology
King's College London
Floor 25 Guy's Tower
Guy's Hospital
London SE1 9RT

Dr P J Moynihan
Child Dental Health
School of Dental Sciences
University of Newcastle
Framlington Place
Newcastle upon Tyne NE2 4BW

Professor J J Murray CBE
Emeritus Professor of Child Dental Health
University of Newcastle
Framlington Place
Newcastle upon Tyne NE2 4BW

Professor J H Nunn
Department of Public & Child Dental Health
Dental School & Hospital
Lincoln Place
Trinity College
Dublin

Dr N M Nuttall
Dental Health Services Research Unit
University of Dundee
Dental School
Park Place
Dundee DD1 4HN

Professor R R B Russell
Oral Biology
School of Dental Sciences
University of Newcastle
Framlington Place
Newcastle upon Tyne NE2 4BW

Professor C Scully CBE
Dean
Eastman Dental Institute for Oral Health Care Sciences
University College London
256 Gray's Inn Road
London WC1X 8LD

Dr L Shaw
Senior Lecturer & Consultant in Paediatric Dentistry
School of Dentistry
University of Birmingham
St Chad's Queensway
Birmingham B4 6NN

Professor A Sheiham
Department of Epidemiology & Public Health
University College London
Gower Street Campus
1-19 Torrington Place
London WC1E 6BT

Dr J G Steele
Restorative Dentistry
School of Dental Sciences
University of Newcastle
Framlington Place
Newcastle upon Tyne NE2 4BW

Professor A W G Walls
Restorative Dentistry
School of Dental Sciences
Framlington Place
Newcastle upon Tyne NE2 4BW

Dr R Watt
Department of Epidemiology & Public Health
University College London
Gower Street Campus
1-19 Torrington Place
London WC1E 6BT

Professor R R Welbury
Department of Child Dental Health
Glasgow Dental Hospital & School
378 Sauchiehall Street
Glasgow G2 3JZ

Dr J M Whitworth
Restorative Dentistry
School of Dental Sciences
University of Newcastle
Framlington Place
Newcastle upon Tyne NE2 4BW

1

Oral health in the twenty first century

Oral health in the twenty first century

John Murray

Introduction

The aim of this book is to draw together current epidemiological and clinical knowledge on the prevention of oral and dental diseases in order to highlight the tremendous improvement in oral health, which would occur if a preventive philosophy underpinned our approach to oral disease.

The mouth contains a number of different tissues, some of which, such as mucous membrane, connective tissue, blood vessels, nerves, muscle, and bone, are found throughout the body. Any of these tissues can suffer from infection, trauma, degeneration, or neoplastic change. Of overwhelming importance to the condition of the mouth are its two specialized tissues—the teeth and the periodontium. Indeed, dental caries and periodontal disease are so widespread that virtually everybody in the world, certainly every adult, has either one or both of these conditions.

A considerable amount is known already about how to prevent both dental caries and periodontal disease, and this is detailed in Chapters 2–7. This would not only affect dramatically their prevalence but also, if this knowledge was applied, there would be a dramatic effect on the rate at which they progress, so that the vast majority of people would be able to keep their mouths in reasonable condition for the whole of their lives. Chapters 2–7 are concerned with dental caries and periodontal disease.

Over the last 20 years marked reductions in the prevalence of dental caries in children have been observed in Britain, and many other industrialized countries, and there is now strong evidence that this reduction in caries has resulted in improvements in the dental condition of young adults. Secular decline in caries is referred to in Chapter 15.

About 2000 new cases of oral cancer occur in Britain each year, although in some countries, particularly in Asia, the prevalence of this disease is much higher. Treatment of oral cancer and other oral mucosal diseases requires specialist hospital services. Chapter 10 considers the prevention of oral mucosal disease and highlights the importance of two of the risk factors, alcohol and tobacco, involved in oral cancer.

A World Health Organization perspective

Although the prevalence of dental diseases and the provision of dental services varies in different countries, the same underlying general principles of prevention must apply throughout the world. The World Health Organization has pointed out the potentially disastrous consequences of a rise in dental caries in developing countries (Fig. 1.1). The provision of dental treatment consumes economic resources and requires highly trained personnel. The only possible way forward in improving oral and dental health for all, is to reduce the prevalence of disease.

The WHO considered the present global situation with respect to oral diseases that occur in and affect the oral cavity in a document *Oral health for the 21st Century,* and also in a Technical Report, *Recent advances in oral health* (1992). These reports examined the trends and advances in oral health research, delivery of oral care, and the education of personnel for oral care related to changes in the attitudes and demands of members of the community. The conclusion was that oral health services and education of personnel will need to be radically transformed. Less technical/manual skills will be needed, due in part to new technology, and more special skills in diagnosis, pathophysiology, disease risk, assessment and management, and communication will be required. The Expert Group identified 12 guiding principles:

1. Oral health is an essential part of human function and the quality of life.
2. Oral health status should be improved and maintained in the most economical manner consistent with quality and access.

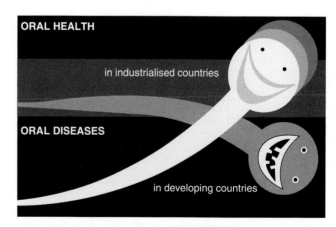

Figure 1.1 'Healthy mouths for all by the year 2002'—part of a World Health Education poster. (World Health Organization 1984.)

3. Prevention is preferable to treatment as a general rule.

4. Individuals should do as much as possible for themselves to achieve and maintain oral health.

5. Caries and periodontal diseases can be prevented and controlled.

6. Community methods of prevention should be supportive of individual and personal care, and in some situations are more efficient.

7. Oral health care should be provided in the context of comprehensive care.

8. Oral health care providers should be prepared and motivated to consider general health, and should participate in the provision of general health care.

9. The type, number, and distribution of oral health care personnel should be maintained at levels consistent with need, quality, cost, and access necessary to achieve desired oral health status.

10. Planning, health care practices, and educational programmes should be appropriate for the population or situation in question.

11. Research, evaluation, and education are essential for the continued advancement of oral heath.

12. Learning must continue throughout the career of the health professional.

These recommendations are comprehensive and should underpin any oral health strategy.

Resources, treatment, and prevention

There is a dynamic relationship between the natural history of any disease and the response by society in trying to combat the problem. As far as dental disease is concerned, in Britain and in many other countries, the historical response to a carious tooth was to extract it. This was usually a painful and hazardous procedure performed by untrained operators. Society's response was to encourage the development of professional skills and to allow the practice of dentistry to be limited to those who had received appropriate training. As knowledge and skill increased, attention turned to the preservation of teeth and the treatment of caries by restoration rather than extraction. This trend from extraction to restoration depended not only on the skill of the dental professional but also on the reaction of society with respect to the economic resources that individuals and government were prepared to commit to dental treatment, and the attitude of individuals to the advice proffered by professionals. Real improvements in health can only occur when both the community at large and the health professionals share the same objectives, which surely should be the primary prevention of disease.

Simplistically, the progress of dentistry can be represented as one in which there is movement from extraction to restoration and onwards to prevention (Fig. 1.2). The main thrust of this book is to gather together information on diet, fluoridation, preventive measures for the individual, and oral hygiene, all of which would have an effect on the prevention of the two main dental diseases, caries and periodontal disease. It would be facile however, to assume that these measures alone can exert a beneficial effect without appreciating that they can only work within a favourable framework agreed by society. Patient's attitude, dentist's attitude, remuneration, and manpower all have a crucial role to play in the prevention of dental disease.

Demographic changes mean that other conditions assume a great significance; for example, as people retain teeth for longer, they become exposed to increasing wear and this is covered more extensively in this edition. Changing priorities, as well as increasing sophistication in care focuses attention on more vulnerable groups in society, like very old people and those with a disability (Chapters 12 and 13).

Clinical governance, evidence-based dentistry

Aspects of a preventive approach are to be found in the increasing attention being paid to clinical governance and evidence-based medicine and dentistry. The UK Government's White Paper 'A First Class Service—Quality in the new NHS' defines clinical

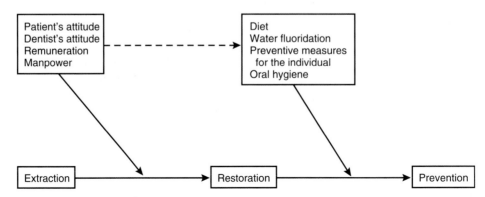

Figure 1.2 Factors affecting changes in dental treatment and prevention.

governance as 'a framework through which NHS Organisations are accountable for continuously improving the quality of their services and safeguarding high standards of care by creating an environment in which excellence in clinical care will flourish'. The drive to identify best practice means that unnecessary treatment is avoided and most appropriate care is provided, reducing the need for further intervention and prolonging the effectiveness of treatment. Chapter 16 summarizes some of the issues impinging on prevention as a result of increasing attention being paid to evidence-based dentistry.

Dental Education

Today, education is evaluated in terms of knowledge, skills, and attitudes. The general dental council uses these terms to focus on the desirable outcomes in its document on a framework for undergraduate dental education, 'The First Five Years'.

In the section on Preventive Dentistry in the second edition of TFFY, the GDC states

> Dental students should be made aware of the successes and limitations of preventive dentistry, and the potential for further progress. The ethos of preventive dentistry should prevail in every clinical dental department, so that new preventive dentistry techniques are taught to students as they become available. Students should be conversant with the practice of preventive care including oral health education and oral health promotion. Students should recognise the increasing evidence-based approach to treatment and should be able to make appropriate judgements. The student should appreciate the need for the dentist to collaborate in prevention, diagnosis, treatment and management of disease with other health care professionals and with patients themselves. The student should be aware of the economic and practical constraints affecting the provision of health care.

This book is concerned with summarizing our knowledge on important topics such as, for example, diet and nutrition, fluoride and plaque and the effect of smoking on oral health. It considers important skills relevant to the prevention of oral disease (e.g., enamel caries, maintenance of pulp vitality, trauma to anterior teeth). The *attitude* of the profession and the public toward dentistry is vital if the prevalence (and severity) of oral diseases are to be reduced, that is why an appreciation of oral health promotion and policy (Chapter 15) is essential. If further progress is to be achieved, the dental profession must extend its horizons beyond the traditional role of clinical, diagnostic and technical expertise for individual patients in the surgery, and become more aware of

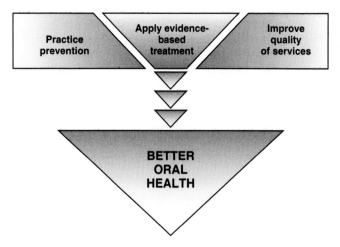

Figure 1.3 Factors involved in improving oral health.

the psychological and social factors relevant to the prevention of oral disease.

Conclusions

Figure 1.2 was first used almost 30 years ago. The movement from Extraction to Restoration to Prevention was in part meant to show the development of dental services, particularly in Britain, from the 1940s and 50s (strong emphasis on extraction and complete dentures), onwards to restoration, especially amalgam restorations in the 1960s and crowns in the 1970s, to the first shoots of prevention, noted from epidemiological studies in the 1970s and 80s.

Figure 1.3 depicts the main thrust of this book, suggesting that practising prevention, applying evidence-based treatment and improving the quality and organization of services, must all coalesce if better oral health is to be achieved.

References

World Health Organization (1987). *Alternative systems of oral care delivery*. Technical Report Series 750, Geneva.

World Health Organization (1992). *Recent advances in oral health*. Report of a WHO Expert Committee. Technical Report Series 826, Geneva.

World Health Organization (1993). *Oral health for the 21st century*. Oral Health Unit, Geneva, Switzerland.

A First Class Service: Quality in the New NHS. HMSO Command Paper 3807, December 1997.

General Dental Council (2002) *The First Five Years*, Second Edition.

2

Diet and dental caries

Diet and dental caries

Paula Moynihan

Introduction

Despite a low mortality rate associated with dental caries, it has a considerable impact on self-esteem, eating ability, nutrition, and health. Teeth are important in enabling consumption of a varied diet and preparing the food for digestion. In modern society the most important role of teeth is to enhance appearance and facial appearance is very important in determining an individual's integration into society. Teeth also play an important role in speech, being essential for making certain sounds. Dental diseases may therefore impact on diet and nutrition, facial appearance and speech. In addition, dental caries cause considerable pain and anxiety. The 1998 Adult Dental Health Survey showed that 40% of adults in the United Kingdom had experienced dental pain in the past year. Almost half of English children aged 8 years have experienced dental pain and this is associated with crying, loss of sleep, stopping playing and not eating. These factors are likely to be exacerbated in less developed societies where pain control and treatment are not readily available. Dental decay ultimately results in tooth loss, which impairs quality of life and reduces the ability to eat a varied diet, and is in particular associated with a diet low in fruits and vegetables and non-starch polysaccharides.

Dental caries is a costly burden to health care services. Dental caries is the most costly human disease in terms of treatment costs, more so than cardiovascular disease, osteoporosis or diabetes. The cost of dental treatment is unlikely to be reduced in westernized countries despite improvements in disease trends in younger people. This is because caries is progressive and requires continued care; so, the trend for increased retention of teeth into older age increases the cost of dental treatment.

The systemic effect of diet on the aetiology of dental caries

In the early half of the twentieth century, it was thought that provision of good nutrition while the teeth were developing was the principal way to prevent dental caries. It is now known that the topical effect of diet in the mouth, after the teeth have erupted plays a much more important role. However, undernutrition and deficiencies of specific nutrients do influence the development of the teeth and the formation, function and secretion of the salivary glands, which in turn influence susceptibility to dental caries.

In populations where undernutrition exists and there is moderate exposure to sugars in the diet, higher levels of caries are found in comparison to experience from developed countries. This has led to the suggestion that undernutrition may exacerbate the cariogenicity of dietary sugars. This is of concern in countries that are undergoing 'nutrition transition', i.e. countries that are moving away from their traditional diets to adopt the 'westernized diet' that is higher in free sugars and fat. It is a common misconception that a diet high in sugar promotes growth, and the importance of limiting sugars consumption in undernourished populations is often overlooked. However, there is no evidence to show that a high sugar intake is associated with growth and increasing sugar intake does not address micronutrient deficiencies.

Diet and Sugar

- A poor diet high in sugars results in dental caries
- Dental caries can result in tooth loss
- Tooth loss reduces the ability to eat a healthy diet high in fruits and vegetables and fibre rich foods
- In many low-income countries, malnutrition coexists with a high sugar intake, such countries are at higher risk of dental caries

Systemic nutritional influences on enamel developmental defects

Poor nutrition is only one of many causes of enamel developmental defects. An enamel defect that is common in undernourished communities is linear enamel hypoplasia (LEH). This usually occurs in primary incisors and is characterized by a horizontal groove usually found on the labial surface that becomes stained post-eruptively. Several investigators have shown that the presence of enamel hypoplasia is associated with undernutrition and its prevalence increases with the severity of undernutrition. However, the specific mechanism for an effect of diet on the development of enamel hypoplasia was not understood until the 1980s when the association between hypocalcaemia and hypoplasia was discovered. Hypocalcaemia is common in undernutrition and is associated with diarrhoea.

The studies of Lady May Mellanby in the early half of the twentieth century showed that vitamin D deficiency had a marked effect on the development of the teeth. Dogs reared on diets that were deficient in vitamin D had delayed development of teeth and teeth that were poorly calcified and poorly aligned. Many of the teeth showed signs of hypoplasia. Mellanby attributed the improvements in the teeth of children in Britain between 1929 and 1943 to improvements in diet and the status of vitamin D, including the introduction of cheap milk in 1934, the provision of vitamin D rich cod liver oil to pregnant and lactating mothers, infants, and young children, and the addition of vitamins A and D to margarine. More recent studies have shown that supplementation with vitamin D to pregnant mothers resulted in higher circulating calcium levels in infants at birth and lower incidence of hypoplasia in infants at age three, compared with controls who did not receive supplements.

Mellanby suggested that hypoplastic teeth were more susceptible to decay and she performed a clinical trial in which the diets of children were supplement either with cod liver oil (high in vitamins A and D), olive oil (low in vitamins A and D) or treacle. The cod liver oil supplemented children developed fewer caries over the two year study period. In more recent trials, classrooms in Canada were installed with full spectrum lighting that has a high UV output and hence promotes vitamin D synthesis in the skin. Children attending schools with the full spectrum lighting were found to develop fewer caries over the two year study period compared with children attending classrooms with conventional lighting.

The studies of Lady May Mellanby

- Showed that vitamin D deficiency impairs tooth development
- Concluded that the improved diet during the war years, with respect to vitamin and calcium intake was responsible for improved dental health
- Showed that enamel hypoplasia increased susceptibility to dental caries
- Showed that vitamin D supplementation reduced the incidence of dental caries in children

Can nutrition during tooth development influence future caries susceptibility?

Undernutrition may exacerbate the development of dental caries in three ways. First, as already mentioned, it contributes to the development of hypoplasia which in turn increases caries susceptibility. Secondly, it causes salivary gland atrophy, which results in reduced saliva flow and altered saliva composition. This reduces the buffering capacity of the saliva and increases the acidogenic load of the diet. There is also evidence that deficiency of vitamin A causes salivary gland atrophy and a consequent reduced saliva flow. Thirdly, undernutrition delays eruption and shedding of teeth which affects the caries experience at a given age. Poorly

nourished children have been shown to have 2–5 less teeth erupted compared to well–nourished children of the same age (Fig. 2.1). Stunted children have been shown to have delayed exfoliation of primary teeth and delayed eruption of permanent teeth. The prevalence of dental caries as a function of time occurs approximately 15 months later in undernourished children compared with well-nourished children (Fig. 2.2). This suggests that

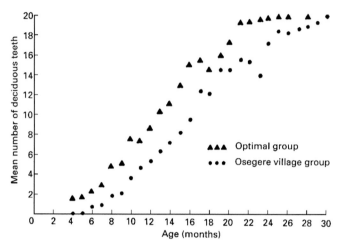

Figure 2.1 The mean number of primary teeth erupted at various ages between 4 and 30 months in well-fed Nigerian children (optimum group) and in underprivileged, malnourished children (Osegere village group). All children were from the Yoruba tribe. (Reproduced from Enwonwu 1973, with permission of the editor of *Archives of Oral Biology.*)

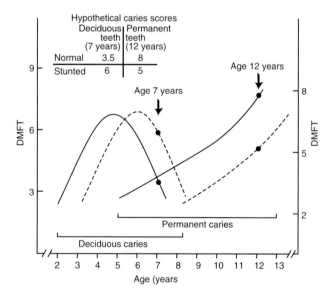

Figure 2.2 Severity of dental caries in primary and permanent dentition as a function of time. The solid lines represent the well-nourished children and the dotted lines malnourished children. (Reproduced from Alvarez and Navia (1989), with permission of the editor of *American Journal of Clinical Nutrition.*)

the higher incidence of dental caries in primary teeth of under-nourished children could partly be explained by the delayed exfoliation of these teeth. At age 12, undernourished children appear to have a lower prevalence of decay in the permanent teeth, but this is due in part to the delayed eruption of the permanent dentition.

The systemic effect of diet on dental caries

- Undernutrition is associated with hypoplasia of enamel which increases caries susceptibility
- Undernutrition results in salivary gland atrophy, reduced salivary flow rate, and reduced buffering capacity—these factors increase caries susceptibility
- Deficiency of vitamin D is associated with enamel hypoplasia and increased caries risk
- Undernutrition results in delayed shedding of the primary teeth and delayed eruption of the permanent teeth. This may influence the caries prevalence at a given age
- In undernourished populations where there is exposure to sugars in the diet, caries prevalence is higher than expected from observations in well-nourished populations

Post-eruptive effect of diet on the development of dental caries: is intake of dietary sugars still an important cause of dental caries?

There is a wealth of evidence to show the role of dietary sugars in the aetiology of dental caries. The evidence comes from many dif-ferent types of investigations, including human studies (both observational and interventions), animal studies, human plaque pH studies, enamel slab, and incubation studies of oral bacteria and dietary substrates *in vitro*. Collectively, information from all the different types of studies provides an overall picture of the car-iogenic potential of different dietary carbohydrates. The strength of the evidence incriminating sugars in the aetiology of dental caries comes from the multiplicity of the studies rather than the power of any one study alone.

Fifty years ago, dietary issues relevant to dental health largely focused on dietary sugar (in particular sucrose) and although sugars are undoubtedly the most significant dietary factor in the aetiology of caries, modern diets also contain an increasing array of fermentable carbohydrates including highly refined starches, fructose syrups, glucose polymers, and synthetic oligosaccharides. More information is also available about the effect of other com-ponents of the diet on the interaction between sugars and dental caries (i.e. protective factors including fluoride). In this chapter the term 'sugars' refers to total sugars in general and the term 'sugar' refers to sucrose.

Evidence for a relationship between diet and dental caries comes from different types of studies

- Human intervention studies (clinical trials)
- Human observational studies
- Animal experiments
- Plaque pH studies
- Enamel slab experiments
- Incubation studies

World-wide epidemiological observational studies

Sugar intake and levels of dental caries can be compared at a between-country level. Sreebny (1982) correlated the dental caries experience of primary dentition (dmft) of 5 and 6-year-olds with sugar supplies data of 23 countries, and dental caries experience (DMFT) of 12-year-olds to sugar supplies data of 47 countries. For both age groups, significant correlations were observed: $+0.31$ for the primary dentition and $+0.7$ for the permanent dentition—meaning that 52% of the variation in caries levels could be explained by the per-capita availability of sugar. From these data it was calculated that for every 25 g of sugar per day, one tooth per child would become decayed, missing or filled. In countries with an intake of sugar below 18 kg/person per year (equivalent to ~50 g/person/day) experience of caries was consistently below DMFT 3. The countries with sugar supplies in excess of 44 kg/person per year (120 g/person/day) had significantly higher levels of caries (see Fig. 2.3).

A later analysis conducted in 1994, did not find such a strong association between per capita sugar availability and mean DMFT of 12-year-olds in developed ($n=29$) and developing ($n=61$) countries. However, the reason for an absence of any relationship between sugar supply data and mean DMFT in developed countries was because with such very high availabil-ity of sugar in these countries, changing the level of sugar intake by a few kilograms per year does not influence the caries chal-lenge. Availability still accounted for 28% of variation in levels of dental caries and 23 of the 26 countries with sugars availabil-ity below 50 g/day had mean DMFT values for 12-year-olds of below 3. Whereas only half of the countries with sugar avail-ability above this level had achieved DMFT<3. The weaker association between per capita sugar availability and levels of caries in industrialized countries may partly be accounted for by the fact that many sugars other than sucrose are contributing to total sugars intake. For example, in the USA there is a signif-icant use of high fructose corn syrup (similar to invert sugar) and in other industrialized countries the use of glucose syrups, fruit juice concentrates, and glucose polymers is becoming widespread.

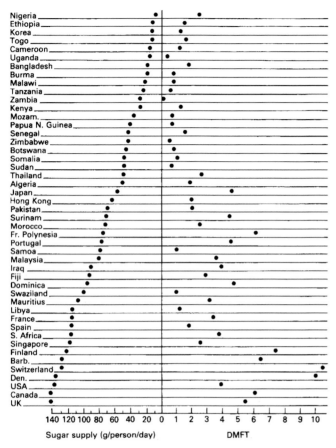

Figure 2.3 Caries experience (DMFT) of 12-year-old children and sugar supply (g/person/day in 47 countries. (Data from Sreebny 1982.)

Table 2.1 Consumption (g/person per day) of Sugar- and Flour-containing Foods in Tristan da Cunha

	1938	1966
Sugar	1.8	150
Cakes and biscuits	0.5	24
Jam and condensed milk	0.2	20
Bread	1.7	
White flour		110
Sweets and chocolates	0	50

intake and this is associated with a marked increase in dental caries. Examples of such populations include the Alaskan Inuit, Sudan and Ethiopia, Ghana and Nigeria, and the Island of Tristan da Cunha (see Rugg-Gunn 1993 for a review). Inhabitants of the Island of Tristan da Cunha had a diet very low in sugar prior to 1940 when a trading store opened on the Island. The store sold imported sugar and sugar-containing foods and the marked increase in the consumption of such imported foods can be seen in Table 2.1. The dental records of the inhabitants from before and after the opening of the store show very low caries in 1937 but a steady increase in dental caries levels in all age groups between 1937 and 1966 (Fig. 2.4).

Do dental caries patterns change following changes in availability of dietary sugars?

Populations that had reduced sugar availability during the Second World War showed a reduction in dental caries, which subsequently increased again when the restriction on sugar was lifted. The annual caries increment in the first molars between 1941 and 1958 has been shown to mirror annual sugar consumption in many countries including Japan, Norway, Scandinavia, Switzerland, and New Zealand. Although these data were collected before widespread exposure to fluoride, a reduction in dental caries was observed between 1943 and 1949 in areas of North England with both high and low water-fluoride concentrations. It should be noted that during the Second World War, a reduction in intake of sugar was not an isolated dietary change and that intake of other carbohydrates, e.g. refined flour, was also restricted.

Isolated communities with a primitive way of life and a consistently low sugar intake have very low dental caries levels. As such societies increase trade with industrialized countries they shift towards habits and diets associated with modern living (known as 'nutrition transition') including a marked increase in sugars

Do people who habitually consume a high sugars diet have higher levels of dental caries?

There is evidence to show that many groups of people with habitually high consumption of sugars also have levels of caries higher than the population average. Examples include confectionery industry workers and children with chronic diseases requiring long-term sugar-containing medicines. Studies have shown up to 71% higher caries in confectionery industry workers than factory workers from other industries. This holds true even in countries such as Finland where there is good exposure to fluoride. Some medical conditions such as phenylketoneuria require diets that are high in refined sugars. There have been few studies of such groups; yet, existing reports do not show an increased level of caries. However, children on long-term sugared medicines have been shown to have higher caries experience compared with healthy children.

Do people who habitually consume a low sugars diet have lower levels of dental caries?

Low dental caries experience has been reported in groups of people who have a habitually low intake of dietary sugars; for example, children of dentists, children in institutions where strict dietary regimens are followed and children with hereditary fructose intolerance (HFI). Despite reports by parent dentists of restricted intake of sugars by their children, the low dental caries experience of these children cannot be assumed to be due to low sugars intake alone as oral hygiene and other preventive care is likely to be greater in these children.

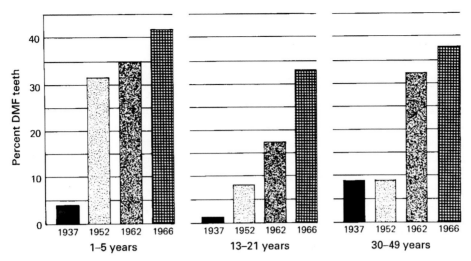

Figure 2.4 Caries severity (per cent DMFT) in three age groups of inhabitants of Tristan da Cunha at four examinations between 1937 and 1966.

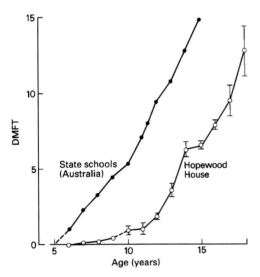

Figure 2.5 Caries experience (DMFT) in children in Hopewood House (with SEM) and children in state schools of South Australia. (Data from Marthaler, 1967 with permission of the editor of Caries Research.)

Children living in the Hopewood House children's home in New South Wales received annual dental surveys between 1947 and 1962. The children followed a strict lacto vegetarian diet that was low in sugars and refined flour, however, oral hygiene was virtually absent and fluoride exposure was low. Dental caries levels were much lower than in children of the same age and socio-economic background attending state schools in New South Wales (Fig. 2.5); 46% of 12-year-olds in Hopewood house were caries-free compared with 1% of the children from state schools. However, after 12 years of age, when the children's association with the home ended, the rate of caries increased to levels observed in children from the state schools.

A weakness of the data from observations of populations is that changes in intake of sugars are often associated with changes in the intake of refined flour, making it impossible to attribute changes in dental caries solely to changes in the intake of sugars. A good exception to this are the data from studies of children with HFI. HFI is a congenital deficiency of fructose-1-phosphate aldolase, and consumption of fructose results in nausea and hypoglycaemia; hence all foods containing fructose and sucrose are excluded from the diet. People with HFI therefore have a low intake of sugars but, as glucose is tolerated they are not restricted on intake of starch. Studies have shown that subjects with HFI have a low intake of sugars and a higher than average intake of starch, yet a low caries experience.

Cross-sectional comparisons of diet and dental caries levels in populations

Numerous cross-sectional epidemiological studies from many countries, have related sugars intake with dental caries levels at one point in time. Those published before the early 1990s have been summarized by Rugg-Gunn (1993). All studies varied widely in methodology and means of reporting the findings, making drawing of overall conclusions complicated. Nine out of 21 studies that compared weight of sugars consumed to caries increment found significant associations and the remaining 12 did not. Twenty-three out of the 37 studies that investigated the association between frequency of sugars consumption and caries levels found significant relationships and 14 failed to find an association. Some cross-sectional studies have also considered tooth brushing habits and exposure to fluoride as well as sugars intake. In most studies, all these factors have been shown to be important determinants of caries levels and in some, level of sugars intake is considered the most important factor. For example Granath et al. (Granath 1978) compared the level of dental caries in over

500 4-year-old Swedish children to sugars consumption, fluoride supplementation and oral hygiene practices. Intake of sugars was the most important factor associated with dental caries, and differences in dental caries experience of children with the highest and lowest in-between meal sugars intake could not be explained by difference in use of fluoride or oral hygiene practices. When the effects of oral hygiene and fluoride were kept constant the children with a low sugars intake in between meals had 86% less buccal and lingual caries and 68% less approximal caries than children with high intakes of sugars in between meals.

The National Diet and Nutrition Survey (NDNS) of young people aged 4–18 years collected information on diet and dental health on a representative sample of children in England, Wales, and Scotland in a cross-sectional survey. No overall relationship between the amount of sugars consumed and levels of dental caries were observed. When children were divided into high, medium, or low bands of sugars consumption, no significant relationship was found between caries experience and band of sugars intake. However, in the 15–18-year-old age group, the upper band of intake of sugars were more likely to have decay than those in the lower band (70% compared with 52%). Children who consumed sugared confectionery (sweets/candies) daily were also more likely to have decay than those who consumed it less frequently and those with a high frequency of carbonated soft drink consumption were more likely than non-consumers to have caries in the primary dentition. However, this relationship was not observed for the permanent dentition. Those that consumed three or more cups of sugared tea or coffee daily were more likely to have caries experience (Walker *et al.* 2000).

When considering the finding of these cross-sectional surveys, it is important to consider that dental caries develops over time and, therefore, simultaneous measurements of disease levels and diet may not give a true reflection of the role of diet in the development of the disease. It is the diet several years earlier that may be responsible for current caries levels. Cross-sectional studies should, therefore, be interpreted with caution. This phenomenon is less of a problem in young children, whose diet may not have changed significantly since the eruption of the primary dentition and several studies of young children have found associations between intake of sugars or high sugars foods and levels of caries. The NDNS of 1.5–4.5 year old children (Hinds and Gregory 1995) showed that the strongest determinants of dental health were social factors such as the level of household income and level of education of mothers. However, when social factors were controlled for, associations were also found between household expenditure on confectionery, frequency of consumption of confectionery and soft drinks, and high average intake of sugar confectionery and soft drinks.

Longitudinal studies of diet and caries incidence

Stronger evidence for a relationship between diet and dental caries is acquired from studies that have assessed sugars eating habits over time in relation to changes in dental caries experience over that time period. This type of study is relatively more costly and time consuming and in comparison to the number of cross-sectional studies in the literature, this type of study is relatively rare. Stecksen-Blicks and Gustafsson measured caries increment over one year in 8 and 13-year-old children and related it to diet at one time point (Stecksen-Blicks and Gustafsson 1996). Despite the short period of observation, a significant relationship between caries development and intake of sugars was found for both the primary and permanent dentition. In a more recent study (i.e. in the era of exposure to fluoride) of the causes of caries in the primary dentition, Grindefjord *et al.* observed caries levels in a cohort of young children between the ages of 1 to 3.5 years (Grindefjord *et al.* 1996). A significant relationship between the consumption of confectionery and sugar-containing beverages and caries increment was found.

In a comprehensive study of caries intake and diet of over 400 English adolescents (aged 11–12 years) (Rugg-Gunn *et al.* 1984) a small but significant relationship was found between intake of total sugars and caries increment over two years (+0.2).

The Michigan Study was carried out in the USA between 1982 and 1985 and studied the relationship between sugars intake and dental caries increment over three years in children initially aged 10–15 years (Burt *et al.* 1988). This study also found weak relationships between the amount and frequency of intake of dietary sugars. Children who consumed a higher proportion of their total dietary energy as sugars had a higher caries increment for approximal caries, though there was no significant association between sugars intake and pit and fissure caries. The frequency of intake of sugars or sugar-containing foods (with >15% sugars) was not related to caries increment but the amount of sugars eaten in between meals was related to approximal caries. When the children were divided into those who had a high, compared with a low, caries increment, a tendency towards more frequent snacking was seen in the high caries children. However, intake of sugars was generally high for all subjects in this study with only 20 out of 499 children consuming less than 75 g/day, and the average intake of the lowest quartile of consumption being 109 g/day or 23.4% of energy intake. The reason for the low relative risk of caries development in the high sugars consumers was that small variances were found both for caries increment and intake of sugars.

A review by Marthaler (1990) pointed out that many older studies failed to show a relationship between sugars intake and development of dental caries because many of these were of poor methodological design, used unsuitable methods of dietary analysis, and were of insufficient power. Correlations between individuals' sugars consumption and dental caries increments may be weak due to the limited range of sugars intake in the study population–variation in sugars intake within populations is too low to show an effect on caries occurrence. There is more between-country variation in intake of sugars which explains the stronger association between sugar availability and dental caries levels found from analysis of world wide data (Sreebny 1982).

Epidemiological studies of the sugars/caries relationship

- A positive relationship exists between per capita sugar availability and DMFT at age 12 years
- A marked increase in the prevalence and severity of dental caries has been observed in populations who move away from their traditional way of eating and adopt a westernized diet, high in sugars
- Sub-groups of the population who habitually consume a high sugars diet have been shown to have higher levels of dental caries compared to the general population
- Sub-groups of the population who habitually consume a low sugars diet have been shown to have lower levels of dental caries compared with the general population
- Caution is needed when interpreting the findings of cross-sectional studies that have compared diet to levels of dental caries at one time point, since caries develops over time. It may be the diet several years previous which is responsible for current disease levels
- Studies with a longitudinal design, that measure diet and relate it to change in levels of dental caries over time provide stronger evidence
- Human intervention studies provide the strongest evidence for an association between diet and diseases, however, these are difficult to conduct from an ethical and logistic point of view

Human intervention studies

Human intervention studies where intake of sugars has been altered and caries development monitored are rare, partly due to the problems inherent in trying to prescribe diets for the long period of time necessary to measure changes in caries development. Those that have been reported are now decades old and were conducted in the pre-fluoride era on highly selected groups of people, before the strong link between sugars and caries was established. Such studies would not be possible to repeat today because of ethical constraints.

The Vipeholm study

The Vipeholm study was conducted shortly after the Second World War in an adult mental institution in Sweden between 1945 and 1953 (Gustafsson *et al.* 1954). The study investigated the effects of consuming sugary foods of varying stickiness (i.e. different oral retention times) and at different times throughout the day on the development of caries by measuring caries increment in subjects who consumed (1) refined sugars with a slight tendency to be retained in the mouth at meal times only (e.g. sucrose solution, chocolate) (2) refined sugars with a strong tendency to be retained in the mouth at meal times only (e.g. sweetened bread) (3) refined sugars with a strong tendency to be retained in the mouth, in between meals (e.g. toffee). The subjects were divided into 6 groups (and two groups were subdivided into male and female); these are listed in Table 2.2. The dietary regimes were given in two periods. The first carbohydrate period was between 1947 and 1949 and the second carbohydrate period in which the regimens were changed slightly ran between 1949 and 1951. The dental caries increments of the 6 groups are shown in Figure 2.6.

Main conclusions of the Vipeholm study

- Sugar intake, even when consumed in large amounts, had little effect on caries increment if it was ingested up to a maximum of four times a day at mealtimes only
- Consumption of sugar in-between meals was associated with a marked increase in dental caries
- The increase in dental caries activity disappears on withdrawal of sugar-rich foods
- Dental caries experience showed wide individual variation

The significance of mealtime consumption of sugars is also that salivary flow rate is greater at mealtimes due to stimulation by other meal components and therefore plaque acids may be more rapidly neutralized.

The study had a complicated design and subjects were not randomly assigned to groups (as groups were determined by wards to separate dietary regimens). A period of vitamin supplementation occurred for 1.5 years prior to the carbohydrate periods as at this time it was thought that dental caries may be a deficiency disease. The period of vitamin supplementation was too short to properly monitor the effects on caries development and was inconclusive. The study was carried out on adults in a situation where it was possible to prescribe dietary regimen. As adults, the subjects may have been more resistant to caries (as enamel is fully mineralized) and a more marked effect may have been observed if children had been studied. The fluoride concentration in the drinking water was 0.4 ppm (low) and the study was carried out before use of fluoride in dentifrices.

The Turku sugar studies

A second important intervention study was the Turku study. This was a controlled longitudinal study carried out in Finland in the 1970s (Scheinin and Makinen 1975). The study investigated the effect of almost total substitution of sucrose in a normal diet with either fructose or xylitol on caries development, but evidence from the control group can be used as indirect evidence for the impact of sugar on the development of caries. Three groups of subjects (n = 125 in total) aged 12–53 years, with 65% being in their twenties, consumed a diet sweetened with either sucrose, fructose, or xylitol for a period of 25 months and dental caries increment was monitored blind at six-month intervals by one person throughout the study and both carious cavities and pre-cavitation lesions were monitored. Foods were specially manufactured for the fructose and xylitol groups and intake of starch was not restricted but subjects were asked to avoid sweet fruits such as dried fruits since sugars in these foods could not be substituted. The xylitol group consumed xylitol-containing foods significantly less frequently than the sucrose or fructose groups consumed their sweetened foods and the overall intake of xylitol in the xylitol group was lower than that of sucrose or fructose in the other groups. An 85% reduction in dental caries was observed in the xylitol group who had removed sugar from their diet. The findings are summarized in Table 2.3 and Figure 2.7. The

Table 2.2 Summary of the Vipeholm Study (Gustaffson *et al.* 1954)

Group	Males (n)	Females (n)	Outcome
Control (low sugar diet)	60		Caries increment almost nil. Increase in sugar in second carbohydrate period was accompanied by a small but significant increase in caries.
Sucrose at meals. 300 g/d reduced to ~150 g in second period	57		No significant increases in dental caries increment. Though slightly higher than in 1946.
Sweet bread at meals 345 g at afternoon coffee in period 1 and then at 4 mealtimes in period 2	41	42	Significant increase in caries increment in second carbohydrate period—significant for males only.
Chocolate 300 g sucrose at meals in first period. Then 110 g at meals and 64 g chocolate (30 g sugar) in four portions between meals	47		Caries increment was low in first carbohydrate period but increased significantly in the second period. In subjects aged < 30 there was a three fold increase in caries.
Caramel Stale sugar rich bread during first year of first period. Second year of first period 22 caramels (70 g sugar) in two between meal portions. First year of second period 22 caramels per day in four portions	62		Dental caries was unchanged during the first year. Consumption of caramels led to a significant increase in caries increment, so much that caramels were with drawn in the first year of second period. Withdrawal resulted in fall in caries increment to previous level.
8 toffees/d First year, first period low carbohydrate high fat diet. Then 8 toffees a day (40 g sugar) in second year first period at breakfast and lunch only. In second period given in between meals. Sucrose solution was taken at meals so sucrose intake was equal to other groups	40		First year, first period caries increment was low. Significant increase in caries in all three years when toffees were consumed. Greatest in third year.
24 toffees/d First period 24 toffees available throughout day. **Toffees stopped at end of first period.**	48		A very marked rise in dental caries increment during first period. Consumption of toffees was higher in females and so was caries increment. Issue of toffees was stopped before end of first period (because of increased caries) and consumption in-between meals was not allowed. This led to marked decrease in caries increment.

conclusions of the Turku study are that substitution of sucrose with xylitol resulted in a markedly lower dental caries increment in both cavities and at the pre-cavitation stage.

Animal experiments

Animal experiments designed to investigate the relationship between dietary sugars and dental caries most commonly use the rat model; however, mice, hamsters, and monkeys have also been used. Animal experiments have enabled study of different types, concentrations, and frequencies of carbohydrates and sugars under specified conditions. It would not be possible to test such dietary regimens in humans due to problems of palatability and compliance.

The importance of the local effect of sugar in the mouth was clearly demonstrated in studies where rats were fed a cariogenic diet either conventionally via the stomach or by a stomach tube (Table 2.4). The salivary glands of some of the animals in each group had been removed. The results demonstrate (1) the importance of the local presence of sugars in the mouth and (2) the important role of saliva in protecting against dental caries.

The precise control of frequency of feeding a cariogenic diet became possible when the Zurich Dental Institute developed an automatic feeding machine. This enabled food to be given to animals at defined times and under-feeding ensured that the animals ate all of the feed provided. In such studies a clear positive relationship between frequency of feeding and caries severity was seen (Table 2.5). Animals fed ad libitum consumed 11.7 g food per day which was nearly twice the 6 g fed to other groups in whom frequency was controlled. The results show that frequency of eating a cariogenic diet is more important than the overall amount consumed.

Another important factor is the amount of time between food intakes. In an experiment where animals received 18 portions of feed per day, one group received 3×6 portions, with no time between consumption of the 6 portions. The second group had a 30 minute interval between each of the 18 portions. Caries development was greater in the latter group.

Animal experiments have also been used to examine the effect of concentration of sugars in the diet. A large number of studies have shown that diets containing some sugar (~10%) cause more caries than sugar-free diets, further increases in caries have not always been seen when the sugar concentration is increased above 10%. Results have varied due to the type of diet used and also according to whether or not the rats were super infected with cariogenic organisms. The non-sugar components of the diet are important; as little as 2–5% sugar causes caries if the base diet

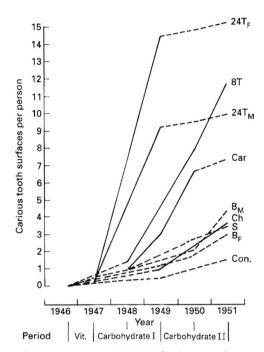

Figure 2.6 Caries experience (DMFT) for the control group and eight test groups as recorded at the seven or eight examinations between 1946 and 1951. Solid line indicates that the subjects ate sugar both at and between meals; interrupted line indicates subjects received sugar only at meals. (Reproduced from Gustaffson *et al.* 1954, with permission of the editor *Acta Odontologica Scandinavica*.)

Table 2.3 The baseline conditions of the 115 subjects who completed the 2-year Turku sugar study

	Group		
	Fructose	Sucrose	Xylitol
Total clinical and radiographic carious surfaces	13.9	11.0	13.4
Filled surfaces	29.4	27.3	29.8
DMFS	48.0	42.1	50.7
Number of subjects	35	33	47
Mean age (years)	26.2	27.2	29.1

contains ~5% starch whereas almost 5 times as much sugar is required when the base diet is high in fat. Caries severity has been shown to increase with increasing sugars concentration up to a level of 40% in rats super infected with *S. mutans* and *Actinomyces viscosus* (Fig. 2.8).

Some animal studies have shown that sucrose is more cariogenic than other mono and disaccharides; however, in these studies animals were inoculated with *Streptococcus mutans*. Some strains of streptococci utilize sucrose preferentially to other sugars and do not thrive in its absence. Experiments in which animals are

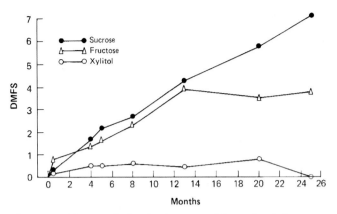

Figure 2.7 The cumulative development of decayed, missing or filled surfaces including cavitation and pre-cavitation carious lesions, diagnosed both clinically and radiographically, but not including secondary caries. At 24 months, differences between all groups were statistically significant ($p < 0.01$). (Scheinin and Makinen 1975, with permission of the editor *Acta Odontologica Scandinavica*.)

Table 2.4 The mean number of carious lesions in rats fed a cariogenic diet either conventionally or by stomach tube. The salivary glands of some of the animals in each group had been removed. Number of animals in each group is given in parentheses

	Conventional	Tube fed
Intact	6.7 (13)	0 (13)
Desalivated	28.8 (4)	0 (3)

infected with such bacteria are likely to exaggerate differences between the carcinogenicity of sucrose compared with other sugars. In three out of four experiments sucrose was more cariogenic than glucose or fructose, but the differences were small. There was no difference in the carcinogenicity of glucose and fructose. In monkeys, sucrose has been shown to have a similar carcinogenicity to glucose/fructose mixes, whereas fructose was less cariogenic than sucrose. Drinking water containing 20% glucose syrup (a product of starch hydrolysis) has been shown to be less cariogenic than 20% sucrose in drinking water.

Animal studies have added to the knowledge of the sugars/caries relationship by showing:

- A clear relationship between frequency of consumption of a cariogenic diet and severity of dental caries
- Increasing caries with increasing sugars concentration
- Little difference in the cariogenicity of glucose, fructose and maltose and increased cariogenicity of sucrose only when animals are super infected with *S. mutans*

Table 2.5 The mean caries severity, daily food intake and weight gain in five groups of rats fed at different frequencies per day; six animals per group

Group	Eating frequency/day	No. of fissure lesions	Daily food intake (g)	Weight gain during experiment (g)
1	12	0.7	6	23
2	18	2.2	6	34
3	24	4.0	6	28
4	30	4.7	6	29
5	*Ad libitum*	4.2	11.7	64

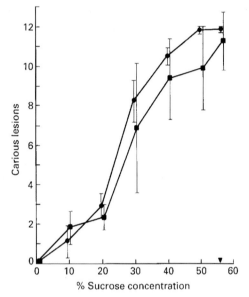

Figure 2.8 Incidence of carious lesions (±SE) in fissures (●) and smooth surfaces (■) in rats fed ad libitum, diets containing 0, 10, 20, 30, 40, 50, and 56 per cent sucrose. (Reproduced from Hefti and Schmid 1979, with permission of the editor *Caries Research*.)

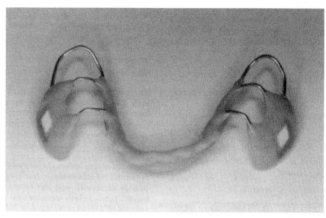

Figure 2.9 An example of an acrylic resin appliance showing two buccal flanges each containing a terylene mesh-covered slab of enamel. (Illustration kindly supplied by E.I.F. Pearce; reproduced with permission of the editor of *New Zealand Dental Journal*.)

Enamel slab experiments

Enamel slab experiments use oral appliances that hold slabs of bovine or human enamel. Plaque forms on the enamel slabs that remain in the mouth for 1 to 6 weeks. The slabs are exposed to the dietary factor being tested, by either consumption with the slabs *in situ* or by removal of the appliances several times a day to dip into vessels containing the dietary test substances. Changes in enamel hardness or degree of demineralization may be measured at the end of the experimental period. An example of an appliance made to fit over mandibular teeth is shown in Figure 2.9. Enamel slab experiments have shown that sugars cause demineralization, while non-fermentable non-sugar sweeteners aid remineralization. Increasing the concentration of sugars, and the frequency of exposure to sugars increases demineralization. The advantage of enamel slab experiments over *in vitro* incubation experiments or *in vivo* plaque pH experiments is that they measure demineralization and

not just acidogenic potential and also account for the protective role of saliva.

Plaque pH studies

Plaque pH studies measure changes in the pH of plaque following consumption of a carbohydrate or carbohydrate-containing food. They measure acidogenic potential, which is taken as an indirect measure of cariogenic potential, although acidogenicity does not take into account protective factors in foods consumed and, salivary factors that may modify the carcinogenicity of a food.

Plaque pH studies usually employ one of four methodologies. First, metal probes are used, (antimony, iridium or palladium), which can be inserted *in situ* into plaque. Secondly, glass probes, which can be inserted in a similar manner. The third method uses miniature glass electrodes built into a partial denture that stays in the mouth for several days to enable plaque to grow on the surface. Recordings of pH are taken from wires coming from the mouth or by radio telemetry. The fourth method is the 'harvesting method' that involves removing small samples of plaque from representative teeth and the measurement of plaque pH on an electrode outside the mouth. Each method has its advantages and disadvantages. The indwelling electrode tends to give an all or nothing response resulting in a maximum drop in pH in the presence of the smallest amount of sugar. This makes the method well suited for testing the non-carcinogenicity of foodstuffs. For example, if a product does not reduce plaque pH to below 5.7 on consumption and for 20 minutes following consumption it may be categorized as 'safe for teeth'. The harvesting method on the other hand is more suited to the ranking of foodstuffs according to their acidogenicity.

Snack foods, meal patterns, and plaque pH

Plaque pH studies that have been used to rank the acidogenicity of snack foods have shown that boiled sweets give the lowest plaque pH (~5.2), sweetened tea and coffee also give low pH values, and foods sweetened with non-sugar sweeteners (e.g. sugar-free chewing gum (pH ~6.8), diabetic chocolate sweetened with sorbitol) and salivary stimulants such as peanuts gave the highest pH values. Figure 2.10 illustrates the difference in the acidogenicity of sucrose-containing and sorbitol-containing chocolate.

Studies using the indwelling glass electrode system have shown starchy staple foods such as wheat-flakes and bread to produce deep pH responses, similar to those produced by sucrose.

Eating hard cheese following a sugar snack (pears in syrup) has been shown to almost abolish the fall in pH that usually accompanies sugar consumption. When sugared coffee was consumed in place of hard cheese, the pH was depressed further. The effect of cheese is probably due to the stimulation of saliva by this highly flavoured food and its low carbohydrate (lactose) content. Peanuts and sugar-free chewing gum are also good salivary stimulants that reduce the pH fall if consumed following a sugar-containing meal or snack. Apples have little benefit compared

with peanuts. It is often advised to consume sugar-rich foods at mealtimes rather than alone, in between meals. This is because, when consumed with other foods the effect on pH is minimized probably due to (1) a dilution effect and (2) the increased salivary flow rate due to mastication of other foods. A study that examined the effect of a three-course breakfast on plaque pH illustrates this. The breakfast consisted of sugar-containing coffee, a boiled egg, and a crisp bread with butter. The smallest drop in pH was observed when all three items were consumed together (Figure 2.11, curve F). The largest drop in pH was observed when the sugared coffee was consumed alone (Figure 2.11, curve E). These studies clearly show how one food can influence the acidogenicity of another.

Plaque pH studies have been used to compare the relative acidogenicity of different mono and disaccharides and to compare the effects of pH of different concentrations of sugars. Using the harvesting method, greater falls in pH have been observed with 50% sucrose compared to 5% sucrose solution. However, using the indwelling glass electrode, no difference in pH drop was observed between 2.5%, 5%, or 10% sucrose and even a very low concentration of sucrose (0.025%) produced a fall in pH of 1.5 units. This demonstrates the 'all or nothing' response from the indwelling electrode, and it is therefore impossible to state, at present, a threshold concentration below which a sucrose solution may be considered safe.

Lactose (10% and 50% solution) produces smaller pH decreases compared with sucrose, glucose, or fructose using either the indwelling electrode or harvesting method. The indwelling electrode method has shown that galactose produces a similar decrease in pH to lactose, and the acidogenicity of maltose is similar to sucrose, glucose, and fructose.

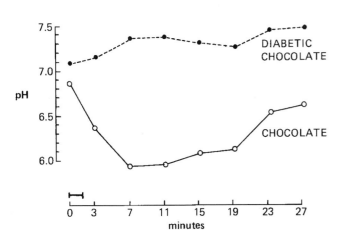

Figure 2.10 Stephan curves produced by dark ('plain') chocolate (containing sugar) and 'diabetic' chocolate (containing sorbitol).

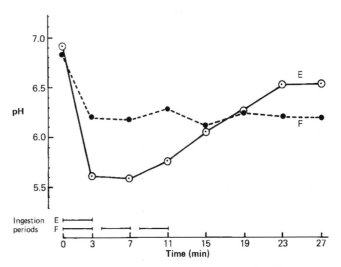

Figure 2.11 Stephan curves produced when sugared coffee was taken alone (E) or taken together with the other two non-acidogenic foods (F). (Reproduced from Rugg-Gunn *et al* 1981, with permission of the editor Journal of Dental Research).

Plaque pH studies

- Measure acidogenic potential, an indirect measure of cariogenicity

- Measure the pH of plaque using either an indwelling electrode that measures pH *in situ* or by removing plaque samples and measuring the pH *in vitro*

- Acidogenicity is expressed as the area of the time/pH graph ('Stephan curve'), the minimum pH reached and/or the time for which pH drops below 5.5 (the 'critical pH')

Incubation experiments

Incubation studies are simple *in vitro* tests that measure if plaque bacteria can metabolize carbohydrate in a test food to produce acid. Pure cultures of micro-organisms may also be used in place of whole plaque. Rapid acid production and/or a low final pH is interpreted to mean that a food is potentially cariogenic, while a slow rate of acid production or higher final pH is likely to be of little clinical significance. All mono and disaccharides (10% solutions) produce a final pH of below 4.5 when incubated with plaque.

In some incubation experiments, teeth, sectioned or powdered tooth enamel, or hydroxyapatite are incubated with the test substance and the plaque micro-organism in order to simulate the caries process. Potential cariogenicity is estimated from the extent of calcium and phosphorus release following incubation. Such studies have indicated that sugars content is an important determinant of the amount of mineral dissolved.

Is dental caries related to the frequency of sugars intake or the amount consumed?

The importance of frequency versus the total amount of sugars is difficult to evaluate as the two variables are hard to distinguish from each other. An increase of either parameter often automatically gives an increase in the other, and likewise a reduction in frequency in intake of sugars in the diet should result in a reduction in the total sugars consumed.

Data from animal studies have indicated the importance of frequency of sugars intake in the development of dental caries, and have shown that dental caries experience increases with increasing frequency of intake of sugars even when the absolute intake of sugars eaten by all groups of rats is the same. Animal studies have also shown that less caries develop as the interval between feeds increases. Some human studies also suggest that the frequency of sugar intake is a more important aetiological factor for caries development than the total consumption of sugar. The primary evidence for the belief that the prevalence of dental caries is directly related to the frequency and to the form, in which sugar is eaten, comes from the Vipeholm study (Gustafsson *et al.* 1954). Many studies have shown a relationship

between the frequency of intake of sugars and sugar-rich foods and dental caries, but many of these have not simultaneously measured the relationship between amount of sugars and caries levels. Studies of preschool children have suggested a threshold of intake of sugars of 4 times a day after which the caries severity markedly increases. For example, Holbrook *et al.* (1995), in a study of 5-year-old children in Iceland, found that in children reporting four or more intakes of sugars per day or 3 or more between meal snacks per day, the caries scores markedly increased. In children that developed 3 or more lesions the intake of sugars averaged 5.1 times per day at age 5 compared with 2.1 times a day for children who developed less than 3 carious lesions (p < 0.01). This confirmed earlier work by the same investigators that showed caries levels to markedly increase at frequency of intake above 30 times a week.

Running contrary to the general perception that frequency of intake is more important than the amount of sugars eaten, several longitudinal studies have shown the amount of sugars intake to be more important than frequency (Burt *et al.* 1988, Rugg-Gunn *et al.* 1984). Animal studies have also been used to investigate the relationship between amount of sugars consumed and the development of dental caries and have shown a significant correlation between the sugar concentration of the diet fed to rats and the incidence of dental caries.

There is, undoubtedly, a strong correlation between the amount and frequency of sugars consumption and the expert consensus is that both are important (Rugg-Gunn 1993). In an analysis of dietary data from over 400 11–12 year old children, Rugg-Gunn found the correlation between frequency of intake of sugar-rich foods and total weight consumed to be + 0.77 (Fig. 2.12) (Rugg-Gunn *et al.* 1984). Similar observations have been found in a number of South African ethnic groups. A very high correlation between frequency of consumption of sugary drinks in between

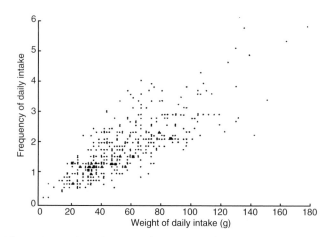

Figure 2.12 The relationship between the frequency and amount of confectionery intake: frequency of intake against (intakes per day) amount of intake (g/day) in 405 12–14-year-old English children. (Reproduced from Rugg-Gunn *et al.* 1984, with permission of the editor of *Archives of Oral Biology*.)

meals and amount consumed has been found in American children (r = +0.97); both increased frequency and amount are associated with higher caries risk. The odds ratios of having a DMFT of above the 80th percentile for age, increased from 1.28 for those having one soft drink per day to 1.87 for twice, and 2.79 for three or more intakes per day.

In summary

- There is evidence to show that both the frequency of intake of sugars and sugars-rich foods and drinks, and the total amount of sugars consumed are related to dental caries
- There is also evidence to show that these two variables are strongly associated, meaning that efforts to control one are likely to control the other
- It is public health policy to reduce the amount of sugars consumed
- At the level of the individual, it is more pragmatic to advise to reduce the frequency of consumption

Are some sugars more cariogenic than others?

Many of the earlier studies investigating the relationship between sugars and dental caries focused on sucrose, which was at that time the main dietary sugar. However, modern diets of populations in industrialized countries contain a mix of fermentable sugars including sucrose, glucose, lactose, fructose, glucose syrups, high-fructose corn syrups and other synthetic oligosaccharides (e.g. fructooligosaccharides). Oral bacteria metabolize all mono and disaccharides to produce acid. Animal studies have shown no clear evidence that the cariogenicity of mono and disaccharide differs, with the exception of lactose. However, plaque pH studies have shown plaque bacteria produce less acid from lactose compared with other sugars. Some animal studies have reported an increased cariogenicity of sucrose but in these studies the rats were super-infected with *S. mutans* which utilizes sucrose in preference to other sugars. It has also been suggested that sucrose is more cariogenic because it is a substrate for extracellular dextran synthesis by *S. mutans*. Consumption of sucrose does, therefore, lead to increased plaque volume. However, the amount of plaque formed is not necessarily related to cariogenicity and high caries development in the absence of significant plaque has been reported (Rugg-Gunn 1993). Studies in humans have also investigated the difference in the cariogenicity of some sugars; for example, the aforementioned Turku study showed no difference between the caries development between subjects on diets sweetened with sucrose compared with fructose (Scheinin and Makinen 1975). Invert sugar (50% fructose + 50% glucose) has been shown to be 20–25% less cariogenic than sucrose.

There is no evidence from epidemiological studies that sugars located within the cellular structure of a food are harmful to teeth; and, therefore, for dental health purposes, it is important to distinguish between these sugars and sugars in the free form. The term 'added sugars' is not ideal as it excludes sugars in fruit juices and honey. The term 'free sugars' has been used by the World Health Organization. In 1989, the UK Committee on Medical Aspects of Food Policy (COMA) classified sugars for dental health purposes into 'intrinsic' and 'extrinsic sugars' (Fig. 2.13) (Department of Health 1989). Extrinsic sugars were sub-divided into 'milk sugars' (as lactose naturally present in milk is not thought

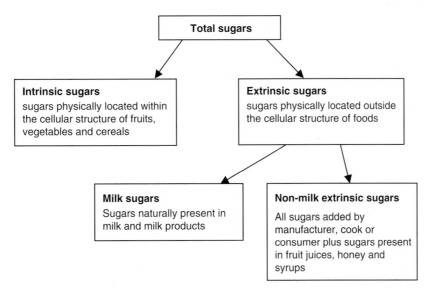

Figure 2.13 Classification of sugars for health purposes: classification of the 1989 Department of Health COMA report 'Dietary Sugars and Human Disease'.

to be harmful to the teeth) and 'non-milk extrinsic sugars (NMES)' which include all sugars added by manufacturer, cook, or consumer, and honey and fruit juices. In terms of dental caries, it is the intake and frequency of intake of NMES (or 'free sugars') that needs to be reduced.

Cariogenicity of sugars

- Sucrose, glucose, fructose, and maltose have similar cariogenicity
- Lactose is less acidogenic/cariogenic
- Physical location of sugars in foods effects their cariogenicity and sugars have been classified into 'intrinsic' and 'extrinsic'
- Intrinsic sugars are located within the cellular structure of the food and are not thought to be harmful to teeth
- Extrinsic sugars are located outside the cellular structure of the food and include 'milk sugars' and non-milk extrinsic sugars'(free sugars)
- Milk sugars, when naturally present in milk or milk products, are not harmful to teeth
- Non-milk extrinsic sugars (free sugars) are the sugars that are harmful to teeth

Does fluoride eliminate the sugars/caries relationship?

The evidence discussed in chapter 3 illustrates that fluoride is the most effective prophylactic agent against caries, its use largely accounting for the decline in dental caries that has been observed in developed countries over the past three decades.

Much of the data that illustrates an association between intake of dietary sugars and dental caries were collected in the pre-fluoride era. More recent studies of the relationship between sugars and caries are confounded by the presence of fluoride but show that a relationship between sugars intake and caries still exists in the presence of fluoride. For example, the oral health survey of the NDNS of children aged 1.5 to 4.5 years in the UK (Hinds and Gregory 1995) found that the association between frequency of intake of sugary foods and dental caries was only partially negated by the frequent use of fluoride. In two major longitudinal studies of the relationship between intake of dietary sugars and dental caries levels in children, the observed relationships between sugars intake and development of dental caries remained even after controlling for use of fluoride and oral hygiene practices (Burt *et al.* 1988, Rugg-Gunn *et al.* 1984). Weaver (1950) reported on the fall in caries levels between 1943 and 1949 in 12-year-olds from areas with naturally high and low water fluoride concentration in North East England. Caries levels were lower in the high fluoride area in 1943, but following the war time sugar restriction, dental caries levels fell a further 54%, indicating that exposure to fluoride did not totally override the effect of sugars in the diet and that exposure to fluoride, coupled with sugars restriction, has added benefits for caries reduction. Marthaler (1990), a leading epidemiologist, reviewed the changes in the prevalence of dental caries and concluded that even when

preventive measures such as use of fluoride are employed, a relationship between sugars intake and caries still exists. After reviewing the literature on declines in caries and associated factors Marthaler concluded that

> within modern societies which are aware and make use of prevention, the relation between sugars consumption and caries activity still exists,

and he also concludes that

> recent studies have demonstrated that sugar—sucrose as well as other hexoses—continues to be the main threat for dental health of 1) whole population in some developed and many developing countries 2) for the individual in both developed and developing countries 3) in spite of the progress made in using fluorides and improved oral hygiene.

Although dental caries levels have declined in many developed countries, a significant relationship between intake of dietary sugars and caries levels persists despite widespread use of fluoride toothpaste.

In a systematic review, Burt and Pai (Burt and Pai 2001) aimed to determine whether with extensive fluoride exposure, individuals with a high level of sugars intake experienced greater caries severity relative to those with a lower level of intake. The review consisted of a search of databases for papers published between 1980 and 2000. The final analysis included 36 studies that are summarized in Table 2.6. Over half of the papers found a moderate relationship and a further sixteen, a weak relationship; no paper failed to find a relationship between sugars intake and caries. The conclusions of the systematic review were:

- Where there is good exposure to fluoride, sugars consumption is a moderate risk factor for caries in most people; and so, preventing consumption of excess sugars is a justifiable part of caries prevention if not the most crucial aspect for most people.
- Sugars consumption is likely to be a more powerful indicator for risk of caries infection in persons who do not have regular exposure to fluoride.

Table 2.6 Distribution of 36 papers showing strong, moderate, and weak relationships between sugars intake and dental caries by type of study design (Burt and Pai 2001)

	Strong	Moderate	Weak	Totals
Cohort studies	1	7	4	12
Case-control studies	0	1	0	1
Cross-sectional studies	0	11	12	23
Totals	1	19	16	36

- With widespread use of fluoride, sugars consumption still has a role to play in the prevention of caries but this role is not a strong as it is without exposure to fluoride.

The evidence of an association between dietary sugars and dental caries comes from a number of different types of experiment. From this body of evidence, the following conclusions may be drawn.

Dietary sugars and dental caries

- Sugars are the most cariogenic item in the diet
- The cariogenicity of sucrose, glucose, fructose, and maltose are similar but that of lactose is lower
- Frequency of eating is important, but frequency of eating sugars-rich foods and amount consumed are highly associated so that efforts to control one will control the other
- Reducing sugars consumption is an important part of caries prevention even when there is widespread exposure to fluoride

Do starches cause dental caries?

Starch constitutes a heterogeneous food group; it varies in botanical origin, it may be highly refined or consumed in its natural state; it may be consumed raw or in a cooked form—all these factors should be considered when assessing the cariogenicity of starches. Some argue that all carbohydrates cause dental caries because starches are broken down by salivary amylase releasing glucose, maltose, and maltotriose that may be metabolized by oral bacteria to produce acids. However, the evidence to support this argument is not strong. In the UK, as in many countries, current dietary guidelines for health promote increased consumption of starch-rich staple foods but recommend limiting the amount of non-milk extrinsic sugars (free sugars) consumed. It is, therefore, important to consider the cariogenic potential of starch-rich staple foods and sugars as separate issues. The following paragraphs will consider the evidence from all types of experiments relating to the cariogenic potential of starch-containing foods.

Human observational studies

Epidemiological studies have shown that starch is of low cariogenicity. People who consume high starch/low sugars diets generally have low caries experience, whereas people who consume low starch/high sugars diets have high levels of caries. In the Hopewood House study, children consumed a high starch, low sugars diet and had low levels of caries. Children with HFI have been shown to have low levels of caries; they cannot consume sucrose or fructose, but can consume unlimited amounts of starch. In a longitudinal study of diet and dental caries in 11–12-year-old English children, Rugg-Gunn et al. found no correlation between intake of starch and caries increment when controlling for sugars intake, and children with high starch and low sugars intakes developed significantly fewer carious lesions than children with low starch/high sugars intake (Rugg-Gunn et al. 1984). Further

evidence that starch is of little importance in the development of caries comes from studies of dietary changes during the Second World War. The intake of starch increased during the war years in Norway and Japan, yet the prevalence of caries was reduced. When sugars intake increased after the war, levels of caries also increased. Populations that habitually consume a high starch/low sugars diet have also been reported to have low levels of dental caries, for example, the Chinese and Vietnamese, Ethiopians, and South American Indians have eaten cooked starches in the form of rice, wheat, and maize but have a low sugars intake and low caries levels.

The ecological study of Sreebny (1982), along with comparing sugar availability and level of caries, compared the cereals availability and levels of caries in 12-year-old children from 47 different countries, using data from the World Health Organization Global Epidemiology Bank and food balance sheets compiled for the Food and Agricultural Organization of the United Nations. Cereal availability was quantified in two ways: (1) as the proportion of energy provided by cereals and (2) as the number of calories provided by cereals per day. Bivariate correlation analysis showed the correlation between total cereals availability and DMFT to be -0.25 (calculated as cal/day) and $+0.45$ (calculated as proportion of energy). For wheat, positive correlations were obtained with coefficients of $+0.45$ and $+0.30$ for cal/day and percent of energy respectively. However, when the data were examined further, using partial correlation analysis (which allows an examination of the caries versus cereal relationship when the effect of differences in sugar availability is removed), the correlations between cereal availability and DMFT were low and not significant. When the correlation between DMFT and sugars availability ($r = 0.7$ from bivariate analysis) was controlled for cereal availability, the correlation fell only slightly to 0.67 and remained highly significant. These findings suggest a much closer positive relationship between dental caries and sugar availability than between cereal availability and dental caries.

Human intervention studies

In the aforementioned Turku sugar studies (Scheinin and Makinen 1975), that investigated the effect on caries of total substitution of sucrose with xylitol or fructose, many foods were specially manufactured replacing sucrose with xylitol or fructose, but the starch content remained unaltered. The mean 2-year caries increments for the sucrose, fructose, and xylitol groups were 7.2, 3.8, and 0.0 respectively. As intake of starch was not limited and all groups ate unlimited starch, dietary starch cannot have contributed significantly to caries development in this study.

Animal experiments

Animal studies have shown that raw starch is of low cariogenicity regardless of the method of feeding. In studies where cooked starches have been fed ad libitum, starches cause caries but only about half the amount caused by sucrose. However, mixtures of starch and sucrose are more cariogenic than starch alone and the amount of caries that develops is related to the sucrose concentration in the mix. Baking of sugars-containing starch foods increases their cariogenic potential. Animal studies have shown that starch-rich foods such as bread cause caries but to a much lesser extent than sucrose. As the frequency of intake of cooked starch or cooked starch-containing foods increases, the level of caries increases. A study using the rat model showed that intake of starch and lactose was not related to caries development, whereas highly significant correlations between intake of glucose ($r = +0.43$), reducing sugars ($r = +0.30$), and sucrose ($r = +0.18$) were found. Caution needs to be applied when extrapolating the results of animal studies to humans due to differences in tooth morphology, plaque bacterial ecology, and salivary flow and composition. The buffering capacity of rat saliva is also less than that of humans. In animal studies the feeds are also usually provided in a powdered form that differs in the way in which starch is habitually consumed by humans. Nonetheless, animal studies have enabled the effect on caries of different types, frequencies, and amounts of carbohydrates to be studied.

Plaque pH studies

Plaque pH studies of starch-containing foods using the harvesting method have indicated that cooked starch or starchy foods are less acidogenic than sugars or sugars-rich foods. However, studies using the indwelling glass electrode method have shown starchy foods to depress plaque pH below 5.5, by a similar extent to sugar, and by these criteria, starch cannot be categorized as 'safe for teeth'. Plaque pH studies that use an indwelling plaque electrode do, however, tend to give an all or nothing response, and are not good at discriminating the acidogenic potential of different carbohydrates. Plaque pH studies that remove plaque from all areas of the mouth and then measure pH (harvesting method) are more discriminating. It must also be considered that plaque pH studies measure acid production from a substrate and do not measure caries development. This means plaque pH studies take no account of the protective factors found in some starch-rich foods.

Enamel slab experiments

There have been two reports of the effect of cooked, starch-rich foods upon the demineralization of enamel slabs under experimental conditions and both have indicated that starch causes approximately 25% of the demineralization seen with sucrose. Enamel slab experiments in humans have shown that raw starch does not cause demineralization.

Incubation experiments

Starch is not transported across the cell membrane of plaque micro-organisms and so cannot be metabolized by oral bacteria to produce acid. However, salivary amylase may hydrolyze starch to produce glucose, maltose, and maltotriose, all of which may be taken up and metabolized by bacterial cells. The rate at which starch is broken down will depend on the nature of the starch and the amount of amylase present.

Summary of starch and dental caries

The UK COMA panel on dietary sugars and human disease concluded that starchy staple foods were a negligible cause of dental caries and that in order to reduce the risk of dental caries NMES consumption should be decreased and replaced with fruit, vegetables, and starchy staple foods (Department of Health 1989). Starches have become more processed and the frequency of eating may have increased in some countries. Many highly processed starchy foods may also be high in fats and or sugars and salt (e.g. corn snacks, sweetened breakfast cereals, cakes, and biscuits). It is not intake of these, but the increased intake of starchy staple foods that is being encouraged.

Starches and dental caries

- Cooked staple starchy foods such as rice, potatoes, and bread are of low cariogenicity in humans
- The cariogenicity of uncooked starch is very low
- Finely ground and heat-treated starch may cause dental caries but the amount of caries is less than that caused by sugars
- The addition of sugars increases the cariogenicity of cooked starchy foods. Foods containing cooked starch and substantial amounts of sucrose appear to be as cariogenic as similar quantities of sucrose

Novel carbohydrates and dental caries risk

Commercial production of polymers of glucose and oligosaccharides of glucose, fructose and galactose, and their use in food products is increasing. Information on the dental health effects of these carbohydrates is therefore of importance. Glucose polymers and non-digestible oligosaccharides are fermentable carbohydrates, however, products that contain them may be labelled as sugar-free (e.g. some chewable 'sugar-free' vitamin tablets contain fructooligosaccharides).

Glucose syrups and maltodextrins are collectively known as glucose polymers and are produced by acid hydrolysis of starch. They vary in composition but contain a mixture of mono, di, tri, tetra, penta, hexa, and hepta-saccharides and alpha limit dextrins (short branched-chain saccharides). The degree of complexity is expressed as the dextrose equivalent (DE); the less complex the glucose polymer, the higher the DE. Glucose syrups have a DE of 20 or more, whereas maltodextrins are more complex and have a DE of less than 20. Glucose polymers are virtually tasteless and odourless and are used to increase the energy content of a variety of foods. They are frequently added to infant food and drinks, sports drinks, desserts, confectionery, and energy supplements for use in clinical dietetics.

Glucose polymers contain traces of mono, di, and trisaccharides that may be metabolized by plaque micro-organisms. Additionally, salivary amylase may hydrolyze the longer glycosidic chains to maltose and glucose. The extent of hydrolysis by amylase will be determined by the retention time in the oral cavity. Therefore, glucose polymers have the potential to cause dental caries but evidence to demonstrate this is sparse. Most data come from animal, plaque pH and *in vitro* laboratory studies. Glucose syrup solutions have been found to be less cariogenic than sucrose solutions; however, when added to the solid component of the rat diet, no difference in caries development has been shown between rats fed glucose syrups and rats fed sucrose. In humans, substitution of sucrose with glucose syrups resulted in markedly reduced plaque scores, but the amount of plaque present is not necessarily related to caries development. Glucose syrups are present, in place of lactose, in soya infant formula, raising concern about the effect of such milks on infant caries. Plaque pH studies show no significant difference in acidogenic potential between soya infant formula and standard infant milk. However, plaque pH studies do not account for the lower content of protective factors in soya milks and the extended time for which infants may need to remain on this formula.

A maltodextrin solution (10%) has been shown to lower plaque pH but to a lesser extent than a 10% solution of sucrose (Fig. 2.14). In the absence of evidence from human clinical trials, advice for the use of glucose polymers should be the same as that for non-milk extrinsic sugars. To safeguard dental health, it is preferable that, if consumed in between meals, maltodextrins are added only to foods and drinks that are cleared from the mouth quickly.

There is an increasing interest in the synthesis of novel oligosaccharides (e.g. prebiotics) and in isolating the transglucosylase enzymes that enable their production, not only for economical reasons but also due to potential health benefits. Many synthetic oligosaccharides are resistant to digestion and pass on to the large intestine where they encourage the growth of bifidobacteria, which are known to reduce the growth of pathogenic microorganisms. They may, therefore, protect against diseases of the bowel. Many of the species of bacteria found in the colon are also present in dental plaque (e.g. bifidobacteria and lactobacilli), and therefore the dental health effect of these novel carbohydrates is of importance.

Isomaltooligosaccharides

- Isomaltooligosaccharides (IMO) contain monosaccharides that are α1-6 linked (but may contain α1-4)

- IMOs include isomaltose (glucose α1-6 glucose), isomaltulose (glucose α1-6 fructose which is also known as palatinose) and panose (glucose α1-6 glucose α1-4 glucose)

- IMOs are produced from starch or sucrose by transglucosylation reactions using transglucosylase enzymes

S. mutans species metabolize IMOs to a much lesser extent than glucose and sucrose, and plaque pH studies in human volunteers have also shown that IMO are less acidogenic compared with glucose or sucrose, but may nevertheless result in a fall in pH to below the critical pH of 5.5. Studies *in vitro* have shown IMO to inhibit glucan synthesis from sucrose and inhibit the sucrose-dependent adherence of *S. mutans*.

Fructooligosaccharides

- Fructooligosaccharides (FOS) are also resistant to digestion in the upper gastrointestinal tract and increase the growth of bifidobacteria

- FOS are widely used in the food industry in Japan and increasingly so in the United Kingdom

- Incubation studies show FOS to be as cariogenic as sucrose, being rapidly metabolized following incubation with several strains of oral streptococci and inducing plaque growth

- Human plaque pH studies support these observations indicating FOS to be as acidogenic as sucrose and thus potentially cariogenic

Does fruit cause dental caries?

Health reports throughout the world encourage increased consumption of fruits and vegetables with a minimum intake quoted as 400 g per day or five portions. The 1989 UK COMA report recommended that in order to reduce the risk of dental caries, consumption of non-milk extrinsic sugars should be decreased and that these sugars should be replaced by fresh fruit, vegetables, and starchy foods. The UK National Food Guide 'The Balance of Good Health' recommends that one-third of dietary volume should be provided by fruits and vegetables (fresh, canned, and frozen). Fresh fruit juices are included amongst fruit and vegetables, but it is recommended that fruit juice consumption may count as only one of the minimum five portions. The preference

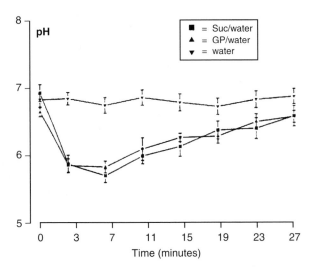

Figure 2.14 Stephan curves (mean values (±SE) of 14 subjects) of 10% (W/V) solutions of maltodextrin, of sucrose and of water alone. (Reproduced from Moynihan *et al.* 1996, with permission of the editor of *International Journal of Paediatric Dentistry*.).

towards whole fruits and vegetables is because these contain more non-starch polysaccharides and plant cell wall materials that benefit health. From a dental point of view, it is also preferable to consume whole fresh fruit as opposed to juices, because their mastication provides a good stimulus to salivary flow. In addition, fresh fruit juices contain non-milk extrinsic sugars, since liquidation releases the fruit sugars from the cellular structure of the fruit. What is the evidence, therefore, for an association between fruit and dental caries?

Human observational studies

There is little evidence from epidemiological studies in humans that consumption of fruit is associated with the development of caries; and indeed, negative correlations between fruit consumption and dental caries have been reported.

A number of cross-sectional studies have compared dental caries experience to levels of fruit consumption. Studies in the USA, UK and Scandinavia have failed to find an association between frequency of fruit consumption and dental caries. When the fruit intakes of children with high caries have been compared to those with low caries, the latter group tend to have a higher fruit consumption. Longitudinal studies in the UK and USA have found a negative association between caries increment and the consumption of fruit. The only epidemiological study, in which an association between fruit consumption and dental caries was demonstrated, compared dental caries experience of South African workers on apple and grape farms with workers on grain farms. The subjects were aged 15 and over and had lived on the farms for a minimum of 8 years. The dental caries experience was higher in the workers from the apple growing farms (DMFT 24) compared with the grape growing farms (DMFT 17), and the caries experiences of both these groups of workers was significantly higher than that of the grain workers (DMFT 10). The levels of intake of fruit by the workers were very high; the workers on the apple farms consumed on average eight apples per day whereas the workers on the grape farms consumed on average three bunches of grapes per day. However, the high DMFT levels were largely due to missing teeth, the cause of which was unknown.

Dried fruit, potentially, may be more cariogenic; since the drying process breaks down the cellular structure of the fruit releasing extrinsic sugars. However, consumption of dried fruit is generally low and there are no epidemiological data to link it to caries development.

Human intervention studies

The only intervention studies of fruit and dental caries have investigated the effect of apples on the development of dental caries with equivocal results. In one study, in children's homes in Liverpool, the children were given a slice of an apple following each meal of the day and after any between meal snacks. Three age groups were studied: under 6 years, 6–10 years and 11–15 years. At the end of a two-year trial, the caries increment was low in both the primary and permanent dentitions in all age groups. In

another dietary intervention study, of older subjects, an apple was provided following the last meal of the day but no significant difference was observed in caries increment compared with a control group not receiving apples. Neither of these studies found that providing extra fruit in the form of apples increased caries levels.

Animal studies

Higher caries scores have been found in rats fed figs, apples, bananas, grapes, and raisins compared with rats fed citrus fruits, peanuts, or dried apricots. However, all fruits consumed resulted in lower caries prevalence than sucrose consumption alone. When the cariogenicity of 22 snack foods including bananas and raisins was scored in relation to sucrose (which was given a score of 1), bananas scored 1.2 and raisins 1.1 indicating they caused more caries lesions than sucrose alone. In general, animal studies have shown that when fruit is consumed frequently (e.g. 17 times a day) in a mashed form (meaning some of the sugars will be extrinsic), it causes caries. However, there are limitations in extrapolating the findings of these studies to humans.

Plaque pH studies

A number of plaque pH studies using the harvesting method have found fruit to be acidogenic (but less so than sucrose) although the extent of this varies according to texture and sugars content. Plaque pH studies using the indwelling glass electrode method have shown apples to depress pH to below 4.5 in experiments using one-day-old and four-day-old plaque. Using the same technique, bananas have been shown to depress pH to below 4 and to remain low for at least 90 minutes. Dates and raisins have been found to result in a low pH for a long period of time, while dried apple or apricot led to small changes in pH. It is important to note that plaque pH studies measure acidogenic potential and do not account for protective factors that are present in fruit or the stimulation to saliva flow from their consumption.

Incubation experiments

Incubation studies have been used to give food products a decalcification score. In a study that tested 96 foods relative to sucrose at

Fruit and dental caries

- Large quantities of grapes and apples have been associated with an increased DMFT, but only in one study
- Bananas appear to have a greater potential than citrus fruits or apples to cause dental caries, but this does not appear to have occurred in man
- Fruit juices contain non-milk extrinsic sugars and cannot be considered safe for teeth
- Based on present evidence, increasing consumption of whole fresh fruit in order to replace non-milk extrinsic sugars (free sugars) in the diet, as recommended by the Department of Health, is likely to decrease the level of dental caries in the population

a score of 231, apple gave the lowest score of 4, pineapple 22, peach 48, pear 130, banana 180, and date 505. Vegetables gave very low scores.

When foods are mixed with saliva and powdered enamel, bananas cause slightly less demineralization than sucrose, apples cause slightly more demineralization, and raisins cause twice as much demineralization as sucrose. Surprisingly, dates only cause around one-third of the demineralization caused by sucrose. In experimental conditions, with fruit as a major dietary constituent, fruits may cause caries. However, as consumed as part of the mixed human diet there is little evidence to show fruit to be an important factor in the development of dental caries.

Factors in the diet that protect against dental caries

Foods and food components that have anti-cariogenic properties are sometimes referred to as 'cariostatic factors'. Fluoride is undoubtedly the most effective of these factors. However, dairy products, plant foods, tea, and even chocolate contain factors that protect against decay. Below is an overview of protective factors and the implications of their consumption for dental health.

Milk

Despite being one of the main sources of sugars in the diet of small children, normal milk consumption does not cause dental caries; and an inverse relationship between the consumption of milk and caries increment has been reported. Cow's milk contains lactose, which is less acidogenic than other mono and disaccharides, and it also contains calcium, phosphorus, and casein, all of which are cariostatic. Calcium and phosphate are present in cow's milk in high concentrations (125 mg/100 ml and 96 mg/100 g respectively) and are able to prevent enamel demineralization. Animal experiments and *in vitro* studies have shown that the phosphopeptide, casein, may protect against demineralization; however, casein is unpalatable to humans and so its practical value may be limited.

Several studies have shown that the fall in plaque pH following milk consumption is negligible. A plaque pH study in human volunteers that compared the acidogenic potential of cow's milk and human breast milk with 7% solutions of lactose and sucrose showed that sucrose caused a substantial decrease in plaque pH while both milks depressed pH only slightly and lactose decreased pH to a much lesser extent than sucrose (Fig. 2.15).

In enamel slab experiments, milk has been shown to produce less enamel dissolution compared with lactose or sucrose solutions. Such experiments have also shown milk to reduce the cariogenic potential of sugar-containing foods.

There is some evidence from animal studies that the addition of milk to a cariogenic diet reduces the caries prevalence. Additionally, in experiments where rats have had their salivary glands removed, making them caries prone, they remained more or less

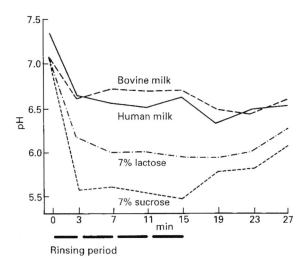

Figure 2.15 Mean Stephan curves (relation between plaque pH and time) for 14 volunteer subjects who rinsed with cow's milk (bovine) human milk, 7% lactose or 7% sucrose four times during 15 minutes. (Reproduced from Rugg-Gunn *et al*. 1985, with permission of the editor of *Caries Research*.)

caries-free when fed milk, compared with those fed sucrose or lactose in water. From this it was concluded that milk can be used safely by patients with low salivary flow as a saliva substitute.

Compared with cow's milk, breast milk contains more lactose (~7% vs. 4–5%) and lower concentrations of calcium and phosphate (34 mg and 15 mg/100 g respectively), and so, in theory, may be more cariogenic. However, epidemiological studies have, in general, associated breast feeding with low levels of dental caries. To what extent this is secondary to socioeconomic status and consumption of other sources of sugars is unknown. Breast feeding provides no opportunity to add additional sugar to milk feeds and breast-fed infants are perhaps less likely to use baby bottles containing sugary liquids. There have been a few reports of cases of severe dental caries associated with prolonged (usually over 2 years), on-demand breast feeding, often with infants feeding during the night when protection from saliva is low.

Milk and dental caries

- Milk is a substantial source of sugars in the diet of young children
- The sugar in milk is lactose, which is less acidogenic
- Milk contains phosphorus, calcium, and casein all of which protect against demineralization
- Animal studies have shown milk to be anticariogenic
- Human breast milk is higher in lactose and lower in phosphorus and calcium; however, normal breast feeding does not cause dental caries
- Prolonged, *ad libitum*, and nocturnal suckling have been associated with increased caries risk

However, these cases are rare and associated with unusual feeding practice. Therefore, human breast milk has a greater potential than cow's milk to cause dental caries but dental caries in human infants due to breast feeding is rare and is always associated with prolonged, on-demand feeding. As formula feeds contain similar amounts of lactose, calcium, and phosphate to breast milk, there are no benefits to dental health of feeding a formula feed. Breast feeding should be promoted since it provides the best infant nutrition.

Cheese

Numerous animal studies and experimental studies have indicated that cheese is anticariogenic. Plaque pH studies have shown that consuming cheese following a sugary snack virtually abolishes the usual fall in pH that is associated with sugars consumption. Cheese stimulates salivary secretion and increases plaque calcium concentration. The calcium concentration within dental plaque strongly influences the balance between de- and re-mineralization of enamel. In experimental studies, cooked, cheese-containing meals have also been shown to increase plaque calcium concentrations in human volunteers. Plaque calcium concentrations were measured in 16 volunteers before and following consumption of cheese-containing meals and cheese-free control meals. Plaque calcium concentrations increased significantly on consumption of a 15 g cube of cheese and on consumption of meals containing 15 g cheese, but did not increase significantly on consumption of cheese-free control meals (Fig. 2.16).

Enamel slab experiments have shown that cheese promotes the remineralization of previously demineralized enamel and, in an epidemiological study, cheese intake was higher in children who remained caries-free over a two-year period than in those who developed caries (Rugg-Gunn et al. 1984). Furthermore, a controlled clinical trial showed that fewer caries developed over a two-year period in children who ate a 5g piece of hard cheese daily, following breakfast, compared with a control group who did not consume the extra cheese.

Plant foods

A lower-than-expected caries level in groups of people known to have high carbohydrate diets—such as the Bantu Tribe of South Africa and sugar cane cutters, led to an interest in the presence of protective factors in foods of plant origin. The effects, on caries, of factors in foods of plant origin including organic phosphates, inorganic phosphates, and phytate have been investigated. It has been postulated that organic phosphates protect the teeth by adsorbing onto the enamel, forming a protective coat. Both organic and inorganic phosphates have been found to be effective in animal studies, but studies in humans have produced inconclusive results. Calcium sucrose phosphate was marketed as a cariostatic food additive in Australia, but its use was never supported by evidence from clinical trials.

Phytate is anticariogenic and acts by adsorbing onto the enamel surface to form a physical barrier that protects against plaque acids. When isolated from foods, phytate is an effective anti-caries factor, but as an intrinsic food component, is not effective. Therefore to be effective, phytate would need to be extracted from grains and then used as a food additive. This would not be desirable since phytate binds minerals (calcium, iron, magnesium, and zinc) in the gastrointestinal tract.

Animal studies have shown that inorganic phosphates are cariostatic and prevent demineralization of enamel. However, studies in humans have produced equivocal results. Sodium trimetaphosphate has been shown to be the most effective inorganic phosphate, but its use would result in undesirably high sodium intakes.

Probably, one of the main reasons why people who consume diets high in unrefined plant foods have fewer carious lesions is due to stimulation of saliva flow that occurs on consumption of fibrous foods. Saliva not only helps to clear food debris from the mouth, but also buffers plaque acid, and therefore, favours remineralization of tooth enamel. Other foods that markedly increase saliva flow include chewing gum (sugar free), cheese, and peanuts.

Do chocolate and liquorice protect against dental caries?

In the Vipeholm study mentioned previously, the group receiving chocolate developed relatively fewer carious lesions than groups receiving similar amounts of sugars at similar frequencies (Fig. 2.6). This led to the suggestion that chocolate contained protective factors. Animal studies also showed that cocoa may have a protective effect. In 1986 cocoa factor was extracted from chocolate and was shown to be effective *in vitro*. Recent studies have shown that theobromide in chocolate is able to increase crystal size in enamel, thus increasing the resistance to acid demineralization. In addition to 'cocoa factor' and theobromide, milk chocolate contains calcium and casein, and is high in fat, which

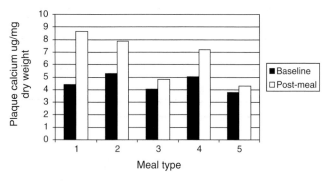

Figure 2.16 Plaque calcium concentration before and following consumption of cheese and cheese-containing meals. Mean values of 16 subjects. 1, 15 g cube of cheese; 2, Test meal: pasta in cheese sauce; 3, Control meal: pasta in mushroom sauce; 4, Test meal: chicken breast with cheese and ham filling; 5, Control meal: chicken breast with mushroom and ham filling.

aids oral clearance. However, the high sugar content of chocolate outweighs these potential benefits. Likewise, honey contains protective esters, the benefit of which is outweighed by its high sugars content.

Glycyrrhizinic acid, a major constituent of liquorice, has cariostatic properties. Glycyrrhizinic acid inhibits bacterial glycolysis preventing the formation of acid from dietary sugars, and it increases the buffering potential of plaque. However, it has a strong taste, may cause staining of the teeth and liquorice may also cause electrolyte disturbances. Its use as an anti-caries factor is therefore somewhat limited.

Tea and apples

There is increased interest in foods that contain polyphenols, as animal and experimental studies have shown that these compounds have antibacterial properties. Apples contain polyphenols and are a good stimulus to salivary flow. Tea also contains polyphenols in addition to fluoride and flavanoids. Black tea extracts have been shown to inhibit salivary amylase activity and reduce dental caries in animal studies. Epidemiological studies have reported lower caries in green tea drinkers in Japan and tea drinkers in Israel. However, in English 5-year-olds no difference in caries levels between tea drinkers and non-drinkers was found, although no account was taken of the possible effect of added sucrose. The protective effect of tea may be due to fluoride or the antibacterial action of polyphenols, or both.

Protective factors and dental caries

- Cow's milk is non-cariogenic, since the protective factors present counteract any cariogenic potential due to the lactose content

- All types of experiment, including a clinical trial, have shown cheese to be cariostatic. Small quantities, that make a negligible contribution to fat intake, are effective

- Plant foods contain phosphates, which have been shown to be effective at preventing caries in animal studies; but human studies have not produced convincing results

- A number of foods including cocoa, liquorice, and honey contain protective factors, but their practical potential in reducing caries is limited

- Foods that are good stimuli to salivary flow protect against dental caries; examples include sugar-free chewing gum, peanuts, and cheese

Non-sugars sweeteners

Sugar substitutes can be separated into two major groups 'intense sweeteners (non-caloric), and 'bulk sweeteners' (caloric). Some of these are naturally occurring compounds; however, the production of synthesized sweeteners has increased steadily due to new technologies and increased demand for sugars-free alternatives. The sweeteners that are permitted for food use varies between countries. Those permitted in the UK are listed in Table 2.7.

Table 2.7 Bulk and intense non-sugars sweeteners permitted for food use in the United Kingdom

Sweetener	Food Uses	Sweetness (x sucrose)	Cariogenicity	Clinical trials	Disadvantages
Bulk					
Isomalt	Chocolate	0.5	Virtually non-cariogenic	no	Excess causes diarrhoea
Lycasin	Confectionery, gums	0.7	Between sorbitol and xylitol	Yes (sweets)	
Maltitol	Chewing gums	0.7	Virtually non-cariogenic	No	Excess causes diarrhoea
Mannitol	Dusting powder on chewing gums	0.7	Virtually non-cariogenic	One	Excess causes diarrhoea
Sorbitol	Confectionery, gums, jams,	0.5	Virtually non-cariogenic	Yes (gums, sweets)	Excess causes diarrhoea
Xylitol	Mints, gums confectionery	1.0	Non-cariogenic. Anticariogenic?	Yes (foods, gums, sweets)	Excess causes diarrhoea
Intense					
Acesulfame potassium	Low calorie drinks, confectionery and preserves	130	Non-cariogenic	No	
Aspartame	Soft drinks, dried and frozen foods, chewing gums	200	Non-cariogenic	No	Cannot be used by those with phenylketonuria
Saccharin	Table top sweeteners, drinks	500	Anticariogenic?	No	Bitter aftertaste
Thaumatin	With other sweeteners in soft drinks	3000	Non-cariogenic	No	Liquorice after taste

Intense sweeteners

Intense sweeteners are used in food products like soft drinks, beer, confectionery, desserts, ice cream, marmalade, and jam. They are also used in dentifrices and in sweetening drops/tablets for use in food, coffee, tea, etc. Currently, about 30% of the carbonated beverages consumed in the USA are sweetened with the intense sweetener aspartame.

Saccharin had been used in foods in the UK for almost a century. It has a bitter taste in concentrations over 0.1%, although the perception of this varies between individuals. Saccharin is widely used in foods such as sweetening tablets. Acesulfame potassium is a chemically synthesized sweetener that is stable over a range of pH values and does not break down on heating. These properties make it a useful sweetener in boiled sweets and preserves. Aspartame is a dipeptide comprising of aspartic acid and phenylalanine. It is marketed under the brand names of 'Nutrasweet' and 'Canderel'. It is used extensively in frozen foods, desserts, drinks, and gums. Thaumatin, a protein extracted from a plant in West Africa is an example of a naturally occurring intense sweetener. It has a liquorice aftertaste and its main use is in pharmaceutical products.

Food labels must declare if a product contains a sweetener and, in the case of aspartame, the label must also say that the product contains a source of phenylalanine, because individuals with phenylketonuria are unable to metabolize this amino acid.

Intense sweeteners are not metabolized to acids by oral micro-organisms and they cannot cause dental caries. Saccharin has been reported to inhibit bacterial growth and metabolism, but animal studies have shown that its caries-inhibiting effects are small. Limitations of intense sweeteners include poor taste quality, instability, and lack of volume. Caution is still needed when recommending products containing intense sweeteners because other ingredients, e.g. citric or phosphoric acids, in beverages may cause dental erosion. In some food products, intense sweeteners are added in addition to sugars, e.g. to fruit flavoured soft drinks, and the naturally occurring sugars in the drink (fructose, glucose, and sucrose) may also cause caries.

Intense sweeteners

- are not chemically related to sugars
- are added in very small quantities to add sweetness and not volume
- are hundreds to thousands of times sweeter than sucrose
- have a negligible energy value (kilocalories)

Bulk sweeteners

Bulk sweeteners provide sweetness and bulk to a food product. Many are sugar alcohols; and, being chemically similar to sugars, their cariogenicity has been tested in many types of experiments and, in some cases in clinical trials. Bulk sweeteners are widely used in confectionery, preserves and sugar-free gums. One of the disadvantages of the bulk sweeteners is that they are only partially absorbed in the small intestine and pass to the colon where they

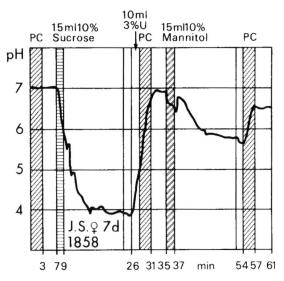

Figure 2.17 Telemetrically recorded plaque pH after rinsing with (a) 15 ml of 10% sucrose solution, (b) 15 ml of 10% mannitol solution. (Reproduced from Imfeld 1997, with permission of the editor of *Helvetica Odontologica Acta*.)

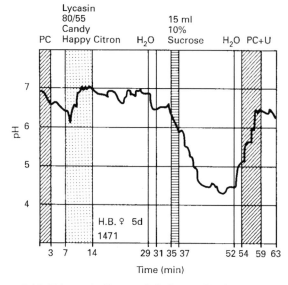

Figure 2.18 Telemetrically recorded plaque pH after (a) eating a hard sweet containing lycasin, (b) rinsing with 15 ml of 10% sucrose solution. (Reproduced from Imfeld, 1977, with permission of the editor of *Helvetica Odontologica Acta*.)

may induce osmotic diarrhoea. Bulk sweeteners are therefore not recommended for children under three years of age and care must be taken with sugar-free medicines containing bulk sweeteners, since high intakes cause gastrointestinal disturbance. The dental health effects, food uses, and specific properties of the bulk non-sugars sweeteners are presented in Table 2.7.

The non-acidogenicity of mannitol and lycasin is illustrated in Figures 2.17 and 2.18.

Bulk sweeteners

- are chemically similar to sugars
- add volume and sweetness to a product
- vary from 0.5 times to 1.0 times as sweet as sucrose
- have an energy value (kilocalories)
- many are naturally found in foods

Does sugars substitution with non-sugars sweeteners prevent dental caries? Clinical trials of polyol-containing chewing gums

Many trials of the effect of sugar-free chewing gum on caries experience have been carried out. Some have compared the effect of giving subjects sugar-free gum with sugared gum and some have compared the effect of giving sugar-free gum to taking no gum. Some of the studies have aimed to compare the relative effectiveness of different non-sugars sweeteners.

The Turku chewing gum study compared the effects of sucrose-containing gum with that of xylitol-containing gum in young adults. The mean caries increment after 1 year was 2.9 DMFT in the sucrose and −1.0 in the xylitol group. In the Ylivieska study, school children were randomly divided into two test groups, using xylitol gums, and a third control group that chewed no gum. The xylitol gum groups developed fewer caries. When the children were re-examined 2–3 years later, a significant caries reduction was found. The authors concluded that xylitol was anticariogenic. However, neither the influence of the chewing action nor the specific effect of xylitol on caries reduction can be measured from this study as it did not include a control group on a placebo gum or a gum containing a sugar substitute other than xylitol. It should also be noted that the dental examination was not carried out blind to the group identity of the children.

In the Montreal study, school children were assigned to one of three groups, two xylitol groups (either 65% xylitol or 15% xylitol) and one control group, who chewed no gum. Children chewed for 5 minutes three times a day. After 1 year the xylitol groups had significantly lower caries increments. The group who chewed the 65% xylitol gum had less caries than those who used the 15% xylitol gum. However, after two years the difference between the two xylitol groups did not remain, but both had a lower caries incidence compared with the control group. A review of clinical trials of xylitol (Imfeld 1994) concludes that the similarity in caries increment between the two xylitol groups means that the caries preventive effect was due to chewing rather than the xylitol content of the gum. However, as the study did not include a control group that chewed a placebo gum, no firm conclusion may be drawn.

In the Belize study, 10-year-old children, initially with moderate to high caries levels, were divided into 9 groups, one of which received sugared gum. Seven groups received either xylitol or sorbitol gums, or gums that contained mixtures of these two sweeteners. One group received no gum. Children chewed for 5 minutes five times a day. After 28 months, the lowest DMFT scores were observed in groups using 100% xylitol gum. The sorbitol gum and the gums containing mixtures of xylitol and sorbitol resulted in higher DMFT scores compared with gum containing only xylitol, the highest mean DMFT scores were found in the two groups using either sugared gum or no gum. The Belize study is the first clinical trial of xylitol that enables a comparison of the caries-preventive action of xylitol to be compared with sorbitol and the results indicate that xylitol is superior in reducing caries.

A recent review of the effect of polyols on the prevention of dental caries concluded that the replacement of sucrose with sorbitol and xylitol may significantly decrease the incidence of dental caries (Hayes 2001). This is in line with the conclusion of the 1989 COMA report 'Dietary Sugars and Human Disease' that concluded

> current evidence suggests that bulk sweeteners have negligible cariogenicity compared with sugars and that substitution of sugars by alternative sweeteners could substantially reduce caries development. The greatest gain would be expected to occur if they were used to replace sugars in foods ingested frequently such as sweet snacks, drinks, and liquid medicines.

Non-sugars sweeteners

- The bulk sweeteners sorbitol, mannitol, lactitol, isomalt, lycasin, and maltitol are non-cariogenic or virtually so
- Xylitol and the intense sweeteners are non-cariogenic
- Chewing gums sweetened with xylitol and/or sorbitol protect against dental caries. This effect is due to the non-cariogenicity of the sweeteners and the stimulation of saliva flow resulting from chewing
- It is important to remember that the usefulness of a sugars substitute has to be looked upon not only from a cariological, but also from a nutritional, toxicological, economic, and technical point of view

Political issues in relation to diet and dental health

Strategies to prevent dental caries: limiting intake of sugars

It is important to have a maximum recommended level for intake of free sugars against which the dental health risks of populations may be assessed and health promotion goals monitored. There is evidence that the relationship between dental caries levels and sugars is an S-shaped relationship (Fig. 2.19). At low levels of sugar intake (10 kg/person/year) caries is very low. At levels of intake around 15 kg/person per year, the line of the graph steeply rises and the level of caries increases with increasing sugar availability. At high levels of sugar intake (~35 kg/person/year) the curve flattens out and a saturation level is reached, so that a further increase in sugars content of the diet does not increase caries to an appreciable extent. The evidence for the sigmoid relationship between sugars intake and dental caries comes from a number of studies. Data from Japan on caries levels following the Second World War, when the availability of sugar was restricted shows an S-shaped dose–effect curve that reaches saturation level at 35 kg/person per year. The annual caries increment was positively related with the annual sugar availability in Japan (r=+0.8) when sugar intakes were between 0.2 kg to 15 kg/person per year and when intakes were above 15 kg/person per year the rate of caries intensified.

Data from Britain and Norway during the war years also support these findings. When Norwegian children consumed less than 10.4 kg/person per year, levels of dental caries were low. Children evacuated from Jersey during the war years were exposed to high intakes of sugar (30 kg/person/year) than those that remained in Jersey. Children in Jersey consumed on average 8.3 kg sugar per year and had a DMFT of 1.8 compared to 5.5 in the evacuees.

The aforementioned data of Sreebny (1982) found that low caries rates were associated with low sugar intake in 12-year-old children; for the 21/47 countries where sugars availability was less that 18.25 kg/year (~50 g/day), DMFT levels were below 3.0, suggesting that this may be the upper safe limit for sugars intake.

In Japan, caries levels increased as sugar intake increased through the years until a peak in sugar intake was reached at 29 kg/person per year in 1973. Thereafter, the intake of sugar decreased and so did the caries experience. The correlation between sugar availability and caries levels was high and significant (r=+0.91).

The above studies were on populations not exposed to the benefits of fluoride. Exposure to fluoride in some countries has altered the sugars–caries relationship. It has been argued that where fluoride is present in drinking water at a concentration of 0.7–1ppm, or over 90% of toothpastes available are fluoridated, the dose–effect curve shifts to the right and raises the safe limit on the level of sugars consumption.

Effects of sugars intake and fluoride on caries experience

- Overall, the studies show that when annual sugar consumption is above 15 to 20 kg per person per year, dental caries increases with increasing sugar intake
- 15–20 kg is equivalent to 41–55 g per day
- A number of studies have shown that caries levels increase with intakes of free sugars above four times a day
- Widespread exposure to fluoride may raise the threshold level of safe intake, and this is reflected in the dietary guidelines adopted by several industrialized countries

Policies on sugars intake in different countries

A number of countries have adopted policies/recommendations for sugars intake based on these data (Table 2.8). In the UK, where there is widespread exposure to fluoridated toothpaste, the Dietary Reference Value for non-milk extrinsic sugars is 60 g/day or <10% of energy intake. Similar recommendations have been adopted by several countries including the Scandinavian countries,

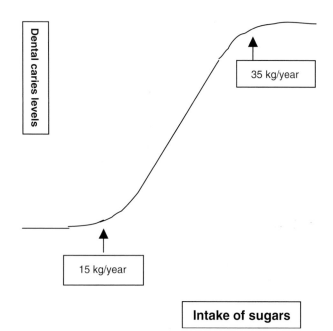

Figure 2.19 Sigmoid curve to illustrate the relationship between intake of sugars and dental caries levels. Figures are based on data from epidemiological studies.

Table 2.8 Policies on intake of free sugars by a number of countries

Year	Country	Recommendation
1986	Netherlands, Ministry of Health	0–10%
1987	Australia, Department of Health	≤12%
1987	Finland, Nutrition Board	≤10%
1989	Poland, National Institute	<10%
1990	WHO	<10%
1991	United Kingdom, Department of Health	≤10%
1996	Nordic Nutrition Recommendations	≤10%
1997	Sweden	≤10%

the Netherlands, and Poland. The 1990 WHO report 'Diet, Nutrition & Prevention of Chronic Diseases' also recommended that free sugars should contribute no more than 10% to energy intake.

Is there an inverse relationship between the intake of sugars and fat in the diet?

The claim that total sugars intake is commonly inversely related to total fat intake has been used as an argument for not setting a recommended limit on sugars consumption, suggesting that decreasing dietary sugars would lead to an increase in fat intake or vice versa. However, data available are not sufficient to support this argument, and there are longitudinal data to show that there is no evidence for such a relationship. The data that theoretically support an inverse relationship use cross-sectional analysis of the diets of populations, and are not based on longitudinal studies of populations following changes in intakes of sugars or fats. Recent evidence from a repeated cross-sectional study of English school children does not support the existence of an inverse relationship between fat and sugars. The study showed that although fat intake significantly reduced between 1990 and 2000, this was not accompanied by an increase in sugars intake (Fletcher, Adamson *et al*. personal communications). In a short-term dietary intervention study aimed at increasing the intake of dietary fibre by dietitians and their households, a reduction in the intake of added sugars was achieved at the same time as reducing the intake of dietary fat. There is no sound evidence to support the existence of a 'sugar/fat seesaw', and permitting unlimited sugars consumption may not lead to a reduction in dietary fat. Health reports have stated that any deficit in energy resulting from a reduction in intake of free sugars may be met by an increase in the intake of fruits, vegetables, and starch-rich staple foods and should not be met by increasing intake of fat.

Recommendations for prevention of dental caries

- In the presence of adequate exposure to fluoride, the intake of free sugars should be limited to 15 to 20 kg/person per year (equivalent to 40–55 g/day). In the absence of fluoride, the intake of free sugars should be below 15 kg/day (<40 g/day). These values equate to 6–10% of energy intake. The frequency of intake of foods containing free sugars should be limited to a maximum of four times a day.

- The potential financial consequence of failing to prevent dental caries needs to be highlighted, especially to governments of countries that currently have low levels of disease, but are undergoing nutrition transition (adopting a westernized diet).

- The detrimental impact on quality of life throughout the life course—the longer-term nutritional consequences of dental caries and tooth loss—need to be highlighted.

- The myth that a high sugars intake is important for energy intake and growth needs to be dispelled, especially in developing countries where undernutrition is prevalent.

- Restricting the intake of free sugars to 10% of energy intake would still enable a sustained production of sugar cane as a cash crop in low-income countries.

- Regular monitoring of the prevalence and severity of dental caries should be encouraged using World Health Organization global guidelines, in different countries in all age groups.

- More national information on the dietary intake of sugars, sugar availability, and soft drink intake should be collected.

- Governments should support research into prevention of dental caries through dietary means.

- Nutrition needs to be recognized as an essential part of training for dental health professionals, and dental health issues, an important component of education of nutritionist and other health professionals. This is essential if advice for dental health is to be consistent with dietary advice for general health.

- Departments of Education must ensure that teachers, pupils, and health professionals receive adequate education on diet and dental health issues. There should be cross-Departmental guidelines for the use and content of educational materials to ensure they are sound, and not biased towards the interests of the food industry.

- International non-govermental organizations (e.g. World Health Organization, Food & Agricultural Organization, FDI, International Association for Dental Research) should recommend fiscal pricing policies for food items that are high in non-milk extrinsic sugars (free sugars) and are otherwise of questionable nutritional value, and should encourage governments to adopt more stringent codes of advertising practice, especially those aimed at children.

- Food manufacturers should continue to develop and produce low sugars/sugars-free alternatives to products rich in free sugars, including drinks. To enable individuals to make informed choices regarding sugars intake, there is a need for clear, unbiased, and non-misleading labelling of foods with respect to sugars contents.

Conclusions

This chapter has provided an overview of the evidence for an association between diet and dental caries. For a more comprehensive account, the reader is referred to Rugg-Gunn (1993) and Rugg-Gunn and Nunn (1999). To conclude: collatively, a multiplicity of different types of studies provide convincing evidence of a causal relationship between the amount and frequency of free sugars intake and dental caries.

Sugars are necessary for dental caries to occur. Other factors such as exposure to fluoride, oral hygiene practice, and salivary flow rate and composition modify the response to sugars. Fluoride is very effective at reducing dental caries; but it does not eliminate caries, and many low income countries do not have adequate exposure to fluoride. In developed countries where exposure to fluoride is adequate, the only way to further reduce caries is to restrict sugars consumption. Therefore, despite excellent progress made by use of fluoride, sugars restriction remains important in caries prevention in the twenty-first century. The evidence suggests that in order to minimize dental caries, the intake of free sugars should not exceed 15–20 kg per person per year.

References

Burt, B. and Pai, S. (2001). Is sugar consumption still a major determinant of dental caries? Consensus development conference on diagnosis and management of dental caries throughout life, Bethesda MD, USA.

Burt, B.A., Eklund, S.A., Morgan, K.J., Larkin, F.E., Guire, K.E., Brown, L.O., and Weintraub, J.A. (1988). The effects of sugars intake and frequency of ingestion on dental caries increment in a three-year longitudinal study. *Journal of Dental Research*, 67, 1422–1429.

Department of Health (1989). Dietary sugars and human disease. Report on health and social subjects No 37. London, HMSO.

Granath, L.-E., Rootzen, H., Liljegren, E., Holst, K., and Kohler, L. (1978). Variation in caries prevalence related to combinations of dietary and oral hygiene habits and chewing fluoride tablets in 4-year-old children. *Caries Research*, 12, 83–92.

Grindefjord, M., Dahllof, G., Nilsson, B., and Modeer, T. (1996). Stepwise prediction of dental caries in children up to 3.5 years of age. *Caries Research*, 30, 256–266.

Gustafsson, B.E., Quensel, C.E., Lanke, L.S., Lundquist, C., Grahnen, H., Bonow, B.E., and Krasse, B. (1954). The Vipeholm dental caries study. The effect of different levels of carbohydrate intake on caries activity in 436 individuals observed for 5 years. *Acta Odontologica Scandinavica*, 11, 232–364.

Hayes, C. (2001). The effect of non-cariogenic sweeteners on the prevention of dental caries: a review of the evidence. *Journal of Dental Education*, 65(10), 1106–1109.

Hinds, K. and Gregory, J. (1995). National diet and nutrition survey: children aged 1.5–4.5 years: *Report of the Dental Survey*, Vol. 2. London, HMSO.

Holbrook, W.P., Arnadottir, I.B., Takazoe, I., Birkhed, D., and Frostell, G. (1995). Longitudinal study of caries, cariogenic bacteria and diet in children just before and after starting school. *European Journal of Oral Sciences*, 103, 42–45.

Imfeld, T. (1994). Clinical caries studies with polyalcohols a literature review. *Schweiz Monatsschr Zahnmed*, 104(8), 941–945.

Marthaler, T. (1990). Changes in the prevalence of dental caries: how much can be attributed to changes in diet? *Caries Research*, 24, 3–15.

Rugg-Gunn, A.J. (1993). *Nutrition and Dental Health*. Oxford, Oxford Medical Publications.

Rugg-Gunn, A.J., Hackett, A.F., Appleton, D.R., Jenkins, G.N., and Eastoe, J.E. (1984). Relationship between dietary habits and caries increment assessed over two years in 405 English adolescent schoolchildren. *Archives of Oral Biology*, 29, 983–992.

Rugg-Gunn, A.J. and Nunn J.H. (1999). *Nutrition, diet and oral health*. Oxford, Oxford University Press.

Scheinin, A. and Makinen, K.K. (1975). Turku sugar studies. I-XXI. *Acta Odontologica Scandinavica*, 33(Suppl. 70), 1–349.

Sreebny, L.M. (1982). Sugar availability, sugar consumption and dental caries. *Community Dentistry and Oral Epidemiology*, 10, 1–7.

Stecksen-Blicks, C. and Gustafsson, L. (1996). Impact of oral hygiene and use of fluorides on caries increment in children during one year. *Community Dentistry and Oral Epidemiology*, 14, 185–189.

Walker, A., Gregory, J., Bradnock, G., Nunn, J., and White, D. (2000). National diet and nutrition survey: young people aged 4 to 18 years. *Report of the Oral Health Survey*, Vol. 2. London, HMSO.

Weaver, R. (1950). Fluorine and war-time diet. *British Dental Journal*, 88, 231–239.

3

Fluoride and dental caries

Fluoride and dental caries

John Murray

Introduction

The history of fluorides in dentistry is over 100 years old. Sir James Crichton Browne made an inspired guess about the importance of fluoride in the diet in 1892. Fluoride was isolated from water supplies in 1931 and has been incorporated into water, milk, salt, tablets, and drops. It has also been included as an active agent for the prevention of dental caries in toothpastes, professionally applied topical fluoride agents and mouth rinses. The purpose of this chapter is to summarize the information concerning the effect of fluorides in the prevention of dental caries.

Fluoride 1890–1930

The use of fluorides for dental purposes began in the nineteenth century. The first entirely speculative ideas led to the development of fluoride-containing pills in the 1890s. This aspect of fluoride and dental health then lay dormant for over 40 years.

The first reference to a prophylactic role for fluoride may well have been made by Erhadt in 1874. In a contribution to Memorabilia—a monthly publication in German for 'rational physicians'—he reported:

> As, for a long time, Iron was given for the blood, Calcium and Phosphorus for the bones, so has it been successful to add Fluoride to the tooth enamel in a soluble and absorbable form. It is Fluoride that gives hardness and durability to the tooth enamel and protects against caries.

Pindborg (1965) and Hunsfadbraten both refer to a pamphlet published in 1902 by Cross and Co. in Copenhagen, Denmark, entitled 'Fluoridens. How to Remedy the Decay of our Teeth'. The Danish Apothecary Society analysed the tablets and found they contained 83.7 per cent calcium fluoride (Fig. 3.1).

The importance of fluorine was emphasized by Sir James Crichton Browne in an address to the Eastern Counties Branch of the British Dental Association in 1892:

> I would name to you, as a specific cause of the increase of dental caries, a change that has taken place in a food stuff of a particular kind, and of primary importance. I mean bread, the staff of life, from which, in the progress of civilisation, the coarse elements—and the coarse elements consist of the outer husks of the grains of which it is composed—have been eliminated. In as far as our own country, at any rate, is concerned, this is essentially an age of white bread and fine flour, and it is an age therefore in which we are no longer partaking to anything like the same amount that our ancestors did of the bran or husky parts of wheat, and so are deprived to a large degree of a chemical element which they received in abundance, namely, fluorine.

In 1908 the British Dental Journal, under the heading 'Calcium fluoride in therapeutics' gave over half a page to an abstract from a French pharmaceutical journal on fluoride dosages. The article referred to the beneficial effect of fluoride in the healing of bone fractures and stated that it was 'generally recognized' that

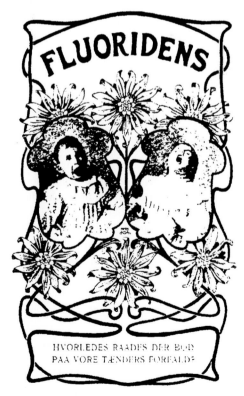

Figure 3.1 Front cover of a leaflet, 'Fluoridens: How to Remedy the Decay of Our Teeth', *c.* 1902 (Pindborg, 1965).

fluoride is necessary for the health of teeth. A powder prescribed by A. Robin included magnesium and calcium carbonate, calcium triphosphate, calcium fluoride and one gram of white sugar.

The man who had the greatest impact on the early history of water fluoridation was Dr Frederick McKay who arrived in Colorado Springs, Colorado in 1901, the year following his graduation from the University of Pennsylvania Dental School. He soon noticed that many of his patients, particularly those who had lived in the area all their lives, had a permanent stain on their teeth, which was known to the local inhabitants as 'Colorado stain'. McKay checked his lecture notes, but found nothing to describe such markings, nor could he find any reference to it in any of the available scientific literature. He called the stain 'mottled enamel', characterized by:

> Minute white flecks, or yellow or brown spots or areas, scattered irregularly or streaked over the surface of a tooth, or it may be a condition where the entire tooth surface is of a dead paper-white like the colour of a china dish.

In the forefront of his mind all the time was the desire to determine the cause of mottled enamel. He established that the occurrence of mottled enamel was localized in definite geographical areas. Within these endemic areas a very high proportion of children were affected: only those who had been born and lived all their lives in an endemic area had mottled enamel; those born elsewhere and brought to the district when two to three years of age were not affected. The condition was not influenced by home or environmental factors: families whether rich or poor were affected. This observation tended to eliminate diet as an aetiological factor. McKay observed that three cities in Arkansas where mottling occurred, although separated from each other by some miles, all received their water supply from one source, Fountain Creek. This, together with many other reports, led him to believe that something in the water supply was responsible for mottled enamel.

McKay's research lasted over 30 years. In 1928 the US Public Health Service asked Dr McKay to accompany Dr Gromer Kempt, one of their medical officers, to carry out examinations in Bauxite. They found that no mottling occurred in people who grew up on Bauxite water prior to 1909, but all native Bauxite children who used the deep well water after that date had mottled teeth. No individual whose enamel developed during residence in Benton had mottled teeth. They reported that the standard water analysis of Bauxite water 'throws little light whatever on the probable causal agent'. Another piece of evidence had been gathered, but McKay seemed no closer to the solution.

Mottled enamel and fluoride concentration in drinking water

The chief chemist of ALCOA, Mr H. V. Churchill, read Kempt and McKay's paper and was greatly disturbed. Certain people in the United States were condemning the use of aluminium-ware

Table 3.1 Fluoride analyses from Churchill (1931)

Location of sample	Fluorine as fluoride (ppm)
Deep Well, Bauxite, Ark	13.7
Colorado Springs, Colo.	2.0
Well near Kidder, S. Dak.	12.0
Well near Lidgerwood, N. Dak.	11.0
Oakley, Idaho	6.0

for cooking. ALCOA mined most of its aluminium supply from Bauxite; if the story of the stain in Bauxite got into the hands of those who claimed that aluminium cooking utensils caused poisoning, ALCOA would have to reply to the charge. When Churchill received a sample of Bauxite water he instructed Mr A. W. Petrey, head of the testing division of the ALCOA laboratory, to look for traces of rare elements—those not usually tested for. Petrey ran a spectrographic analysis and noted that fluoride was present in Bauxite water at a level of 13.7. Churchill wrote to McKay on 20 January 1931:

> We have discovered the presence of hitherto unsuspected constituents in this water. The high fluorine contet was so unexpected that a new sample was taken with extreme precautions and again the test showed fluorine in the water.

He also asked McKay to send samples of water from other endemic areas with a 'minimum of publicity'. McKay quickly arranged for dentists in Britton, South Dakota, Oakley, Idaho, and Colorado Springs to send samples of the water in their areas. The results of these analyses were published in 1931 (Table 3.1). Churchill emphasized the fact that no precise correlation between the fluoride content of these waters and the mottled enamel had been established. All that was shown was the presence of a hitherto unsuspected common constituent of the waters from the endemic areas.

Fluoride in water

The work of H. Trendley Dean

The study of the relationship between fluoride concentration in drinking water, mottled enamel, and dental caries was given an impetus by the decision of Dr Clinton T. Messner, Head of the US Public Health Service, in 1931, to assign a young dental officer, Dr H. Trendley Dean, to pursue full-time research on mottled enamel. Dean was responsible for the research unit within the US Public Health Service and was the first dental officer of the service to be given a non-clinical assignment. His first task was to continue McKay's work and to find the extent and geographical distribution of mottled enamel in the United States. He reported that there were 97 localities in the country where mottled enamel was said to occur and this claim had been confirmed by a dental survey.

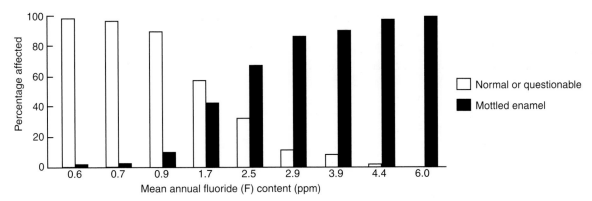

Figure 3.2 The prevalence of mottled enamel in areas with differing concentrations of fluoride in the water supply. (From Dean 1936.) (Reproduced from *Fluoride drinking waters*, edited by F. J. McClure, by kind permission of the US Department of Health, Education and Welfare 1962.)

Many of these confirmatory surveys were carried out by Dean himself. He developed a standard of classification of mottling in order to record quantitatively the severity of mottling within a community so that he could relate the fluoride concentration in the drinking water to the severity of mottling in a given area. His aim was to find out the 'minimal threshold' of fluorine—the level at which fluorine began to blemish the teeth. He showed conclusively that the severity of mottling increased with increasing fluoride concentration in the drinking water (Fig. 3.2).

Dean continued his studies into the relationship between the severity of mottled enamel and the fluoride concentration in water supplies. He presented additional evidence to show that amounts of fluoride not exceeding 1 ppm were of no public health significance. On 25th October, 1938, in conjunction with Frederick McKay, he summarized the knowledge of mottled enamel in a paper to the Epidemiology Section of the American Public Health Association. He reported that in the United States there were now 375 known areas, in 26 states where mottled enamel of varying degrees of severity were found. He also stated that the production of mottled enamel had been halted at Oakley, Idaho, Bauxite, Arkansas and Andover, South Dakota, simply by changing the water supply, which contained high concentrations of fluoride, to one whose fluoride concentration did not exceed 1 ppm. This information was 'the most conclusive and direct proof that fluoride in the domestic water is the primary cause of human mottled enamel'.

The story of fluoridation now entered a new and, from a public health point of view, a most important phase. Dean was aware of the reports from the literature that there may be an inverse relationship between the level of mottling and the prevalence of caries in a community. He knew of McKay's observations, first made in 1916, that mottled enamel was no more susceptible to decay than normal enamel. During his study to determine the minimum threshold of mottling, Dean had, in some cities, also examined the children for dental caries. Taking a selected sample of 9-year-old children, he found that of 114 children who had continuously used a domestic water supply comparatively low in fluoride

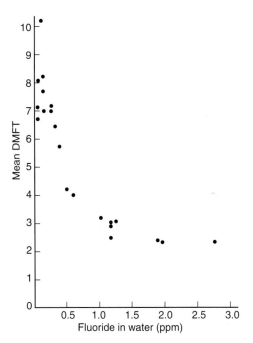

Figure 3.3 The relation between caries experience of 7257 12- to 14-year-old white schoolchildren of 21 cities in the USA and the fluoride content of the water supply. (From Dean et al. 1942.) (Reproduced from *Fluoride drinking waters*, edited by F. J. McClure, by kind permission of the US Department of Health, Education and Welfare 1962.)

(0.6–1.5 ppm) only five, or 4 per cent, were caries-free. On the other hand, of the 122 children who had continuously used domestic water containing 1.7–2.5 ppm fluoride, 27 (22 per cent) were caries-free.

This study paved the way for a much larger investigation of caries experience of 7257 12–14-year-old children from 21 cities in four states. The results (Fig. 3.3) show clearly the association between increasing fluoride concentration in the drinking water and decreasing caries experience in the population. Furthermore, this study showed that near maximal reduction in caries experience occurred with a concentration of 1 ppm F in the drinking water. At this concentration fluoride caused only 'sporadic instances of the mildest forms of dental fluorosis of no practical aesthetic significance' (Dean *et al.* 1942).

Why 1 ppm F in water?

Dean's work formed the basis of the decision to fluoridate at 1 ppm in the United States of America. His original observations have been substantiated by a number of investigators. Moller (1965) showed that data from Denmark and Sweden followed the same trend as that reported by Dean *et al.* (1942) (Fig. 3.4). In addition, studies in Great Britain, Hungary, Austria, Spain, and the United States show a decrease in caries experience with increasing fluoride content of the water supply up to about 2 ppm.

The relationship between caries experience in the deciduous dentition and the fluoride concentration in the drinking water

History of fluoride in dentistry 1874–1942

- 1874, role of fluoride as a nutrient first recorded in Germany
- 1916, Frederick McKay noted 'mottling' of teeth in Colorado
- 1931, Fluoride identified in significant amounts in water from areas with mottling
- 1939, Trendley Dean demonstrated relationship between water fluoride and enamel mottling
- 1942, Dean's survey demonstrated inverse relationship between fluoride and dental caries

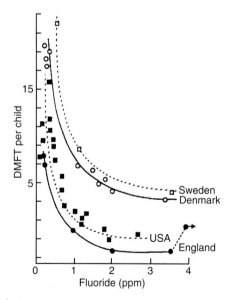

Figure 3.4 Caries experience in 12- to 13-year-old children from Denmark, Sweden, and the USA in relation to concentration of fluoride in water supplies. (From Moller 1965.) (Reproduced with permission.)

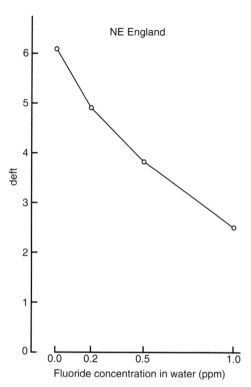

Figure 3.5 The relationship between caries experience (deft) in 1038 5-year-old children living in four areas of NE England and the fluoride concentration in their drinking water. (Rugg-Gunn *et al.* 1981.) (Reproduced by courtesy of the editor *British Dental Journal.*)

was investigated by Rugg-Gunn *et al.* (1981). They examined 1038 5-year-old children from four areas in the north-east of England and showed a progressive decrease in caries experience with increasing concentration of fluoride in the water, up to 1.0 ppm (Fig. 3.5), thus following the same trend as that reported for the permanent dentition.

Temperate and tropical climates and fluoride concentration

Reports in the 1940's from the United States of America showed that mottling increased with the F concentration in the water supplies and the mean annual temperature (Fig. 3.6). Countries in tropical areas should reduce the F content in their water. For example, Hong Kong fluoridated their water at 0.7 ppm F and have since reduced this to 0.6 ppm F.

Is artificial fluoridation as effective as natural fluoridation?

Grand Rapids–Muskegon study

The crucial step was to see if dental caries could be reduced in a community by adding fluoride at 1 ppm to a fluoride-deficient

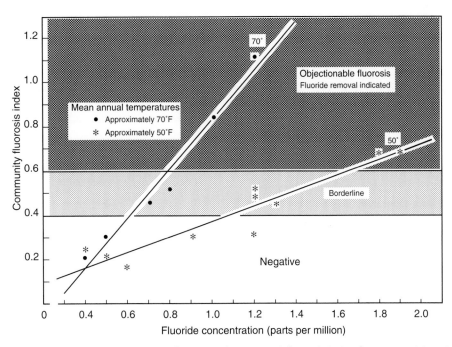

Figure 3.6 Relationship between fluoride concentration of municipal waters and fluorosis index for communities with mean annual temperatures of approximately 50° F. (Midwest) and 70° F. (Arizona).

water supply. The US Public Health Service was ready to embark on such an experiment. In December 1942 the service began talks with city officials of two cities in the Lake Michigan area, Grand Rapids and Muskegon. Both city councils agreed to carry out a study, with Grand Rapids becoming the experimental town and Muskegon the control town. Baseline studies showed that caries experience in the primary and permanent dentition in Grand Rapids was similar to that of Muskegon. In addition children continuously resident in the natural fluoride area of Aurora Illinois (F = 1.4 ppm) were examined to provide further baseline information.

On 25 January 1945 sodium fluoride was added to the Grand Rapids water supply. This was an historic occasion, because for the first time a permissible quantity of a beneficial dietary nutrient was added to the communal drinking water. The effects of six-and-a-half years of fluoridation in Grand Rapids were clear: caries experience of 6-year-old Grand Rapids children was almost half that of 6-year-old Muskegon children. The city officials of Muskegon, convinced of the efficacy of fluoridation, decided to fluoridate their own water supply in July 1951, so from this date Muskegon could no longer be used as a control town.

The only control left for Grand Rapids was a retrospective comparison with baseline data. Results after 10 years of fluoridation and 15 years of fluoridation are recorded in Figure 3.7. They indicate that caries experience in 15-year-old Grand Rapids children had fallen from 12.5 DMF teeth per mouth in 1944 to 6.2 DMF teeth per mouth in 1959, a reduction of approximately 50 per cent. Furthermore, caries experience in the fluoridated

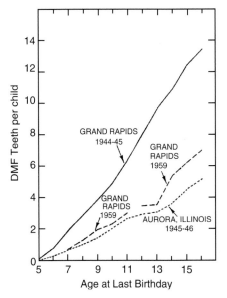

Figure 3.7 Dental caries in Grand Rapids children after 10 and 15 years of fluoridation (From Arnold *et al.* 1962; copyright by the American Dental Association, Reprinted by permission.)

community of Grand Rapids was very similar to that occurring in the natural fluoride area of Aurora. This was the experimental proof that the previously observed inverse relationship between fluoride in drinking water and dental caries experience was a cause and effect relationship.

The feelings that Trendley Dean and his co-workers had when they started the Grand Rapids experiment were recalled in an article by John Knutson in 1970:

> It is now 25 years ago that the late Trendley Dean and I journeyed by train from Washington, D.C., to Grand Rapids, Michigan, to be joined by Philip Jay for a meeting with the mayor to gain his approval for a water fluoridation experiment. … There were no signs of apprehension of daring or of pioneering. There were no implications or inferences that we were being foolhardy in subjecting a population of 160,000 people to a procedure which might have either short or long-range hazards. We were merely replicating nature's best, based on an extensive background of study data in nature's laboratory, a laboratory which was extremely large. In the United States alone, some seven million people in 1,900 communities had throughout life used drinking water which was naturally fluoridated with a fluoride concentration of 0.7 ppm or greater. We knew what too much did, we knew what too little did, we knew what the optimum amount was and we had assurance that one part per million fluoride in the drinking water had the same biological effect whether it got there from flowing over rocks or from a feeding machine.

Newburgh–Kingston study

In addition to the Grand Rapids–Muskegon study, two other fluoridation studies were carried out in the USA. On 2nd May 1945, sodium fluoride was added to the drinking water of Newburgh, on the Hudson river. The town of Kingston, situated 35 miles away from Newburgh, was chosen as a control town. Baseline studies were carried out in the two communities in 1944–46. Clinical examinations after 10 years of fluoridation were carried out in 1954–55. They reported that while caries experience in 10–12-year-old Kingston children had changed little from 1945 (23.1 per cent of teeth were carious) to 1955 (26.3 per cent), in contrast in similarly aged Newburgh children over the 10-year period, the DMF rate had fallen from 23.5 per cent to 13.9 per cent.

Evanston–Oak Park study

A third American fluoridation experiment began in January 1946 in Evanston, Illinois; the nearby community of Oak Park acted as the control town. The findings after 14 years of fluoridation in Evanston were published in 1967. Whereas the DMF values of 14-year-old Evanston children fell from 11.7 to 6.0 between 1946 and 1960 (a reduction of 49 per cent) no change was observed in the DMF values of 14-year-old Oak Park children over the intervening years.

The strength of the experimental proof of the caries-inhibitory property of fluoride drinking water lies not only in the conclusion of one study, but also in the fact that the three American studies, carried out by different investigators in different parts of the country, reached similar conclusions: addition of 1 ppm fluoride in the drinking water reduced caries experience by approximately 50 per cent.

Artificial fluoridation

- First scheme in Grand Rapids (T) and Muskegon (C), 1945, DMF reduction 12.5 per cent to 6.2 per cent
- Second experimental scheme, Newburgh (T) and Kingston (C), 1945, DMF reduction, 23 per cent to 13.9 per cent
- Third experimental scheme, Evanston (T) and Oak Park (C) 1946, DMF reduction 11.7 per cent to 6.0 per cent

British Studies

In the UK, the studies by Weaver had shown that caries experience in South Shields (natural fluoride content 1.4 ppm) was approximately 50 per cent lower than in North Shields (fluoride content 0.25 ppm), thus confirming Dean's findings in Galesburg and Monmouth, Macomb, and Quincy (Dean *et al.* 1939).

In addition, Weaver (1950) carried out a second investigation in 1949, in the North-East of England, including a survey of West Hartlepool children, where fluoride content of the water supply was 2 ppm. He examined 500 5-year-old children and reported that the mean dmft was 1.76 and that 53.6 per cent of the children were caries-free. A similar number of 12-year-old children were examined: the mean DMF was 0.96 and 59.8 per cent were caries-free. He commented: 'There can be few, if any, other areas in this country where the average DMF figure for uns-elected 12-year-old children is less than 1, as it was found to be in West Hartlepool'.

Forrest studied 324 12–14-year-old children in other parts of Britain with concentrations of fluoride in the drinking water varying from 0.9 to 5.8 ppm. She compared the caries prevalence with 259 children of the same age in non-fluoride areas. Caries was markedly lower in the high-fluoride regions.

A further study of areas with varying concentrations of fluoride in drinking water was carried out by James, who examined 1027 children aged 11–13 years from three areas in East Anglia: Norwich and Yarmouth (Norfolk) (F = 0.17–0.2 ppm), Chelmsford (intermittent fluoride content), and Colchester (F = 1.2–2 ppm). Children from Colchester were further divided into 'continuous' and 'non-continuous' residents. This study showed that the DMF of those children continuously resident in the high-fluoride area was less than half that of corresponding children in the low-fluoride area. Children aged 11–13 years who were continuous residents of Colchester had nearly double the proportion of sound first permanent molars found in the non-continuous residents.

In 1952, the British Government sent a mission to the USA and Canada to study fluoridation in operation. The mission concluded that fluoridation of water supplies was a valuable health measure, but recommended that in this country fluoride should be added to the water supplies of some selected communities before its general adoption was considered (Report of the United Kingdom Mission 1953). The selected communities chosen were Watford, Kilmarnock, and part of Anglesey. Fluoride was added to these drinking waters in 1955–1956. Sutton, Ayr, and the remaining part of Anglesey acted as the control towns. The results after 5 years of fluoridation (Department of Public Health and Social Security 1962) showed that caries experience in 5-year-old children was 50 per cent lower in the fluoride areas than the non-fluoride areas. Inspite of this, fluoridation was discontinued in Kilmarnock in 1962, on the instructions of the local council. However, dental examinations continued to be carried out in all areas and the findings after 11 years' fluoridation were reported in 1969. The report confirmed the main findings of 1962, that fluoridation of water supplies is a highly effective method of reducing dental decay.

In addition to demonstrating the beneficial effects of fluoridation, the report also confirmed its complete safety. 'During the eleven years under review, medical practitioners reported only two patients with symptoms which they felt might have been associated with fluoridation. Careful investigation in both instances failed to attribute the symptoms to the drinking of fluoridated water.' (Department of Public Health and Social Security, 1969).

Major fluoridation schemes began in the West Midlands in 1964 and on Tyneside in 1968.

surveys of 5-year-old children in fluoridated Newcastle and low-fluoride Northumberland. The results for this 1987 study are compared with the findings of the 1976 and 1981 surveys shown in Figure 3.8. Caries experience fell in both areas between 1976 and 1981, but no further decline was noted between 1981 and 1987. In all three studies the difference between the two communities was 54–60 per cent.

Data for 5-, 12-, and 15-year-old Hartlepool children are available since the 1940s (Weaver 1950, Murray 1969; Murray *et al.* 1991) and are summarized in Table 3.2. There are certain differences in epidemiological methods over the last 20 years. In 1969 a sharp probe was used, replaced or re-sharpened after every tenth examination. Nevertheless, if in doubt about a diagnosis, the surface was recorded as sound. The surveys carried out in 1989–90 based their criteria for diagnosis mainly on visual signs, using a ball-ended probe, diameter 0.5 mm in accordance with the national surveys. This difference in the level of diagnosis may be in part responsible for some of the differences between the 1969 and 1989 surveys. A slight shift in diagnosis, or reduction in dental disease, can affect the per cent caries-free value quite markedly, in that it only takes one diagnosis of a 'sticky fissure' to a carious cavity to remove an individual from the caries-free group.

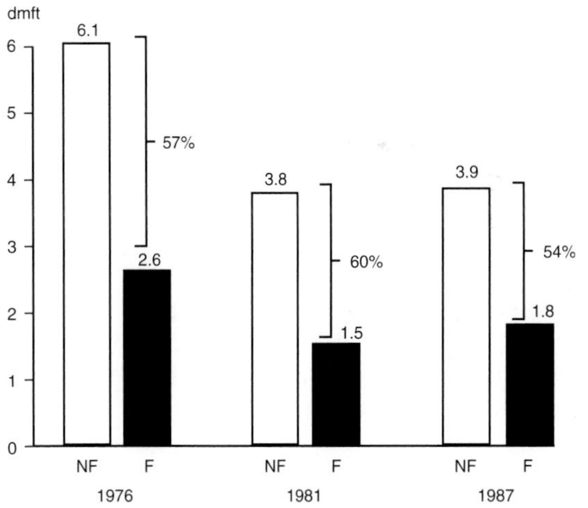

Artificial fluoridation in the UK

- 1955—3 experimental areas: Kilmarnock + Ayr
  Watford and Sutton
  Anglesey—two halves of the island

- Further schemes: West Midlands 1964,
  Tyneside 1968
  West Cumbria
  Leeds

Secular changes in fluoride areas

A great deal has been written about the secular decline in caries in many countries in the 'developed' world, particularly since the 1970s. This secular decline in caries in fluoridated area has been noted in Britain, in Anglesey and in Newcastle (Rugg-Gunn *et al.* 1988). Rugg-Gunn *et al.* (1988) have been involved in three

Figure 3.8 Caries experience (mean DMFT) of 5-year-old children in fluoridated (F: dark columns) and non-fluoridated (NF: open columns) areas of the North East of England in 1975, 1981, and 1987. (From Rugg-Gunn *et al.* 1988, with permission.)

Table 3.2 Caries experience in Hartlepool children 1949–89 (Weaver 1950; Murray 1969; Murray *et al.* 1991)

	5-year-old children			12-year-old children			15-year-old children		
	Weaver (1950)	Murray (1969)	Murray *et al.* (1991)	Weaver (1950)	Murray (1969)	Murray *et al.* (1991)	Weaver (1950)	Murray (1969)	Murray *et al.* (1991)
Mean dmf/DMF	1.8	1.5	0.8	1.0	2.0	0.7	2.1	4.9	1.7
Per cent caries-free	54	51	67	60	30	59	37	26	39

In spite of the secular changes in dental caries that have been referred to so often in the last few years, caries experience in Hartlepool remains one of the lowest recorded of any part of Great Britain.

There is no doubt that in the 1960s and 70s when there was an 'epidemic of caries' in Britain, Europe, and America, water fluoridation was seen to have a major impact on the dental health of a community. A reduction of 5 or 6 DMF teeth in 15-year-old children between Grand Rapids and Muskegon or Hartlepool and York was an obvious tangible benefit. The results from Anglesey and Newcastle/Northumberland show that water fluoridation is still beneficial, but the size of the benefit has been reduced because the total problem of caries has diminished.

Effect of cessation of fluoridation

Mansbridge showed that after cessation of the fluoridation scheme in Kilmarnock, in 1962, the prevalence of caries increased in children aged 3–7 years. By 1968, the proportion of children free from decay approximated to the pre-fluoridation level of 1956 and to that of the control children in Ayr.

Stephen *et al.* (1987) reported the results of clinical and radiographic examinations of 5-year-old children who had been born and raised in the fluoridated town of Wick, compared with similar subjects 5 years after Wick water was defluoridated in 1979 because of a decision taken by Highland Regional Council. The results are summarized in Table 3.3 and show that a substantial rise in dental caries had occurred. The authors concluded that this localized caries increase, which is against all national, local, and social class trends, resulted from the 1977 decision to deprive Wick inhabitants of fluoridated water supplies.

In 1980, a comparison had been made between the dental health of 10-year-old children in Stranraer, 10 years after the introduction of water fluoridation, and those in Annan, which had a negligible concentration of fluoride in the public water supply. In 1986, the opportunity was taken to examine 10-year-old children again, employing the same diagnostic criteria and one of the examiners involved in the previous study (Attwood and Blinkhorn 1988). Only lifetime residents were included in the analysis. The results show that whereas DMFT values had fallen by 16 per cent in Annan, they had risen by 4 per cent in Stranraer after fluoridation had been withdrawn. Although 10-year-old children in Stranraere may still have some residual benefit from earlier fluoridation, their study suggested that dental health had started to deteriorate.

Table 3.3 Caries experience in 5-year-old Wick children in 1979 and 1984 (Stephen *et al.* 1987)

	1979	1984	Per cent increase (1979 base)
Number of children	106	126	
Clinical mean dmft	2.63	3.92	49
Clinical and radiographic dmfs	8.42	13.93	67

One contrary result was reported recently by Kunzel and Fischer (2000), following the cessation of fluoridation in Cuba, in 1990. DMFT values were reported in La Salid before fluoridation (1973), after 9 years of fluoridation (1982) and 7 years (1997) after the cessation of fluoridation in 1990.

The largest reduction in caries occurred between 1973 and 1982. Values for 1997 were similar to the results recorded in 1982 for 8/9 and 10/11-year-old children. However, when water fluoridation ceased in 1990 a fortnightly mouth rinsing programme for all children was instituted, using a 0.2 per cent NaF solution and this may have confounded the results.

Fluoridation and the law

Legislation authorizing water fluoridation is of two types. It may be mandatory, requiring a Ministry of Health or communities of a certain size to fluoridate their public water supplies, or the legislation may be permissive or enabling, giving the 'Ministry of Health' or a local government the authority to institute fluoridation. Such legislation does not automatically bring about fluoridated water supplies, but paves the way for health officials or units of local government to act.

Mandatory laws requiring fluoridation of public water supplies that are fluorine-deficient have been enacted in Brazil, Bulgaria, Greece, Ireland, and five states of the United States of America.

Examples of countries with enabling legislation are several states of the USA, and also Australia, Israel, New Zealand, Canada, and the United Kingdom.

The existing fluoridation schemes in Britain were implemented in the 1960s when the bulk of the water supply industry was in public ownership i.e. under the management of local government. Both private and state owned water suppliers were persuaded, at the time, to fluoridate water for the public good under a non-profit-making arrangement whereby the state met all the appropriate costs.

There was great optimism in public health circles when the 1985 Water (Fluoridation) Bill went through Parliament. The Bill was brought forward by the then Conservative government to rectify a lack of legislative framework to allow new fluoridation schemes to be introduced. This followed a ruling by the High Court in Scotland in 1983 that fluoridation was 'ultra vires' and that existing schemes, in Scotland at least, were found to be unlawful.

It was thus considered by public health practitioners that it would be only a matter of time before fluoridation of public water supplies would be extended throughout the UK. The subsequent Act was not only the mechanism to introduce new schemes, but also set out the respective roles for the health authority, the water undertaker and the Secretary of State. (Lowry and Evans 1999)

However, no new water fluoridation schemes have been introduced under the 1985 (and later consolidating) legislation, but it was only on December 15, 1998, following a judicial review brought by Newcastle and North Tyneside Health Authority, that the legislation was finally proved in court to be inadequate.

Newcastle and North Tyneside Health Authority had requested a judicial review of the decision by Northumbrian Water Company Ltd following a refusal of their original request to the company to extend fluoridation in 1994 (five years after privatization). The aim of the judicial review was to clarify the responsibility of the water company in the local decision making process.

After an extensive publicity and consultation campaign in 1993–94, Newcastle and North Tyneside Health Authority (with all the other health authorities in the Northern health region) asked Northumbrian Water to introduce water fluoridation to a further 1.7 million people, 1 million people having already benefited from water fluoridation in the North East for over 25 years.

The Health Authority contended that Northumbrian Water was acting unlawfully in declining the Health Authority's request to extend fluoridation, and that the reasons given were illogical. The Health Authority argued that the relevant parliamentary acts governing water fluoridation were intended to encourage it, not merely enable it to be implemented if requested to by the Health Authority. The main argument against the Health Authority challenge to Northumbrian Water's decision was that the water company had absolute discretion to proceed or not with new water fluoridation schemes, and that this discretion was wide and unfettered. The presiding judge, Mr Justice Collins, concluded that as a private company (which did not possess power solely for the public good), Northumbrian Water had unfettered discretion for the purposes of the (fluoridation) statute. The Judge concluded that, regrettable though the water company decision was, because of the existing law, the application to have the decision challenged must fail.

The Judicial Review has shown that current legislation is ineffective as far as new water fluoridation schemes are concerned, as the water industry itself agrees. Health professionals cannot justify any more effort under existing regulations. If the present government want improved dental health, and fluoridation is the method of choice, then new (and effective) regulation is the only route.

It is also possible that existing schemes will come under increasing threat if water companies are forced to defer to shareholders (Lowry and Evans 1999).

Political progress of fluoridation in the UK

- 1970s   12% of population fluoridated
- 1980s   Court case in Scotland
- 1985   Water (fluoridation) bill
- 1998   Judicial Review finds legislation inadequate
- 2000   York Centre for Reviews—review of efficacy and safety of fluoridation

Why advocate fluoride dietary supplements?

When introduced, dietary fluoride supplements were perceived to be a reasonable alternative where water fluoridation was not possible. They were regarded as valuable both for individuals and as a public health measure. More recently, it has been concluded that the cariostatic effect of supplements may be less than was suggested in early trials. The initial dosage schedules were introduced before fluoride toothpastes were widely available. They were set to emulate the effects of drinking 1000 ml of water fluoridated at 1 mg per litre, but it would appear that children rarely drink as much as half this amount. More than one study has shown an association between use of fluoride supplements and enamel opacities. Supplements also demand a high degree of co-operation over a long period and it has been suggested that recommendations should not only be reduced but also simplified in order to encourage co-operation.

It is agreed that dietary supplements are not generally suitable as a public health measure and that they should be directed towards children who require them and who live in areas with suboptimal water fluoride levels. Children who stand to benefit include those for whom caries or its treatment may pose an additional hazard, as well as children thought likely to develop caries. For many of these children the potential disadvantage of mild enamel opacities may be outweighed by the benefits of fluoride supplements. It is also agreed that, when given as tablets, supplements should be allowed to dissolve slowly in the mouth to provide topical as well as systemic effect. Both to reduce the risk of opacities and to maximize their effectiveness, supplements should not be given at the same time as teeth are brushed.

There has been less consensus as to the most appropriate dosage schedule. A summary of current schedules used in different parts of the world is given in Fig. 3.9. It may need to be accepted that any dosage schedule which includes the critical period of enamel formation will carry some degree of risk of mild enamel opacities, particularly if fluoride ingestion from other sources occurs at the same time. The risk of opacities varies with time; the age of the child is critical, with permanent teeth at risk up to the age of 6 years, and permanent incisors during the first 3 years of life. The caries risk status of a child may also change with time, so that regular reassessment is needed. Parents must be fully involved in the decision and, where a dentist or doctor wishes to prescribe supplements, the risks and benefits need to be clearly explained to allow parents to make an informed choice.

The British Society of Paediatric Dentistry (BSPD) made the following recommendations with respect to fluoride supplements in a recent policy document:

- Dietary fluoride supplements are not generally a public health measure. They should be recommended only for individual children who are at risk and who live in areas with less than optimal water fluoride levels.

  Each case should be decided on its merits, and the risks and benefits of supplements should be fully explained to parents before prescription. A flexible approach should be adopted and a child's risk status regularly reassessed.

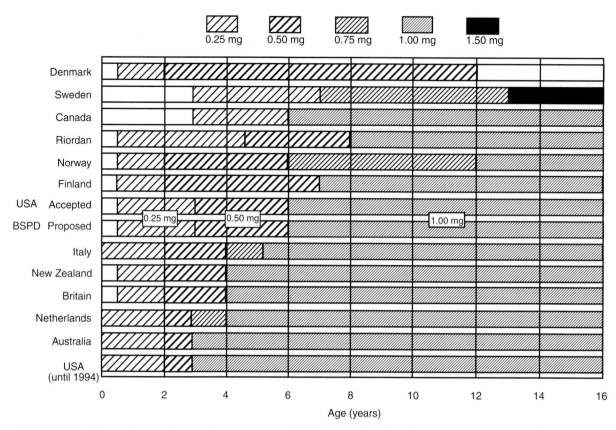

Figure 3.9 Daily fluoride supplement dosages, by age, recommended for use in low-fluoride areas (<0.33 ppm) in different countries. (After Riordan, 1993.)

- For children living in areas with water supplies containing less than 0.3 ppm fluoride and who are considered to be at high risk, the recommended dosage schedule should be:

Age	mg F per day
6 months up to 3 years	0.25
3 up to 6 years	0.50
6 years and over	1.00

In areas with water supplies containing fluoride at or above 0.3 ppm F dentists should consider a lower dosage.

Alternative systemic agents: Fluoride supplements

- Original dosage regimes to mimic fluoridated water levels
- Advent of fluoride toothpastes reduces dosage recommended (BSPD Policy Document)
- Prescribing practitioner needs to weigh up risks and benefits—fluorosis v caries
- Not advocated as a public health measure

Fluoridized salt and milk

As a dietary vehicle for ensuring adequate ingestion of fluoride, domestic salt comes second to drinking water: Salt's enrichment

with iodide already provides an effective means of preventing goitre. Indeed it was a medical practitioner concerned with prevention of goitre in Switzerland who, over 40 years ago, pioneered the addition of fluoride to salt as a caries-preventive measure. Fluoridated salt has been on sale in Switzerland since 1955, and by 1967 three-quarters of domestic salt sold in Switzerland was fluoridated at 90 mg F/kg salt (or 90 ppm F). Since 1983, the amount of fluoride added to salt has been 250 mg F/kg salt (250 ppm F). This is available in 23 Swiss cantons with 5.5 million inhabitants and is used voluntarily by 70 per cent of the population.

Despite the widespread use of fluoridated salt in Switzerland, its effectiveness is not easily measured since, in many Swiss communities, other preventive programmes (fluoride tablets or fluoride brushing) have been operating in many schools for over 20 years.

Interim results were published by Marthaler *et al.* from which they concluded that the caries-preventive effectiveness of fluoridized salt in Vaud was greater than the 25 per cent or so reduction observed following the addition of 90 mg F/kg in other Swiss cantons (Marthaler and Schenardi 1962). The results after 12, years are given in detail by de Crousaz *et al.* (1985). Dental examinations of 100–200 children in four age groups—8, 10, 12, and 14 years—were conducted on an examiner-blind basis in 1970, 1974, 1978, and 1982, although the numbers of children aged 14 years in the control area were too small to analyse. Results for DMF

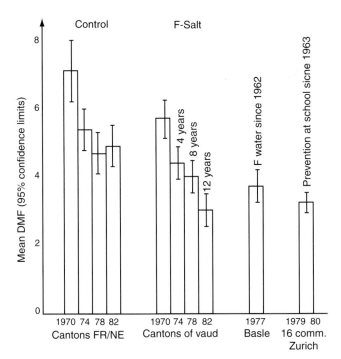

Figure 3.10 Mean DMFT for 12-year-old Swiss children in the control Cantons of Fribourg and Neuchâtel; receiving salt fluoridized to 250 mg F/kg in Vaud; in fluoridized Basle; and in 16 communities in Zurich Canton. (After de Crousaz *et al.* 1985; reproduced with kind permission of editor, *Helvetica Odontologica Acta.*)

sites are given in Fig. 3.10. The authors concluded that (a) there was a decline in caries experience in children in the control communities; (b) a similar decline occurred in 12 and 14-year-old children living in the test communities—this was not the case for 8 and 10-year-olds where a low caries prevalence already existed in 1970, probably due to earlier use of fluoride tablets; (c) caries experience was consistently lower in children who consumed salt fluoridized to 250 mg F/kg compared with children in the control communities. Caries experience of children in Vaud in 1982 was similar to those recorded for children in Basle who had consumed water fluoridated at 1.0 ppm F, and similar to children in Zurich Canton who had benefited from a school-based dental programme, which had been operating for the past 16 years.

Other studies in children have been reported from Hungary, Columbia and Spain. The studies were carried out in the 1960s and 1970s, when caries levels in Europe were very different from what they are now. Furthermore, most of these studies have been carried out over a limited period of time. One study of Swiss military conscripts (age 20) supports the hypothesis of continued effectiveness Menghini *et al.* (1985). Among conscripts from western Switzerland those who had not benefited from fluoridated salt had 10.2 DMF (decayed, missing, or filled) teeth (*n* = 153), while those from the canton of Vaud who had consumed fluoridated salt from the age of 5 years onwards showed only 7.1 DMF (*n* = 56). In Switzerland as a whole, there is a strong general

decline in caries prevalence. This is a small study carried out in 1985 and published in 1991, and is indicative, rather than conclusive, of a long-term beneficial effect due to salt fluoridation.

Fluoridated salt, when well-accepted by the public, has some parallels to water fluoridation in terms of wide coverage, little conscious action by the individual and low expense. It also requires systems of monitoring quality at the processing plants.

The political attractiveness of fluoridated salt, as opposed to water fluoridation, is in the element of choice for consumers. In most places using fluoridated salt, it appears alongside non-fluoridated salt on the supermarket shelves. This makes fluoridated salt more palatable from the social policy viewpoint, but its community-wide caries-preventive impact is clearly related to the extent of public acceptance (in Switzerland, fluoridated salt claimed 75 per cent of the national domestic salt market in 1987 to 1991). The introduction of fluoridated salt, therefore, needs to be accompanied by public education and promotion. When only some domestic salt is fluoridated, consumers retain more choice, but public health effectiveness is diminished. The Swiss canton of Vaud, interestingly enough, removes that choice by fluoridating all salt on the supermarket shelves as well as the salt delivered in bulk to restaurants, bakeries, food processors, hospitals, and other institutions. Oral health should benefit as a result, though consumer choice is curtailed. In France and Germany, which only accept fluoride uses which permit consumer choice, the fluoridated salt programme is limited to domestic salt, which is available alongside non-fluoridated salt. But in both Costa Rica and Jamaica all domestic and institutional salt, except that for bakeries, is fluoridated. Despite the extensive studies carried out in Colombia and Hungary, salt fluoridation has not become established in either country.

Salt fluoridation is not recommended in countries where there is extensive water fluoridation. Further research in salt fluoridation should be in its acceptance and effectiveness in the different countries now adopting the measure, and further refinement of country-specific concentrations with a variety of dietary practices. There is also little information on fluorosis resulting from salt fluoridation; that too requires documentation.

The evidence for the effectiveness of salt fluoridation is based on a limited number of observational studies; the nature of the procedure does not lend itself readily to randomized, double-blind clinical trials. Other uses of fluoride also make it difficult to ascribe specific effects to any one method of using fluoride. Positive results were also reported from studies in Hungary and Spain in the 1970s.

Other dietary vehicles for fluoride

- Fluoridized salt
- Represents 75 percent of table salt in Switzerland
- Available since 1955
- Significant reductions in caries despite background fluorides
- Gives consumer choice—politically advantageous

Fluoridized milk

Both bovine and human milk contain low levels of fluoride—about 0.03 ppm F. Because milk is recommended as a good food for infants and children, it was considered, over 30 years ago, to be a suitable vehicle for supplementing children's fluoride intake in areas with fluoride-deficient water supplies. Ericsson (1958) showed that fluoride was absorbed in the gut just as readily from milk as from water, refuting the suggestion that the high calcium content of milk would render the fluoride unavailable. However, the binding of added fluoride to calcium or protein might reduce the topical fluoride effect in the mouth compared with fluoride in water. All the reported trials have shown caries-preventive effects, especially when milk consumption began before the eruption of permanent teeth. Clinical data are still limited, however. Milk fluoridization requires considerable logistic effort and, as yet, it has not been introduced on a community basis, although studies have been carried out in Glasgow and Cheshire.

Developments in fluoride toothpastes

Developments in Britain between 1960 and 1990

Clinical trials of the effectiveness of fluoride in toothpaste began in England in the 1960s. Four independent studies into the effect of stannous fluoride toothpaste were carried out by Jackson and Sutcliffe, James and Anderson, Naylor and Emslie, and Slack and co-workers and were published in 1967. In addition to investigation of stannous fluoride pastes, Naylor and Emslie, and later Hargreaves and Chester were involved in trials of sodium monofluorophosphate (MFP) toothpaste.

In marketing terms, two commercial products (Colgate MFP and Gibbs F) were launched in the late 1960s alongside standard, non-fluoride toothpastes produced by the same company. Initially the impact of the fluoride toothpastes was small, with these products capturing only 5 per cent of the market share by 1970.

A further critical development in marketing occurred in 1973 when MFP was added to the toothpaste which was then the brand leader (Colgate Minty), with over 20 per cent of the market share. Two further manufacturers (Beechams and Unilever) followed suit, either by converting their main brand to an MFP paste or by introducing a new paste containing fluoride. The fourth major toothpaste manufacturer (Procter and Gamble), entered the British market in 1976, when they launched a new toothpaste (Crest) containing Fluoristan (stannous fluoride). Sales of fluoride toothpastes had increased rapidly and by this time fluoride containing pastes accounted for 75 per cent of the market. Growth continued and by the end of the 1970s this figure had increased to about 95 per cent.

With the increase in sales, competition among the manufacturers became intense and a wide range of fluoride toothpastes was developed and marketed. Products varied in fluoride concentration and in the type of fluoride compound used. Mixed fluoride systems (NaF and MFP) were employed in some toothpastes, and other active agents were included in others.

A number of clinical trials were carried out to investigate the effects of varying fluoride concentrations, with pastes tested containing from 250 to 1000 to 1500 ppm F or higher. Results of these are summarized in Table 3.4. From findings in these studies it has been suggested that a dose response may be seen with each increase of 500 ppm F above 1000 ppm F resulting in an additional reduction in caries increment of 6–7 per cent.

In summary, studies have shown that fluoride in toothpaste at a concentration of 1000–1500 ppm F result in reductions in caries increments in 3 year clinical trials of approximately 30 per cent compared with control groups using non-fluoride formulations.

Table 3.4 DMF increments and percentage differences reported in caries increments—studies involving mainly sodium monofluorophosphate dentifrices of different concentrations

Study	ppm F (approx.)				
	250	500	1000	1500	2000
Koch et al. (1982)	7.5[1] —	[13.4] →	6.7		
Mitropolous et al. (1984)	4.29 —	[18.8] →	3.61		
Winter et al. (1989)		2.52[2] — [10.0] →	2.29		
Triol et al. (1987)			3.21 — [8.8] →	2.95	
				2.95 — [5.7] →	2.79
Stephen et al. (1988)			6.80 — [7.4] →	6.33	
				6.33 — [10.9] →	5.71
Conti et al. (1988)			2.39 — [27.8] →	1.87	
Fogels et al. (1988)			2.36 — [16.8] →	2.02	

[1]NaF dentifrice
[2]0.209 MFP + 0.060 NaF
[]Percentage reduction

Fluoridated toothpaste

- Available commercially in late 1960s
- Fluoridated pastes occupied 75 percent of market by mid-1970s, 95 percent by late 1970s
- Initially based on MFP, followed by Sn(F)2 and later a combination of NaF and MFP.
- Toothpaste containing 1000–1500 ppm reduces caries prevalence by 30 percent

In considering the current status and the future role of fluoride toothpastes, the following issues will be discussed:

- low dose/low concentration formulations;
- fluoride ingestion and the risk of fluorosis;
- toothpaste delivery systems, dispensing instructions and labelling;
- fluoride toothpaste and oral clearance;
- the effect of fluoride toothpastes on root caries;
- the addition of other therapeutic agents.

Low dose/low concentration formulations

Toothpastes containing lower concentrations have been designed primarily to reduce the risk of fluorosis, and are therefore, most often directed towards children. However, fluoride content in toothpastes for children varies and although some do so, not all have a fluoride concentration below the 1000 ppm F—found in the majority of standard pastes. Children's pastes may contain fluoride in the form of sodium fluoride or of sodium monofluorophosphate.

Five clinical studies into the effectiveness of pastes with lower fluoride concentrations have been reported. In four the effectiveness of pastes containing 250 ppm or less was investigated and in the case of the fifth the test paste contained 550 ppm (Winter et al. 1989). Overall, these studies showed that caries inhibition increased with increasing F content of the toothpaste.

Clinical trials of low concentration fluoride toothpastes varied not only in the fluoride concentration employed but also in the age of the children taking part in the trial. Low fluoride toothpastes are designed to reduce the risk of enamel opacities and there would appear to be little justification for using them for teenage children when there is no risk of fluorosis in anterior teeth. The study carried out by Winter et al. in Norwich was large, involving more than 2000 children who were initially aged two years. Children in the test group used a low concentration paste containing 550 ppm of fluoride, and those in the control group used a standard 1050 ppm F paste.

The small difference in mean DMFs at the end of the three year trial seen between the groups amounted to less than 0.1 DMFs per child per year in favour of the controls and was not significant on

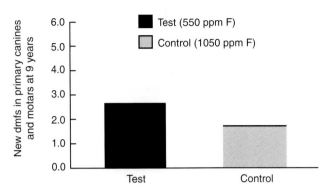

Figure 3.11 Three year low F toothpaste trial in children aged two years—follow-up study at nine years of age.

statistical testing. It was therefore, difficult to infer that there was a difference between the groups at the end of the trial. However, a follow up study was carried out when the children were nine years of age (Holt 1995); no further test or control pastes had been available during the four year interval. Findings at follow up showed that the difference between groups had increased with time. Difference in mean DMFs now amounted to an average of 0.8 of a primary tooth surface per child (Fig. 3.11).

The same result is apparent when increment is considered in relation to caries experience at five years. Figure 3.12 shows the increment for children who had no caries experience at five years, for those with DMFs of between 1 and 5 and for those who had DMFs of more than 5 at this age. In both test and control groups the number of new carious surfaces increased with increasing levels of caries experience at five years.

Low fluoride toothpastes

- In the range 100–550 ppm
- Confine use to children under 6 years of age (at low caries risk) to protect from opacities on anterior teeth
- Dentists to consider the balance between risk of caries versus enamel opacities

Fluoride ingestion and the risk of fluorosis

The trial carried out in Norwich not only provided information about caries but the follow-up study also provided information on enamel opacities in children who had used a low fluoride paste (Holt et al. 1994). The authors in the follow-up study photographed the upper permanent incisor teeth of the children when they were nine years of age. The teeth were scored using the TF index for fluorosis and the Modified Developmental Defects of Enamel (DDE) index. Compared with findings in the standard controls, the child and tooth prevalence of opacities were significantly lower in the children who had used the test paste with a

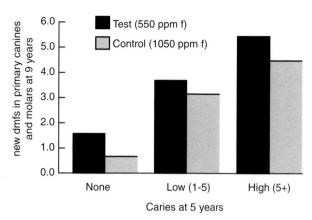

Figure 3.12 Three year low F toothpaste trial in children aged two years—follow-up study at nine years of age.

lower fluoride content. The trend was seen not only with the TF Index but also in the case of diffuse defects measured using the modified DDE index. A third group was included in the study, children who had not participated in the original study and some of whom may therefore, have been exposed during their early years to pastes containing 1000–1500 ppm F. This latter group had the highest proportion of children with a TF1 or TF2 score.

Other workers have reported on fluoride ingestion, toothpaste use, and the risk of fluorosis in fluoride areas. Osuji *et al.* (1988) reported that children who started toothbrushing before the age of 22 months were eleven times more likely to develop fluorosis than those children who began brushing later. Milsom and Mitropoulos (1990) considered the relationship between the age of onset of toothbrushing and residence in a fluoride area. More children in the fluoride community (60 per cent) had enamel defects compared with those in the non-fluoridated community (44 per cent). In the fluoridated community more children whose parents claimed to begin brushing at an early age exhibited enamel defects.

Thus, the risks and benefits of low dose formulations may be seen to be balanced in that there is a higher risk of dental caries against a lower risk of dental fluorosis (Fig. 3.13). However, fluoride ingestion may be from several sources. Whilst investigations reported above employed analysis related solely to toothpastes, three more recent studies have included multivariate methods and have reported odds ratios for more than a single fluoride source. Pendrys *et al.* investigated the risk factors for enamel fluorosis in a fluoridated community and reported that inappropriate fluoride supplements (odds ratio 23.7), soya-based and milk-based infant formula use (OR = 7.2 and 3.3) and frequent toothbrushing (OR = 2.8) were significant risk factors. Broadly similar findings were reported by Lalumandier and Rozier and Riordan; dietary fluoride supplements (OR = 6.5), age at the start of toothbrushing (OR = 3.0), early weaning (OR = 2.8) and swallowing toothpaste (OR = 2.6) were identified as risk factors by these authors. Fluoride toothpastes are very widely used. The potential for

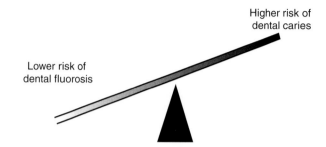

Figure 3.13 Low F toothpaste formulations—risks and benefits.

inappropriate use to result in fluorosis was emphasized in a very recent study, where it was reported that 71 per cent of a series of cases diagnosed as fluorosis were explicable in terms of a history of having brushed more than once per day with more than a pea sized amount of toothpaste throughout the first eight years of life (Pendrys, 1995).

From these reports it may be concluded that risk factors for dental fluorosis may be ranked in the following order:

Risk factors for dental fluorosis

- Inappropriate fluoride supplements
- Age of child when toothbrushing started
- Frequency of brushing/swallowing toothpaste
- Residence in an optimum fluoride area

Toothpaste delivery, dispensing instructions, labelling

How toothpaste is delivered, in terms of the type of packaging and containers used, the instructions given for its use and the way in which it is labelled are important in determining efficacy. These factors may also strongly affect toothpaste ingestion, and so influence the ingestion of fluoride.

There has been much debate as to the quantity of paste that should be used. Instructions have varied, one children's toothpaste, sold in France, advises one to 'cover the brush'. Advertisements as posters or in newspapers or magazines often provide the same message by implication through their artwork. The Health Education Authority recommends that a pea-sized amount be used; this advice has become widespread and is now printed on many toothpaste tubes and cartons. Rock (1994) suggested that the brush should be smeared, rather than using a pea sized amount which may be too much. It is unhelpful to have disparity between exhortations to use small amounts and the images of toothpaste generously applied to the brush. Rock has pointed out that the amount used can radically affect total fluoride ingestion. As an example, a strip of toothpaste containing 1000 ppm F and covering the brush head contains fifteen times the amount of fluoride of a blob of paste of one third the length at a concentration of 200 ppm fluoride.

The amount of toothpaste used will be influenced by the consistency. Paste with low viscosity may be difficult to measure accurately onto the brush head before it flows between the filaments. More conventional pastes show greater coherence, allowing a more accurate estimate to be made. More recently, nozzle designs have been introduced which allow a reduced amount of toothpaste to be dispensed for a given length. Tubes for one children's paste have a star shaped nozzle design in contrast to a round one for example. In the case of some others currently on the market, containers have very small sized round nozzles.

One current recommendation is that children under the age of seven years and at low risk of caries should use a low fluoride toothpaste (British Society of Paediatric Dentistry). However, choosing an appropriate paste may be difficult at present because of the system of labelling used. Labels may give no indication of the level of fluoride contained, or the amount of fluoride may be given only in the form of percentage sodium fluoride or sodium monofluorophosphate. The great majority of consumers and of the dental profession may well be unaware of the amount of fluoride present in either of these two fluoride compounds. On the basis of available information it seems unlikely, therefore, that many consumers could make an informed choice, or that many dentists could make specific recommendations.

Fluoride toothpaste and oral clearance

Chesters et al. (1992) drew attention to the fact that the method of oral rinsing after using F-toothpaste, and the frequency of toothbrushing, can both have a relationship with caries increments in clinical trials. The DMFs increment in this study was highest (6.9) when a beaker was used to rinse away toothpaste followed by 'using a brush' (5.9), putting 'head under tap' (5.8) and 'using hand' (5.5.). The caries increment for those who brushed once per day or less was higher (7.0) than those who brushed twice per day or more (5.4). From these results it may be concluded that the greatest reduction in DMFs increment occurs when brushing at least twice per day and rinsing by means of hand under the tap (Fig. 3.14) Similar findings have been reported by Ashley et al. 1999.

Effect on root caries

In reviewing the development of toothpaste, there has been particular concern about fluoride ingestion by children. However, toothpastes also need to be considered in relation to the needs of the middle-aged and elderly. In these older age groups, fluoride toothpaste may be an important means of reducing root caries. A high prevalence of root caries has been reported in several studies, Katz et al. (1982) reported that 40–60 per cent of the dentate population had at least one root caries lesion, and according to Banting one in nine of exposed root surfaces is carious. Results of a recent study by Steele et al. (1996) illustrated that, in dental adults aged 60+ years, in Salisbury, Darlington, and Richmondshire, the mean number of carious root surfaces was approximately 3.0. The adult dental health survey reported a similar finding (Todd and Lader 1991). It must be recognized that these estimates

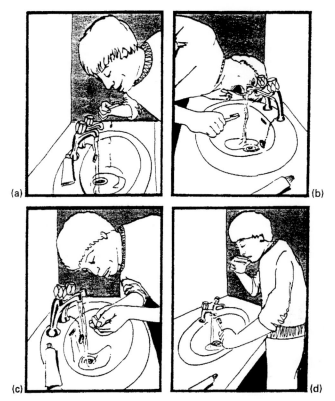

Figure 3.14 Sketches of alternative rinsing methods. (a) using a toothbrush to transfer water to the mouth: (b) putting the mouth under the tap: (c) transferring water using cupped hands: (d) using a beaker to transfer water to the mouth. (From Chesters et al. 1992.)

of root caries in the elderly are higher, in numerical terms, than DMFs values in 5-year-old children. There may well be a case for increasing the fluoride content of toothpaste, specifically for use in the dentate elderly, in order to prevent root caries (Fig. 3.15).

One study by Jensen and Kohout (1988) reported on the benefits of a 1000 ppm F toothpaste in reducing root caries over a very short (one year) period but the most appropriate F concentration for preventing root surfaces represent exposed dentine, toothpastes suitable for the elderly may not only need to have increased fluoride but would also require different abrasive systems. Pastes with low abrasivity may be more appropriate in this context. Recently, Baysen et al. (2001) concluded that a dentifrice containing 5000 ppm F was significantly better at remineralizing primary root surface carions lesions than one containing 1100 ppm F.

Additional therapeutic agents

Several types of fluoride toothpastes include other agents in addition to fluoride. A variety of agents has been added intended to enhance effectiveness and appeal to the consumer. One manufacturer (Smith Kline-Beecham) has added calcium glycerophosphate to monofluorophosphate, claiming that this results in a greater reduction in caries. In the case of some other products, sodium pyrophosphate has been added as an anti-calculus agent. Because of its unpleasant taste, this agent requires complete reformulation to make the product acceptable.

Zinc citrate is used by one manufacturer (Unilever) as an antiplaque agent, Triclosan has also been shown to reduce plaque and gingivitis and is used for example in Colgate Total. Chlorhexidine, used for many years as a mouthrinse or gel, has now been incorporated in some toothpastes, such as Crest Specialist Gum Care. More recently, particularly in Scandinavia, pastes have been introduced which contain Xylitol.

Until recently there was only a limited number of toothpastes aimed at reducing sensitivity, but with a greater proportion of the population retaining their teeth, and an increased prevalence of exposed root surfaces, there has been a marked increase in the numbers of pastes of this type marketed. Pastes designed to reduce sensitivity may contain a variety of different active agents.

In Britain a new toothpaste claiming to 'lock in high fluoride' has been marketed. This product can only be purchased on prescription. The toothpaste contains sodium fluoride 0.619% (2800 ppm F) and is said to be ideal for the management of high risk patients such as the elderly and those with rampant caries,

early, existing or recurrent caries, compromised oral health (Fig. 3.15).

Are topical fluorides effective?

Topical fluoride therapy

Topical fluorides fall into two categories: those applied by the dentist in the surgery and those applied by the patient at home. In practice those employed by the dentist are of high fluoride concentration and are applied generally at regular but infrequent intervals, perhaps twice a year. Those used by the patient are of low fluoride levels and are applied at frequent intervals, often daily.

Fluorides applied by the dentist

Such fluoride agents mainly include simple aqueous solutions of sodium fluoride and stannous fluoride, and low pH solutions and gels of an acidulated phosphate fluoride system. Other agents comprise fluoride prophylaxis pastes and fluoride-containing varnishes. Little change has occurred in this area in the last five years, and for that reason this topic will not be considered further in this chapter.

Toothpastes containing fluoride were first introduced over 30 years ago. Clinical trials have demonstrated their effectiveness in reducing caries and because they have been so widely used in many westernized countries fluoride toothpastes have come to play a major part in dental health.

Topical fluorides have been used as caries-preventive agents in dental practice for over fifty years. During this period four main types of preparations have been advocated: neutral sodium fluoride solutions, stannous fluoride solutions, acidulated phosphate agents, and fluoride varnishes.

Additional therapeutic agents

• Prevention of caries	Calcium glycerophosphate
	Xylitol
• Anti-calculus	Sodium pyrophosphate
• Anti-plaque	Zinc citrate
	Triclosan
	Chlorhexidene
• Desensitising	Potassium citrate
	Strontium chloride

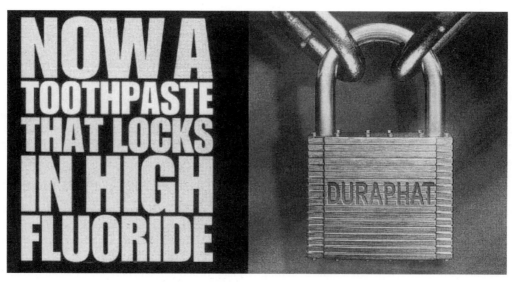

Figure 3.15 Advert for high fluoride toothpaste (2800 ppm).

The minutiae of the results of clinical trials with topical fluoride therapy, and possible advantage of one preparation over another, have been considered elsewhere (Murray, Rugg-Gunn, and Jenkins 1991).

The purpose of this section is to describe briefly some of the fashions in topical fluoride therapy over the last fifty years and to consider the effectiveness of this aspect of preventive dentistry.

In 1940 it was shown that in vitro the solubility of enamel could be reduced by treating it with a fluoride solution. Bibby and Knutson were among those who carried out clinical trials using sodium fluoride solutions. Knutson concluded that maximum reductions in caries was achieved from four treatments of 2 per cent acqueous NaF at weekly intervals (approximately 8000 ppm F) at the ages of 3, 7, 10, and 13 years, to coincide with the eruption of teeth. The problem with this method was that it was not easy to integrate it into routine re-call examinations for children.

In the 1950s attention changed to stannous fluoride, because it had been claimed that this agent was superior to sodium fluoride in achieving fluoride absorption into enamel. Stannuous fluoride is unstable in solution and so it was suggested that an 8 per cent stannous fluoride solution should be freshly prepared each day and would be active for five to eight hours. The agent should be applied every six months. A disadvantage of stannous fluoride is that it causes brown pigmentation of teeth and can also cause gingival irritation.

In 1947 Bibby had found that lowering the pH of a fluoride solution enabled more fluoride to be absorbed into enamel. In the 1960s researchers turned away from stannous fluoride back to sodium fluoride in an acid solution, 0.1 M phosphoric acid, so giving rise to acidulated phosphate (APF) solutions and gels. These agents typically yielded 1.23 per cent F (12,300 ppm F). APF solutions were applied to the teeth with cotton wool for 4 minutes, during which time the teeth had to be isolated from saliva. Some workers introduced a gelling agent (usually methyl cellulose or hydroxy ethyl (cellulose) so that an APF gel could be applied in a tray, which was held in place for 4 minutes. The patient (usually a child) is then instructed not to rinse out for 30 minutes, in order to keep the fluoride agent in contact with the enamel surface for a prolonged period of time.

The need to keep the fluoride agent in close proximity to the tooth surface for as long as possible gave rise to the development of fluoride varnishes, in particular Duraphat, which yields 2.26 per cent F (22,600 ppm) from a suspension of sodium fluoride in an alcoholic solution of natural varnish substances. It is claimed that this material tolerates water well, so that it covers even moist teeth with a film of varnish. A comparison of topical fluorides, based on the work of Horowitz and Ismail 1996 is given in Table 3.5.

Two systematic reviews of the effectiveness of gels and varnishes have been published recently in The Cochrane Library. Twenty five studies of fluoride gels, involving 7747 children, were included. The best estimate of the magnitude of the caries-inhibiting effects of fluoride gel was a 21% reduction in DMFS scores. As many as one in two children with high levels of tooth decay, and one in twenty four with the lowest levels, would have less decay.

Nine studies of fluoride varnish application, involving 2709 children were considered. A substantial caries-inhibitory effect of fluoride varnish in both the permanent (46%) and the primary dentitions (33%) was observed. The reviewers concluded that future trials should be placebo-controlled randomized studies and should include the assessment of other relevant outcomes, including acceptability of treatment and information on possible side effects (Marinho *et al.* 2002 a, b).

All the topical fluorides discussed in this section require professionals, either dentists or hygienists, to apply them. They were extremely popular especially in the United States of America and in Scandinavia in the 1970s, when the prevalence of caries was very high and substantial reductions in DMFs values could be achieved in one or two year clinical trials. These studies were often also carried out in conjunction with fortnightly mouth rinsing programmes at school.

As caries rates have declined, particularly in the permanent teeth of children and adolescents, the cost effectiveness of using professionally applied fluoride agents has been questioned both on effectiveness and economic grounds, especially when the availability of another self-applied topical fluoride agent—toothpaste—increased from around 5 per cent in 1970 to 95 per cent in 1980. Today it is recognized that professionally applied topical fluoride agents are not cost effective as a population measure, but should be targeted at patients at increased risk of developing caries—for example, those who show white spot enamel lesions, or patients undergoing fixed appliance treatment, or those receiving radiotherapy for head and neck malignancy.

Table 3.5 Characteristics of topical fluoride agents (After Horowitz and Ismail 1996)

Characteristic	NaF	SnF$_2$	APF	Duraphat
Percent and ppm F	2%	8%	1.23% F	2.26%
	9,200	19,500	12,300	22,600
Frequency of application	4 at weekly intervals at ages 3, 7, 10 & 13	1 or 2/year	1 or 2/year	1 or 2/year
Taste	Bland	Disagreeable	Acidic	Banana
Stability	Stable	Unstable	Stable in plastic container	Stable
Tooth pigmentation	No	Yes	No	No
Gingival irritation	No	Occasional, transient	No	No

Professionally applied topical fluorides

- 1940s Sodium fluoride 2 percent = 9200 ppm
- 1950s Stannous fluoride 8 percent = 19,500 ppm
- 1960s Acidulated phosphate fluoride 1.23 percent = 12,300 ppm
- 1970s Sodium fluoride in natural varnish 2.26 percent = 22,600 ppm

What about dental fluorosis?

Dental fluorosis is a hypoplasia or hypomaturation of tooth enamel or dentine produced by the chronic ingestion of excessive amounts of fluoride during the period when teeth are developing (Fig. 3.16). The major cause of dental fluorosis is the consumption of water, containing high levels of fluoride, by infants and children during the first six years of life. Although both primary and permanent teeth may be affected by fluorosis, under uniform conditions of fluoride availability fluorosis tends to be greater in permanent teeth than primary teeth. This disparity may be due to the fact that much of the mineralization of primary teeth occurs before birth and the placenta serves as a barrier to the transfer of high concentrations of plasma fluoride from a pregnant mother to her developing fetus, thus controlling to a certain extent the delivery of fluoride to the developing primary dentition. Other reasons may be that the period of enamel formation for primary teeth is shorter than for permanent teeth and that the enamel of primary teeth is thinner than that of permanent teeth.

Interest in dental fluorosis has increased over the past 10 years or so, not only in areas like India and Kenya, where there are communities with high levels of fluorosis associated with high concentrations of fluoride in the water supply, but also in temperate climates with optimal or low fluoridated water supplies where fluoride uptake from other sources, in particular fluoride supplements and fluoride toothpaste, in early infancy, have resulted in

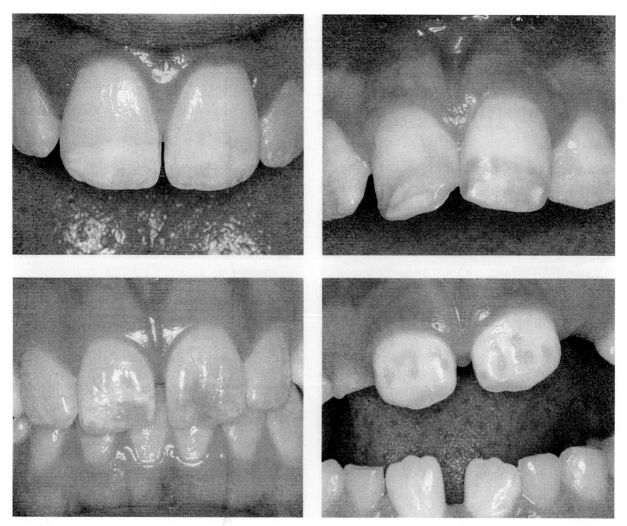

Figure 3.16 Degrees of fluorosis

an increase in the prevalence of enamel mottling. With the decline in caries, following fluoride therapy, increasing attention is now being given to levels of dental fluorosis. In a sense, history is turning full circle, because the history of water fluoridation really started with attempts to ascertain the cause of 'Colorado stain' in the early 1900s.

In the last 10 years a number of workers have drawn attention to the possibility of an increase in the prevalence of dental fluorosis. For example, Osuji and Nikiforuk (1988) presented two cases which exhibited classical dental fluorosis in the permanent dentition, both of whom had received more fluoride supplement than recommended in the dosage schedules. The first received 0.5 mg F/day from infancy and 1.0 mg F/day from the age of 2 to 6 years in an area that has a natural water fluoride concentration of 0.42 ppm. The second case received 1.0 mg F/day from birth to 7 years of age in an area with a natural water fluoride concentration of 0.1 ppm F. Riordan (1993) called for a reconsideration of existing recommendations concerning fluoride supplements in order to reduce the risk of fluorosis. He proposed that fluoride supplements should be aimed only at identifiable high caries-risk individuals and should start at 6 months of age or later. Pang and Vann (1992) quoted an NIDR sponsored international workshop on 'changing patterns of systematic fluoride intake', where it was agreed that the inadvertent ingestion of toothpaste could be a cause of increased dental fluorosis in children.

In an editorial entitled 'Too much of a good thing?' Mason (1991) reported that:

> The available evidence points to an increase in dental fluorosis in both fluoridated and non-fluoridated communities. Increased fluoride exposure from a variety of fluoride-containing dental products is the most likely source. In some cases, health professionals may be prescribing fluoride dietary supplements inappropriately, or failing to advise parents to teach their small children to spit out, not swallow, fluoride toothpaste. (In this regard, government regulations and the manufacturers of dental products need to look at the label instructions to see if they need to be more specific.) Increases in dental fluorosis are an indication that total fluoride exposure is increasing and may be more than necessary to prevent tooth decay. Prudent public health practice dictates using no more than the amount necessary to achieve a desired effect.

Water Fluoridation: a Systematic Review

A systematic review of water fluoridation was commissioned by the Chief Medical Officer of the Department of Health for England to 'carry out an up to date expert scientific review of fluoride and health' (Para 9.20 Our Healthier Nation).

A forest plot of the bone studies (Fig. 3.17) showed that there was no association between water fluoridation and fracture incidence.

The findings of cancer studies were mixed, with small variations on either side of no effect. Individual concerns examined were bone cancer and thyroid cancers, where once again no clear pattern of association was seen. Overall, from the research evidence presented, no association was detected between water fluoridation and mortality from any cancer, or from bone or thyroid cancers specifically.

With regard to changes in caries experience, fifteen studies found a statistically significantly greater mean change in dmft/DMFT scores in the fluoridated areas than the non-fluoridated areas (Fig. 3.18). Studies in which fluoridation was discontinued were also included in the systematic review (Fig. 3.19), with all but one of the studies suggesting that stopping water fluoridation had led to a greater increase in the previously fluoridated area than in the non-fluoridated area.

The systematic review concluded that the best available evidence suggests that fluoridation does reduce caries prevalence, both as measured by the proportion of children who are caries free and by the mean dmft/DMFT score. An effect of water fluoridation was still evident in studies completed after 1974 in spite of the assumed exposure to fluoride from other sources of the populations studies. The available evidence on social class effects of water fluoridation in reducing caries appears to suggest a benefit in reducing the differences in severity of tooth decay between classes among 5- and 12-year-old children.

Systematic reviews

- Systematic reviews locate, appraise, and synthesize evidence from scientific studies in order to provide informative answers to scientific research questions
- They are valuable sources of information for decision makers
- Systematic review adhere to a strict scientific design, with the aim of making them more comprehensive, minimizing the chance of bias and improving reliability
- A systematic review should contain a comprehensive assessment and summary of the available evidence

Reports from the World Health Organization

A conference in 1982 on the appropriate use of fluorides for human health, under the auspices of the International Dental Federation, the Kellogg Foundation, and the World Health Organization, reached the following conclusions and recommendations (WHO 1986).

1. The International Conference on Fluorides reviewed the findings of recent experimental, clinical, and epidemiological research on the use of fluorides in promoting dental health. While welcoming the reports of declining caries experience in many developed countries, it was greatly concerned about the sharp increase in dental caries in some developing countries. As there is no possibility of treating

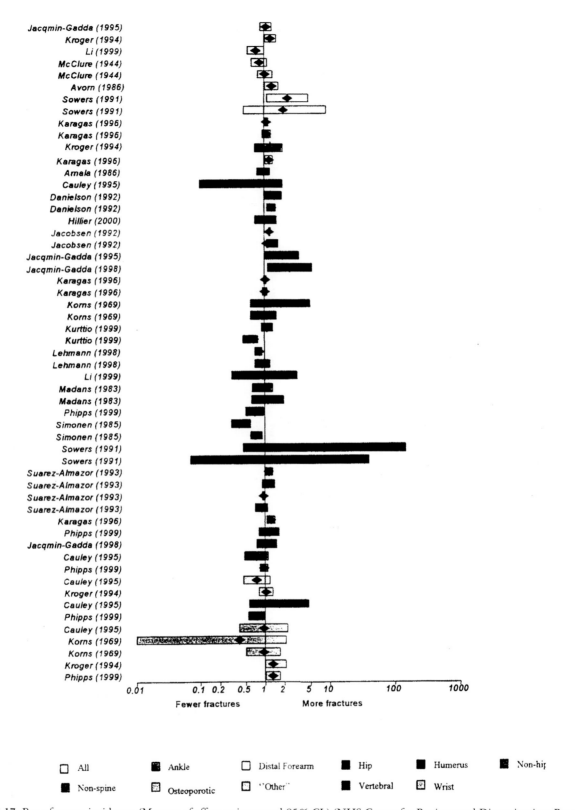

Figure 3.17 Bone fracture incidence. (Measure of effect estimate and 95% CI.) (NHS Centre for Reviews and Dissemination: Report 18.)

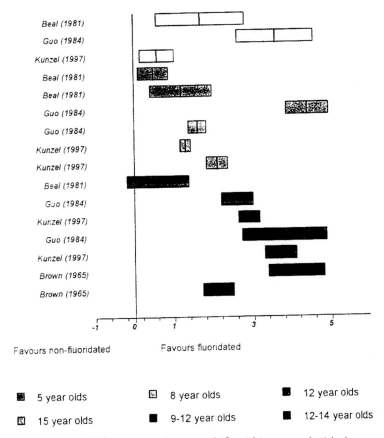

Figure 3.18 Mean difference of the change in dmft/DMFT in the exposed (fluoride) compared with the control group (low fluoride), separately by age (color coded) for the four studies reporting dmft/DMFT, with 95% CIs. Fifteen studies found a statistically significantly greater mean change in dmft/DMFT scores in the fluoridated areas than the non-fluoridated areas. The range of mean change in dmft/DMFT score was from 0.5 to 4.4, median 2.25 teeth (interquartile range 1.28, 3.63 teeth). (NHS Centre for Reviews and Dissemination: Report 18.)

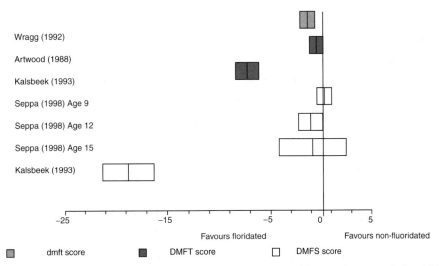

Figure 3.19 Mean difference of the change in the dmft/DMFT and DMFS score in children in the exposed (fluoride) group compared with the control group (low fluoride), in studies in which fluoridation was discontinued after the baseline survey. (NHS Centre for Reviews and Dissemination: Report 18.)

so many decayed teeth with the dental resources available at present in the developing countries, the only hope is to contain the caries problem by preventive measures.

2. The Conference agreed that community water fluoridation is an ideal measure for the prevention of dental caries in countries with well-developed, centralized public water supplies. It was in agreement with the view of the FDI, WHO, and the medical and dental professions throughout the world that community water fluoridation is an effective, safe, and inexpensive preventive measure, which has the virtue of requiring no active compliance on the part of the persons benefited. The Conference recommended that community water fluoridation be introduced and maintained wherever possible.

3. Unfortunately, the vast majority of the world's population live in rural and urban areas with few large water installations. In these situations, community water fluoridation is not feasible and alternative strategies need to be adopted. There is evidence from three long-term studies in both developing and industrialized countries that fluoridized salt may be nearly as effective as water fluoridation in reducing the incidence of dental caries. Consequently, the Conference stressed the need for more long-term field trial of salt fluoridization.

4. There is no justification for using more than one systemic fluoride measure at any one time.

5. Various topical fluoride methods, or combinations of such methods, may be beneficial in communities that have a source of systemic fluoride that is used widely.

6. Wherever possible, when combinations of fluoride therapy are considered, it is best to choose those that are self-administered or group-administered because they are less expensive.

7. Professionally applied fluorides are particularly appropriate for individuals who have been identified as at high risk of dental caries.

8. The conference was concerned about the problems of dental fluorosis in areas with high concentrations of fluoride in the public water supply and urged research to develop effective, simple, and economical defluoridation methods for water supplies of varying sizes. It recommended that, in children under the age of 6 years, brushing with a fluoride toothpaste should be supervised in order to prevent excessive ingestion. For similar reasons, fluoride mouth rinsing should not be considered for children under 5 years of age.

9. Current knowledge of the effectiveness of various methods of using fluorides led the Conference to conclude that each country should review its own dental needs and take legislative action to adopt those methods of using fluorides that best suit its needs in different regions. In view of the proven value of fluorides in promoting dental health, their use should be extended without further delay to all populations throughout the world.

WHO considered the subject again in 1993. The expert working group made a number of recommendations, including the following

- The effectiveness of all caries preventive programmes should be monitored on an ongoing basis.

- Community water fluoridation is safe and cost-effective and introduced and maintained wherever socially acceptable and feasible. The optimum water fluoride concentration will normally be within the range 0.5–1.0 mg/L.

- Salt fluoridization, at a minimum concentration of 200 mg/L F, should be considered as a practical alternative to water fluoridation.

- Encouraging results have been reported with fluoridization of milk but more studies are recommended.

- Fluoride supplements have limited application as a public health measure. In areas with medium to low caries experience a conservative prescribing policy should be adopted; a dose of 0.5 mg F/day should be prescribed for at-risk individuals from the age of 3 years. In areas with high caries experience a regimen starting at 6 months of age, taking into account the fluoride content of the drinking water, should be used.

- Only one systemic fluoride measure should be used at any one time.

- Because fluoride toothpaste is a highly effective means of caries control, every effort must be made to develop affordable fluoride toothpastes for use in developing countries. Measures should be taken to exempt fluoride toothpastes from duties and taxation.

- Fluoride toothpaste tubes should contain advice that, for children under 6 years of age, brushing should be supervised and only a minimal amount (less than 5 mm) should be placed on the brush or chewing stick. Toothpastes with lowered levels of fluoride, manufactured especially for use by children, should be fully studied.

- Toothpastes with candy-like flavours, and toothpaste containing 1500 ppm or more are not recommended for use by children under 6 years of age.

- In low fluoride communities, school-based brushing and mouthrinsing programmes are recommended, but their adoption should be based on the cost of implementation and the caries status of the community. Fluoride mouthrinsing is contraindicated in children under 6 years of age.

- Further research on the effectiveness of fluoride on root surface caries is recommended.

- Dietary practices that increase the risk of infants and young children being over-exposed to fluoride from all sources should be identified and appropriate action taken.

- Dental fluorosis should be monitored periodically to detect increasing or higher than acceptable levels of fluorosis. Action should be taken when fluorosis is found to be excessive by adjusting fluoride intake from water, salt, or other sources. Biomarkers should be used to assess, where practical, current fluoride exposure to predict further risk of fluorosis.

Conclusions

The study of the systemic and topical effects of fluoride has produced a tremendous outpouring of research, particularly over the last 50 years, and our knowledge of dental epidemiology, clinical trials, community dental health, dental plaque, physiology, and biochemistry has increased enormously as a result. This chapter has concentrated on water fluoridation, fluoridization of salt and milk, fluoride supplements, fluoride dentifrices, and dental fluorosis. The incorporation of fluoride in its various forms as a caries-preventive agent for both the individual and the community, is one of the most important factors responsible for the decrease in dental caries in children observed in many industrialized countries.

References

A Systematic Review of Water Fluoridation NHS Centre for Reviews and Dissemination. University of York Report 18.

Arnold, F.A. Jr, *et al.* (1962). Fifteen year of the Grand Rapids fluoridation study. *J. Am. Dent. Assoc.*, **65**, 780–785.

Ashley, P.F., *et al.* (1999). Toothbrushing Habits and Caries Experience. *Caries Res.*, **33**, 401–402.

Attwood, D. and Blinkhorn A. S. (1988). Trends in dental health of ten-year-old school children in south-west Scotland after cessation of water fluoridation. *Lancet.*, ii, 266–267.

Baysan, A., Lynch, E., Ellwood, R., Davies, R., Petersson, L., and Boorsboon, P. (2001). Reversal of primary root caries using dentifrices containing 5,000 and 1,100 ppm fluoride. *Caries Res.*, **35**, 41–46.

Chesters, R.K., Huntington, E., Burchell, C.K., and Stephen, K.W. (1922). Effects of oral care habits on caries in adolescence. *Caries Res.*, **26**, 299–304.

Churchill, H.V. (1931). Occurrence of fluorides in some waters of the United States. *Ind. Engng. Chem.*, **23**, 996–998.

Conti, A.J., Lotzkar, S., Daley, R., Cancro, L., Marks, R.G. and McNeal, D.R. (1988). A 3-year clinical trial to compare efficacy of dentifrices containing 1.14% and 0.76% sodium mono-fluorophophate. *Community Dent. Oral Epidemiol.*, **16**, 135–138.

Dean, H.T., Arnold, F.A. Jr., and Elvove, E. (1942). Domestic water and dental caries, V. Additional studies of the relation of fluoride domestic waters to dental caries experience in 4425 white children aged 12–14 years, of 13 cities in 4 states, *Publ. Hlth. Rep.*, **57**, 1155–1179.

DHSS (1969). *The fluoridation studies in the United Kingdom and the results achieved after eleven years. A report on the Committee on research into fluoridation*, Department of Health and Social Security Reports on Public Health and Medical Subjects No. 122.

de Crousaz, P., *et al.* (1985). Caries prevalence in children after 12 years of salt fluoridation in a Canton of Switzerland. *Schweiz. Mschr. Zahnmed.*, **95**, 805–815.

Fogels, H.R., Meade, J.J., Griffith, J., Miragliuolo, R., and Cancro, L.P. (1988). A clinical investigation of a high-level fluoride dentifrice. *J. Dent. Child.*, May–June, 210–215.

Holt, R.D. (1995). The pattern of caries in a group of 5-year-old children and in the same cohort at 9 years of age. *Comm. Dent. Hlth.*, **12**, 93–99.

Holt, R.D., *et al.* (1994). Enamel opacities and dental caries in children who used a low fluoride toothpaste between 2 and 5 years of age. *Int. Dent. J.*, **44**, 331–341.

Horowitz, H. and Ismail (1996). Topical fluoride in caries prevention. In: Fejecstor, O., Erkstrand, J., and Bart, B. A. (Ed.) *Fluoride in Dentistry, 2nd Edition*. Copenhagen: Munksgaard.

Jensen, M.E. and Kohout, F. (1988). The effect of a fluoridated dentifrice on root and coronal caries in an older adult population. *J. Am. Dent. Assoc.*, **117**, 829–832.

Katz, R.V., Hazen, S.P., Chilton, N.W. and Mumma, J.R. (1982). Prevalence and intraoral distribution of root caries in an adult population. *Caries Res.*, **16**, 265–271.

Koch, G., Petersson, L.G., Kling, E. and Kling L. (1982). Effect of 250 and 1000 ppm fluoride dentifrice on caries: a three-year clinical study. *Swed. Dent. J.*, **6**, 233–238.

Künzel, W., and Fischer, T. (2000). Caries prevalence after cessation of water fluoridation in La Salud, Cuba. *Caries Res.*, **4**, 20–25.

Lowry, R. and Evans, D. (1999). The privatised water industry and public health: back to square one. BDJ Vol. 186, 12, 597–598.

McClure, F.J. (ed.) (1962). *Fluoride Drinking Waters*, US Department of Health Education and Welfare, National Institute of Dental Research, Bethesda, Md.

Marinho V.C.C., Higgins, J.P.T., Logan, S., and Sheiham, A. (2002a). Fluoride gels for preventing dental caries in children and adolescents (Cochrane review). *The Cochrane Library*, **Issue 2**, Oxford: Update Software.

Marinho V.C.C. Higgins, J.P.T., Logan, S., and Sheiham, A. (2002b). Fluoride varnishes for preventing dental caries in children and adolescents (Cochrane review). *The Cochrane Library,* **Issue 3**, Oxford: Update Software.

Menghini, G.D. *et al.* (1991). Caries prevalence and gingival inflammation in conscripts in 1985. *Schweizer, Monatsschrift fur Zahnmedizin*, **101**, 1119–1126.

Milsom, K. and Mitropoulos, C.M. (1990). Enamel defects in 8-year-old children in fluoridated and non-fluoridated parts of Cheshire. *Caries Res.*, **24**, 286–289.

Mitropoulos, C.M. *et al.* (1984). Relative efficacy of dentifrices containing 250 or 1000 ppm F in preventing caries – report of a 32 month clinical trial. *Commun. Dent. Hlth.*, 1, 193–200.

Moller, I.J. (1965). *Dental Fluorose og Caries.* Copenhagen: Rhodes International Science Publishers.

Murray, J.J. (1969). Caries experience of 15-year old children from fluoride and non-fluoride communities. *Br. Dent. J.*, 127, 128–131.

Murray, J.J., Rugg-Gunn, A.J. and Jenkins, G.N. (1991). *Fluorides in Caries Prevention*, 3rd edn. Wright, Butterworth Heinemann.

Murray, J.J., Breckon, J.A., Reynolds, P.J., Tabari, E.D. and Nunn, J.H. (1991). The effect of residence and social class on dental caries experience in 15-16 year old children living in three areas (natural fluoride, adjusted fluoride and low fluoride) in the North-East of England. *Br. Dent. J.*, 171, 319–322.

Murray, J.J., Rugg-Gunn, A.J., and Jenkins, G.N. *Fluorides in Caries Prevention,* 3rd edn. London: Wright 1992.

Ossuji, O.O. and Nikiforuk, J. (1988). Fluoride supplements induced dental fluorosis—case reports. *Paed. Dent.*, 10, 48–52.

Pang, D.T. and Vann, W.F. Jr. (1992). The use of fluoride containing toothpastes in young children: the scientific evidence for recommending small quantity. *Paed. Dent.*, 14, 384–387.

Pendrys, D.G. (1995). Risk of fluorosis in a fluoridated population. Implications for the dentist and hygienist. *J. Am. Dent. Asso.*, 126, 1617–1624.

Pindborg, J.J. (1965). En Dansk Fluorideringspjeca FRA 1902 *Tandlaegebladet*, 69, 557–561.

Riordan, P.J. (1993). Fluoride supplements in caries prevention: a literature review and proposal for a new dosage schedule. *J. Publ. Hlth. Dent.*, 53, 174–89.

Rock, W.P. (1994). Young children and fluoride toothpaste. *Br. Dent. J.*, 177, 17–20.

Rugg-Gunn, A.J., *et al.* (1981). Caries experience of 5 year old children living in four communities in N.E. England receiving different water fluoride levels. *Br. Dent. J.*, 150, 9–12.

Rugg-Gunn, A.J., Carmichael, C.L., and Ferrell, R.S., (1988). Effect of fluoridation and secular trend in caries in 5-year old children living in Newcastle and Northumberland. *Br Dent. J.*, 165, 359–64.

Steele, J.G., Walls, A.W.G., Ayatoilahi, S.M.T. and Murray, J.J. (1996). Major clinical findings from a dental survey of elderly people in three different English communities. *Br. Dent. J.*, 180, 17–23.

Stephen, K.W., McCall, D.R., and Tullis, J.I. (1987). Caries prevalence in North Scotland before, and 5 years after, water defluoridation. *Br. Dent. J.*, 163, 324–326.

Stephen, *et al.* (1988). A 3-year oral health dose response study of sodium monofluorophospshate dentifrices with and without zinc citrate: anti caries results. *Commun. Dent. Oral Epidemiol.*, 16, 321–325.

Todd, J.E. and Lader, D. (1991). *Adult Dental Health 1988 United Kingdom.* London: HMSO.

Triol, C.W., Graves, R.C., Webster, D.B. and Clarke, B.J. (1987). Anticaries effect of 1450 and 2000 ppm F dentifrices. *J. Dent. Res.*, 66 (Spec. Issue), 216 (Abstr. 879).

Weaver, R. (1950). Fluorine and wartime diet. *Br. Dent. J.*, 88, 231–239.

Winter, G.B., Holt, R.D. and Williams, B.F. (1989) Clinical trial of a low fluoride toothpaste for young children. *Int. Dent. J.*, 39, 227–235.

World Health Organization (1986). *Appropriate use of fluorides for human health.* Geneva: WHO.

World Health Organization (1992). *Recent advances in oral health.* WHO Technical Report Series No. 826, Geneva.

World Health Organization (1994). *Fluorides and oral health.* Geneva: WHO.

4

Microbiological aspects of caries prevention

- Introduction
- Oral streptococci
- Dental plaque as a biofilm
- Preventing infection
- Replacement therapy
- Inhibition of mutans streptococci
- Caries vaccines
- Microbiological prediction of caries
- Conclusions
- References

Microbiological aspects of caries prevention

Roy Russell

Introduction

Modern developments in dentistry have given us a wide range of options for the effective treatment of dental disease, but it is only by understanding the details of the events that lead to the diseased state that we can hope to design rational methods of prevention. Insights into the disease will help us to achieve the ultimate aim of prevention and also lead to methods for prediction of disease and new approaches to treatment. In this chapter therefore, we shall first consider what is known of the way in which bacteria are involved in the dental caries process and then how this knowledge can be exploited.

The history of oral microbiology can be traced right back to the origins of microbiology as a science. Antonie van Leeuwenhoek, a seventeenth century Dutch draper who was developing his microscopes so that he could check the quality of his textiles, examined scrapings from his teeth out of curiosity. He was fascinated by the seething activity he could observe, and took great delight in the variety of shapes, sizes, and movement of the 'little animalcules' that he saw. However, not everyone shared his enthusiasm for these tiny fellow-travellers and, indeed, many were horrified at the thought of such monsters in their mouths. From his drawings and descriptions, we now know that van Leeuwenhoek saw spheres, rods, and spirals, which we now recognize as streptococci, fusobacteria, and spirochaetes. We shall return to this theme of a complex oral microflora later but some of van Leeuwenhoek's other observations set the scene for subsequent developments in oral microbiology—for example, he found that everyone he examined harboured a similarly diverse collection of organisms in the dental plaque, but that the mixture of types was not constant. At no time, however, did van Leeuwenhoek appear to have made any connection between what he observed and dental disease. Such discoveries were not to come for another two hundred years.

The fundamentals of our understanding of the pathogenesis of caries date back to the period when specific bacteria were being linked to specific diseases, and researchers such as Pasteur and Koch were developing the 'germ theory' of disease. Pasteur's great edict was 'Cherchez le microbe' and the latter half of the nineteenth century saw rapid advances in the quest to identify the causative organisms of infectious diseases. Over a few decades, the bacteria responsible for diseases such as anthrax, plague, dysentery, cholera, and tuberculosis were isolated and cultured in the laboratory. It was natural, therefore, that interest was aroused in determining the specific aetiology of other diseases, including dental caries. The first report that we have of such investigations comes from the records of the International Medical Congress held in London in 1881. This was clearly a major event, as both Pasteur and Koch attended it. Joseph Lister, the pioneer in the field of antisepsis, invited them both to dinner, perhaps tactfully keeping the conversation only to science as their countries were at war at the time. At that same congress two London dentists, Underwood and Milles, presented a paper describing the microscopic observation of 'germs' in decaying teeth, and the experiments in which they incubated extracted teeth in test tubes and looked for damage to the enamel. They found that enamel dissolution occurred only if there was both a source of carbohydrate—they used chewed bread—and live germs. Killing germs using phenolic solution, introduced by Lister, prevented any damage to the enamel. Underwood and Milles published their work in 1884 but nothing more is known of their investigations. Their concept of the three-way interaction between bacteria, carbohydrate, and teeth was developed and firmly established by W. D. Miller, an American working in the same institute as Koch in Vienna. Miller proposed his 'chemicoparasitic theory' of caries in a book published in 1890, identifying the essential conjunction of bacteria and fermentable carbohydrate to generate the acid that resulted in the demineralization of enamel. Miller's book was an important step in the description and classification of the variety of bacteria found in dental plaque, and helped establish two of the main themes that have dominated research in caries microbiology—what bacteria are involved and how they use carbohydrate. A third major theme that did not emerge until the latter half of the twentieth century concerns the issue of how the bacteria attach to and colonize the tooth.

With the development of bacteriology, it became possible to study the properties of bacteria isolated from carious teeth in the laboratory. Since it was now clear that bacterial acid production was a central feature of enamel attack in the development of caries, interest was focused on those plaque bacteria that produce acid. Miller and subsequent researchers favoured bacteria that produced lactic acid as the causative agents of caries, and for many

Changing concepts of caries microbiology

• Van Leeuwenhoek (1600s)	First microscopic observation of oral bacteria
• Pasteur, Koch (late 1800s)	Germ Theory of disease
• Underwood and Milles (1884)	Association between 'germs' and enamel decay
• Miller (1890)	Chemicoparasitic theory of caries
• Clarke (1924)	Identification of *Streptococcus mutans* and association with initial caries
• Loesche (1986)	Association of mutans streptococci with caries (specific plaque hypothesis)
• Marsh (1994)	Ecological plaque hypothesis emphasizes balance between bacterial species

years *Bacillus acidophilus odontolyticus*, a species name that no longer has any formal recognition, was the favoured culprit. Rod-shaped lactic acid-producing bacteria (now identified as members of the genus *Lactobacillus*) could readily be isolated from established caries lesions; but in 1924 Clarke, working at St. Mary's Hospital in London, described a different approach where he examined the bacteria present in initial 'white-spot' enamel lesions. He identified a bacterium he named *Streptococcus mutans*—the name of the organism reflects the fact that it alters shape depending upon the growth conditions—which was present in a high proportion in such early lesions. Clarke proposed *S. mutans* as the important organism in the initiation of disease. We now think that there is a process of microbial succession so that the lactobacilli move in later, their proliferation being favoured by the low-pH conditions set up by the streptococci. Clarke's work went largely unregarded until the late 1950s, when new approaches to animal models of caries, based on the selective use of antibiotics to modify the oral microflora, refocused attention on the streptococci. The introduction of isolation chambers where germ-free animals could be raised and infected with specific bacteria also clarified a hierarchy of cariogenicity, in which various species of streptococci could be ranked according to their ability to induce caries in rats or hamsters fed on a sugar-rich diet. An animal model of caries could thus be developed, and a streptococcus known first as *S. mutans* 6715 (the fifteenth isolate from an experiment at NIH in 1967), which was later reclassified as *S. sobrinus* became the focus of attention. While such model systems are essential for taking research forward, there is a need for continual vigilance to ensure that the various components of the system—bacterium, animal, diet—truly represent the features of the human disease in which we are interested. Taking the first of these, it is crucial for the exploration of preventive strategies that the true identity of the causative organism(s) of caries is known. It is, therefore, necessary to address the problem of bacterial identification and classification.

Oral streptococci

Taxonomy of oral streptococci

One of the difficulties that has bedevilled investigations into the contribution of oral streptococci to plaque formation has been that of resolving taxonomic relationships between the different types observed. Indeed, many routine diagnostic medical laboratories still lump all the oral streptococci together under the descriptive term 'viridans streptococci', which refers to the greening reaction, or α-haemolysis, produced on blood agar. This classification is clearly limited, as not all the oral streptococci are α-haemolytic, and α-haemolytic species such as *S. pneumoniae* are not normal inhabitants of the oral cavity. More importantly, there is extensive heterogeneity of physiological properties within the group, so one would anticipate different virulence properties. Many attempts have, therefore, been made over the years to develop schemes for identifying streptococci to the species level by laboratory tests. These have largely been based on biochemical properties such as the ability to utilize a range of carbohydrate substrates. Serotyping schemes have also played a part in identifying taxonomic boundaries, but none of the approaches based on bacterial phenotype (i.e. the properties the bacteria display in laboratory culture) has proved entirely satisfactory. It was only with the introduction of molecular methods based on bacterial genotype that the full diversity of streptococcal species came to be recognized, first with DNA–DNA hybridization experiments and later with sequencing of ribosomal RNA genes. By the mid 1980s, it was formally recognized that a group of bacteria that had all been previously described as *S. mutans*, in fact, contained a number of different species, which had various properties in common but, nevertheless, had distinct features. These are collectively referred to as the 'mutans group' or Mutans Streptococci (MS). As a corollary of having different properties, the various species have different hosts and favour different environments. It also became clear that some types that had been the object of study in animals (*S. cricetus*, *S. rattus*) were rarely, if ever, found in humans. Table 4.1 shows the current taxonomic status of the human oral streptococci.

The taxonomy of the mutans group of streptococci now seems to be firmly established, with general agreement over the species definition. Before anyone heaves a sigh of relief, it has to be noted that even the concept of a 'species' for bacteria has been thrown into dispute by further developments in our understanding of bacterial population structures, brought about by new genome sequencing approaches. For a long time we were familiar with the idea that all members of a species such as *S. mutans* were the same, based on our understanding of binary division, so that all descendants of a dividing bacterium are identical and thus formed a homogenous clone. It now seems that this is very far from being the case. The problem is well illustrated by the mitis group, which contains the largest number of named species of oral streptococci. Data from rRNA sequencing shows that *S. pneumoniae* also lies in this group, though its habitat is considered to be the

Table 4.1 Human oral streptococci

Group	Species	Properties
Mitis group	S. mitis S. oralis S. sanguis S. parasanguis S. gordonii S. peroris S. infantis S. australis	Pioneer species in plaque formation. Common causative agents of infectious endocarditis
Mutans group 'mutans streptococci'	S. mutans S. sobrinus	Late colonizers of plaque, increased numbers associated with caries
Salivarius group	S. salivarius S. vestibularis	Found mainly on mucosal surfaces, rarely pathogenic
Anginosus group	S. anginosus S. intermedius S. constellatus	Favour anaerobic environments. Frequently isolated from abscesses

naso-pharynx rather than the oral cavity. *S. pneumoniae* is closely related to *S. mitis* and *S. oralis*, and there is now a substantial body of evidence showing that there is extensive exchange of genetic information between the species. This was first reported for a penicillin-binding protein, when genes in penicillin-resistant isolates of *S. pneumoniae* were shown to have a mosaic structure, with segments clearly identical to genes of *S. oralis*. The commensal oral streptococci thus offer a pool of genetic material, which can undergo gene-shuffling with an important pathogen and lead to the emergence of resistant strains. Other genes show the same mosaicism; so, there is reason to think that there may be extensive mixing of genetic traits within the mitis group. This raises the question as to whether the currently defined species can be separated by clear boundaries, or whether they represent a continuum with many mosaic isolates displaying a mixture of properties now regarded as characteristic of individual species. The existence of heterogeneity and gene exchange within populations of bacteria has important implications for certain preventive strategies that target distinctive features.

Which species are associated with caries?

As should be clear from the above discussion, the technical ability to identify and enumerate particular species has been a crucial factor in allowing an investigation of their association with caries. It has been estimated that some 500 different types of bacteria can be isolated from dental plaque. These comprise our normal oral flora, for the most part living in harmony as commensals. The vast majority of these are not directly implicated as causative agents of caries. They may, nevertheless, influence the properties of plaque and the conditions conducive to caries. Following Pasteur's hunt-the-microbe precept, efficient methods for identifying the likely culprits are essential. The development of selective media such as Mitis-Salivarius agar supplemented with bacitracin, which

inhibits the growth of most oral bacteria but allows mutans streptococci to grow and form colonies that can be counted, was an important advance that led to the finding that presence of high numbers of these organisms at a tooth site was associated with a high risk of subsequent development of caries (Loesche 1986). A substantial number of cross-sectional and longitudinal studies have demonstrated a strong association between mutans streptococci and caries (a recent systematic review found 2730 papers on the topic). One limitation of these studies is that the selective media used for counting the streptococci do not allow accurate identification to the species level—*S. mutans* and *S. sobrinus* cannot reliably be distinguished by colony morphology alone—so it is still not entirely clear what the relative contribution of the two species may be. However, *S. mutans* is by far more common and is carried by over 98% of adults; so, its association with caries is clear. *S. sobrinus* shows a range of properties similar to *S. mutans* and, indeed, is even more cariogenic in animal models. It has been reported to be found in 5–35% of individuals in different countries, but it remains unclear whether *S. sobrinus* can cause caries on its own or is the major or minor partner when it occurs in co-existence with *S. mutans*. It has been suggested that it may be more strongly associated with smooth surface lesions or rapidly advancing caries (and its *in vitro* properties would support this). Nevertheless, all the available evidence indicates that any preventive strategy should have *S. mutans* as its principal target.

It is important to note that the evidence implicating mutans streptococci as major causative agents of caries comes from studies of specific caries-prone sites on teeth. There is a close correlation between the levels of mutans streptococci in saliva and the levels in plaque. Since it is much easier to obtain samples of saliva than of plaque, there has been much interest in using salivary levels as a proxy measure of numbers of bacteria in plaque. This is discussed further in the section on Prediction but it must be recognized that the mere presence of mutans streptococci in the mouth, or even high numbers of mutans streptococci, does not inevitably lead to caries as other conditions must be satisfied for the disease process to advance. The intrinsic resistance of the tooth enamel (perhaps strengthened by the incorporation of fluoride) is one factor, but, returning to Miller's original concept, readily fermentable carbohydrate is also essential. As a consequence, many individuals, particularly those with good general health, good oral hygiene practices, exposure to fluoride, and suitable dietary habits can harbour relatively high levels of *S. mutans* ($>10^5$ colony-forming units/ml of saliva), yet have a lifetime free of caries. We must also note that the majority of the studies that linked levels of mutans streptococci to caries risk were carried out in North America or Scandinavia. It is now apparent that these findings cannot necessarily be applied to other parts of the world. For example, in many African populations, high levels of mutans streptococci are found (possibly due to a starch-rich diet) but the sugar intake, and hence the caries level, remains low. In such populations, attempts to use measurements of mutans streptococci to predict future caries risk are doomed to failure.

When he first described *S. mutans*, Clarke made it clear that caries, sometimes, develops in the absence of any detectable *S. mutans*. He could find *S. mutans* in only 78% of his white-spot lesions, and this suggests that other species, or combinations of species, can produce amounts of acid similar to *S. mutans* and hence cause damage. These other 'non-mutans streptococci', capable of generating a low pH, have been identified as atypical strains of common plaque species such as *S. mitis*, *S. sanguis*, and *S. intermedius* (van Ruyven *et al.* 2000). A corollary of the recognition of strongly acidogenic species other than *S. mutans* is that even if *S. mutans* were to be eradicated, it is unlikely that caries risk would be reduced to zero.

The link between mutans streptococci and caries

- Animal experiments: mutans streptococci cause caries in gnotobiotic animals in the presence of sugar
- Virulence properties: mutans streptococci possess properties that contribute to cariogenicity. They are acidogenic, aciduric and produce extracellular glucans and intracellular storage polysaccharide
- Cross-sectional studies in humans: increased proportion of mutans streptococci are found at sites of initial caries lesions
- Longitudinal studies in humans: high numbers of mutans streptococci at a tooth site correlate with subsequent caries
- Other 'non-mutans streptococci' with similar properties may also be cariogenic

Acquisition of oral streptococci

The oral cavity is sterile *in utero*, but although during birth the neonate is exposed to all the complex microflora of the birth canal, these organisms fail to colonize illustrating the highly selective environment of the mouth. A distinctive oral flora is rapidly established soon after birth. Streptococci are numerically dominant, particularly *S. salivarius*, *S. mitis*, and *S. oralis*, which colonize the mucosal surfaces and dorsum of the tongue. Since the normal habitat of all these species is in humans, it seems most likely that the source of these will be an adult, most probably the mother or other primary carer. However, so far it is only in the case of *S. mutans* that any detailed study has been made of the source of infection. Earlier work based on bacteriocin typing had indicated the mother as the source of an infant's *S. mutans*, but a major advance was made when Caufield and his colleagues (1993) used Restriction Fragment Length Polymorphism (RFLP) to obtain genetic fingerprints of *S. mutans* isolated from mother–infant pairs. *S. mutans* preferentially colonizes hard surfaces and hence, its appearance is delayed until the eruption of the first molar teeth. A majority of infants, therefore, acquire *S. mutans* during a 'window of infectivity' around the age of

two. Because of the great variability of RFLP types amongst isolates, it was possible to accept the conclusion that matching patterns in mothers and children had not occurred by chance, and that maternal transmission was must be the source of *S. mutans* in 80% of the children. While an infant may initially carry only one clonal line of *S. mutans* (identified by ribotyping or RFLP), by adulthood there may be up to seven different clonotypes, though these seem to be remarkably stable once established. The basis for this successful long-term colonization is not clear, but it does illustrate the perfect equilibrium that can be achieved between a particular bacterial type, its host, and its neighbouring bacteria that coinhabit plaque. Despite the fact that most people will have enjoyed a certain amount of intimate oral contact with other people, it is clearly extremely difficult for another person's *S. mutans* to superinfect. This also poses a considerable challenge to preventive strategies that seek to replace a cariogenic bacterial population with one less likely to cause disease.

A variety of molecular typing techniques are now available for fingerprinting *S. mutans* and these are being applied to studies of transmission. It is becoming apparent that social differences in child rearing and feeding practices in different countries can influence the source and the frequency of transmission. Identification of the source of infection with the bacteria responsible for caries provides us with a potential way of developing a preventive strategy, because, as with any infectious disease, identifying the source of infection lays open the possibility of interrupting the chain of transmission. It may not be feasible to achieve a lifetime free of *S. mutans*, but delaying the age at which a child becomes infected can reduce their subsequent caries risk.

Acquisition of *S. mutans*

- Mutans streptococci are undetectable in pre-dentate infants
- Most children become infected around the age of 2 years
- The principal source of infection appears to be the mother
- Mothers who carry high levels of *S. mutans* are more likely to infect their children
- Reducing mutans levels in mothers can delay infection of their child

Dental plaque as a biofilm

The Biofilm concept has become firmly established in the last 20 years, and an appreciation that the vast majority of bacteria live on surfaces and in intimate association with other bacteria, has influenced our understanding of microbial growth on surfaces as diverse as indwelling catheters, oil pipelines, and sewage farms. The oral cavity has been compared to a tropical coral reef in that it is warm, moist, rich in nutrients, and supports an abundant variety of species. These conditions sound idyllic, but challenge an organism to resist the vagaries of current flow and to make the choice between life in the fluid phase and colonization of a hard surface. In order to occupy a niche within such an ecosystem, an organism must have evolved a strategy to avoid being washed away, to live in some sort of balance with others, and to cope with the constant variations in temperature and pH, and the availability of oxygen and nutrients. Dental plaque is, therefore, not a static entity but should be regarded as constantly subject to forces for change—reforming and changing in composition and properties under the influence of environmental stresses. It is our understanding of this dynamism that helps us to explain how plaque bacteria can contribute to caries, and the 'Ecological Plaque Hypothesis' has replaced earlier arguments about the specificity of different plaques associated with disease (Marsh 1994). The emphasis on the balance between different types of bacteria means that we should pay much greater attention to physiological properties of bacterial populations than simply to the presence or absence of particular species (Kleinberg 2002). From our knowledge of the complex process of plaque formation, it is clear that there are numerous points at which intervention might disturb the normal process of plaque build-up. Interference at any of these points could be sufficient to provide a way of reducing plaque, either by delaying plaque formation or by altering its composition, in such a way that it contains lower numbers of mutans streptococci or other cariogenic species. The next section considers what we now know about the molecular mechanisms of plaque formation.

Consequences of the biofilm mode of growth

- Physical stabilization due to coaggregation and extracellular polymers
- Exclusion of invading bacteria (colonization resistance)
- Protection against host defences
- Metabolic stabilization (microbial homeostasis) due to balance of synergistic and antagonistic interactions
- Increased metabolic efficiency due to co-operative effects
- Overall properties of the biofilm are determined by the balance of activities of different species present

Plaque formation

Current models of supragingival plaque formation envisage a succession of stages, each of them involving a different range of bacterial species, but all stages being characterized by a set of specific molecular interactions. This microbial succession, which is common to the formation of biofilms in many situations in nature, may be summarized as follows: in the initial stage, 'pioneer' species of bacteria colonize the tooth surface by binding to components of the salivary pellicle. Predominant among these initial colonizers are believed to be *S. sanguis*, *S. oralis*, and *S. mitis*.

Plaque then develops both by growth of the pioneer species to form microcolonies and by the further accretion of more bacterial cells of the same or other species. This accretion can be direct bacterium–bacterium binding in coaggregation pairs due to specific receptor–ligand binding or may be mediated by salivary macromolecules which crosslink because they are bound by more than one bacterium. Along with these processes, plaque build-up is facilitated by the production of bacterial extracellular polymers, which serve to entrap the cells. The polymers of particular interest are those synthesized from sucrose by various species of streptococci, which will be considered in the next section. Mature plaque, with its 'climax community' of microbial species, is dependent upon the maintenance of a fine balance between the many species present, with metabolic interactions and food-chains taking an increased importance over adhesive interactions. It must be noted that the mutans streptococci are not considered to be amongst the pioneer species and only represent a very minor proportion of the total number of bacteria present, generally less than 1%. Such a level poses no problems so long as the plaque population is maintained in a state of equilibrium, but the relative proportions of different species (and hence the pathological potential of the plaque) can be altered drastically by shifts in the environmental conditions. Prevention of dental caries can only be achieved by keeping the levels of mutans streptococci low, or finding other means of preventing acid production.

Events in plaque formation

- Pioneer species (*S. mitis*, *S. oralis*, *Actinomyces* spp.) colonize tooth surface
- Pioneers multiply to form microcolonies and other species become established by coaggregation with pioneers
- Extracellular polysaccharides help to stabilise plaque
- The relative proportions of different species in the 'climax community' is affected by environmental factors, particularly dietary sugars
- The amount of acid accumulating in plaque depends on the availability of sugars and the balance between activity of acid-producing and acid-neutralizing bacteria

Streptococcal adhesins

Because of the daunting complexity of the eventual plaque microflora, individual bacterial species can only become members of the community if they are partners in some specific binding interaction that prevents them from being swept away by the flow of saliva. It is probable that the surface of any particular bacterium displays a number of different binding molecules with differing specificity and strength of binding, but we, as yet, have detailed information on only a few of theses molecules and we are particularly concerned here with what is known of the species associated with dental caries.

The components of bacteria that bind to receptor molecules are called adhesins and one major family of adhesins has been found to be widespread amongst the oral streptococci. The first, and best characterised, member of this family was identified independently by two research groups working on a caries vaccine in the mid-1970s. It is a major antigen of *S. mutans* that is found both bound to the cell wall peptidoglycan and free in the culture medium. To the original names of I/II and antigen B, other researchers subsequently added the synonyms Pac, SpaP, SR for the *S. mutans* protein, while a further set of names has been applied to the corresponding proteins from other streptococci. A distinctive feature of the I/II proteins is their high molecular weight; and since the cloning and sequencing of a number of their genes, it has been possible to identify common features of their structure (Fig. 4.1a). All have a motif characteristic of wall-anchored proteins in Gram-positive bacteria at the C-terminus. A common feature of these proteins is the possession of stretches of tandem amino acid repeats and all I/II proteins have one block of alanine-rich repeats and another of proline-rich repeats. Repeat regions often are associated with binding and several research groups have implicated the alanine-rich region in binding to a salivary glycoprotein that is responsible for agglutinating streptococci (Jenkinson and Demuth 1997). The importance of I/II in adhesion was first demonstrated by showing that antibody raised against the purified protein could block attachment of *S. mutans* to saliva-coated hydroxyapatite, a laboratory model of adhesion to the tooth surface. Subsequently, gene knockout experiments confirmed its importance in this system but loss of I/II was not sufficient to prevent *S. mutans* becoming established in the mouths of rats. However, deletion of the gene resulted in a reduced level of caries. Furthermore, mutants with the gene deleted are less able than the wild type to invade dentinal

tubules, and this has been attributed to a reduced ability to bind collagen.

The evidence from antibody and gene knockout experiments thus provides a rational basis for the design of strategies that might be expected to reduce, if not entirely abolish, caries caused by *S. mutans*. Antigen I/II was the first pure protein used as an experimental caries vaccine in monkeys and was demonstrated to be effective (see section Caries Vaccines). In another line of attack based upon competition between free adhesin and whole bacteria, it has been reported that a synthetic peptide mimicking a stretch of just 19 amino acids of I/II can block attachment of *S. mutans* to a salivary agglutinin and interfere with colonization by *S. mutans* in volunteers who had the peptide applied to their teeth (Kelly *et al.* 1999).

Adhesion of *S. mutans*

- Surface proteins such as antigen I/II bind to salivary glycoproteins on tooth surface
- Glucosyltransferase enzymes synthesize sticky glucans from sucrose
- Glucan-binding proteins help consolidate plaque
- Molecules involved in adhesion are targets for preventive strategies

Sucrose-dependent adhesion

While any fermentable carbohydrate may be utilized by plaque bacteria to generate the acids which attack enamel substance, sucrose is recognized as being particularly important in the caries process because not only can it be fermented, but it also serves as a substrate for extracellular enzymes of plaque bacteria, which synthesise sucrose-derived polymers. These polymers are of central importance in adhesive interactions in plaque, where they mediate attachment of bacteria to the tooth surface and to other bacteria. Thus they stabilise the plaque biofilm, serve as energy stores aiding the survival of plaque bacteria, and modulate the permeability of plaque and hence the level of acid at the enamel surface. The enzymes catalyzing formation of polymers from sucrose, particularly the glucosyltransferases (GTF) making water-soluble and insoluble glucans, as well as the glucan-binding proteins (GBP), have thus attracted considerable interest as potential targets for inhibition of the processes which can lead to caries.

Glucosyltransferases are extracellular enzymes produced by several species of oral streptococci that synthesize, from sucrose, polymers consisting solely of glucose (glucans). Streptococcal GTF are capable of synthesizing either α-1,6- or α-1,3-linkages between the glucose units, and the relative proportions of these two linkages and the degree of branching determines the ultimate properties of the glucan. A glucan, which is essentially a linear α-1,6-linked chain, is referred to as a dextran and is water-soluble (the trivial name 'dextransucrase' is often applied to GTF which produce dextran); in contrast, mutan is a water-insoluble glucan

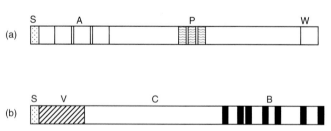

Figure 4.1 Schematic structure of (a) surface antigen I/II and (b) glucosyltransferase, the two major components of *S. mutans* against which protective agents have been targeted.

Key: S, Signal peptides are well-conserved and similar to those found in other proteins secreted by gram-positive bacteria; **A,** Alanine-rich repeats involved in binding salivary glycoprotein; **P,** Proline-rich repeats; **W,** Wall anchor motif.

V, Variable region of which appears to be unique to each GTF but is of unknown function; **C,** Catalytic domain is highly-conserved and similar in all GTF; **B,** Binding domain essential for glucan-binding. Contains multiple tandem repeats of amino acid sequence.

with a high proportion of α-1,3-linkages. Both types of glucans are believed to be important in dental plaque, with dextran mediating bacterial aggregation and serving as a storage polymer, while mutan has been shown to be the major contributor to adherence. In addition to this function of producing glucan, GTF at the surface of bacteria, or adsorbed to the tooth surface, act to bind bacteria and thus consolidate plaque. GTFs thus contribute in a variety of ways to plaque formation and the dental caries process and there is now a substantial body of experimental evidence to support their importance as virulence determinants (Colby and Russell 1997).

While most of the species of streptococci found in plaque produce GTF, attention has been focused on those considered to be most closely associated with dental caries, which belong to the mutans group (*S. mutans*, *S. sobrinus*). Biochemical studies of GTF are greatly complicated by the fact the each species produces a number of different GTF; but the finding that GTF genes could be cloned and expressed in *E. coli* represented a major advance, as it became possible to study each of the GTF in isolation. It is now known that *S. mutans* produces three distinct GTF while *S. sobrinus* produces four. Each GTF is encoded by a separate gene and each enzyme has distinctive properties, varying in the proportion of α-1,6- and α-1,3-linkages and hence the degree of branching it introduces into the glucan, and the total length of the glucan chain produced. Little is yet known about the regulation of the proportions of the different GTF in a single species, but their relative activity determines the eventual properties of the glucan produced. Within dental plaque, the situation will be vastly more complex because the overall properties of the glucan represents the combined action of a dozen or more different GTF and also of their interactions, since one GTF may modify the product of another. Furthermore, glucans will be modified by the action of dextranase, which is produced by various plaque bacteria and which degrades the α-1,6-linked chains.

As nucleotide sequences of GTF became available, it was possible to carry out multiple alignments of the deduced amino acid sequences in order to identify conserved and unique features which may explain which amino acid residues or domains are responsible for common actions of all GTF (such as sucrose hydrolysis) and which determine distinctive activities (such as type of linkage or chain termination). The basic organization of GTF could be discerned as soon as more than one sequence became available; but the gene sequences of over a dozen streptococcal GTF, and several from *Leuconostoc mesenteroides*, are now available to us and this has confirmed the earlier model for a basic common organization for all GTF. All GTF are of high molecular weight and composed of distinct domains, illustrated in Figure 4.1b. Identification of the reaction mechanism and location of the active site is essential for the rational design of GTF inhibitors that mimic the sugar substrate and for targeting antibodies against the catalytic region.

The terminal one-third of GTF consists of a series of related but non-identical tandem amino acid repeats, each about 33 amino acids long. In at least some GTF, this domain contributes to the synthesis of the glucan chain and it appears to be important in binding GTF to preformed or nascent glucan, thus mediating bacteria–bacteria or bacteria–surface adhesion. The mutans streptococci also produce a number of other glucan-binding proteins besides GTF. The functions of these proteins are not yet entirely clear but it seems probable that they contribute in some way to the 'stickiness' of dental plaque and so provide further potential molecular targets for inhibition.

Metabolism of dental plaque

Once the bacteria have managed to become established in dental plaque, they contribute to the overall balance between the species and help to determine the plaque properties. The streptococci are of central importance in the metabolism of plaque not only because they are well-equipped to survive in the fluctuating conditions, but also because they facilitate the survival of other strictly anaerobic species. The various species of streptococci differ both in their ability to generate acid from dietary carbohydrate and in their acid tolerance. A consequence of this is that frequent exposure to carbohydrate and the consequent fall in pH, to values which may go as low as pH 4.0 in carious lesions, serve to enrich the population of aciduric species and particularly of the mutans streptococci. The production of acids by fermentation of dietary carbohydrates has long been recognized as a central element of the caries process, but its importance in determining the microbial composition of plaque has been appreciated only in the recent years. Specific adhesive interactions are the major determinants in selecting which bacteria can establish a toehold in plaque, but, once any particular bacterial species has become a member of the plaque microbial community, its survival depends largely upon its metabolic versatility. Within plaque, it has been estimated that the glucose concentration may vary over a 10 000-fold range, the pH may shift from 7.5 to 4.0 and, while oxygen is freely available at the plaque surface, conditions are entirely anaerobic close to the tooth surface. As facultative anaerobes, the streptococci are well suited to flourishing under varying conditions of oxygen availability. With regard to acid, different plaque species differ in the range of pH that they can tolerate *S. mutans* is notable in combining the properties of being extremely acidogenic and also aciduric. As a consequence, when there is a good supply of carbohydrate, *S. mutans* will produce a large amount of acid (mainly lactic acid) that will lower the plaque pH. *S. mutans* continues to metabolize under the low-pH conditions while other competing species are disadvantaged, with the net result that the relative proportions of *S. mutans* in the plaque population increase. This phenomenon has been demonstrated both by using chemostats in the laboratory and by monitoring the plaque composition in volunteers on a sugar-rich diet. Frequent exposure to fermentable carbohydrates thus has the effect of repetitively enriching the proportion of *S. mutans* in plaque. This, of course, is one of the reasons for the advice against frequent snacking. Longitudinal studies of plaque microbiology have shown that the probability of caries occurring at a particular tooth site rises dramatically once *S. mutans* reaches 50% of the bacterial population—at healthy, caries-free sites *S. mutans* may be present at a level below 0.1% (Loesche 1986). In the absence of a cariogenic dietary challenge, mutans streptococci are harmless commensals in balance with other plaque bacteria and the host defences. The most straightforward way to avoid a disturbance in this balance, which may lead to disease, is therefore dietary control.

Preventing infection

Identifying the course of infection is the first step in control of infectious disease and all dentists are fully familiar with the concepts of cross-infection control in their clinics, where they sterilise contaminated instruments and use physical barriers in the form of gloves and masks to prevent transmission. Since we now have the evidence that an uninfected infant acquires *S. mutans* from their mother or other carer, what can we do to reduce the risk of infection? The best we can hope for is disinfection of the source, i.e. reducing the level of the bacteria in the mother so as to reduce, as far as possible, the risk of cross-infection of the infant.

That this approach is practicable was first demonstrated by treating expectant mothers to reduce their carriage of *S. mutans* by intensive professional oral hygiene, including chlorhexidine treatment, and giving dietary advice during pregnancy and after the birth of the child. A reduction in the salivary levels of mutans streptococci could be demonstrated in the mothers and this dramatically reduced the likelihood of their babies becoming colonized with *S. mutans*, so that most did not become infected during the usual 'window of infectivity' but remained uninfected until they were at least 4 or 5 years old. More importantly, this resulted in a reduction in their subsequent caries attack rate (Kohler and Andreen 1994). These positive benefits have been demonstrated in a number of subsequent studies. In microbiological terms, the results can be explained by the fact that the dental plaque microflora that became established in the early years of life did not include cariogenic species; and the phenomenon of colonization resistance makes it increasingly difficult for superinfection by mutans streptococci to occur at a later date. Of course, it remains essential for the child to maintain good oral hygiene and dietary habits to avoid conditions that would favour invasion by *S. mutans*, but getting a good start in life by reducing the risk of infection by paying attention to the mother can pay rich dividends (Thorild *et al*. 2002).

Replacement therapy

An extension of the theme of establishing a benevolent plaque microflora had led us to an alternative approach to caries control that is still in the experimental stage but has attracted considerable publicity. Ideally, we might like to have no infection with *S. mutans*; but, if we cannot achieve that, can we at least render the bacteria harmless? Starting from the premise that undesirable species in plaque perform particular functions, this approach depends upon constructing 'good' variants of those species, which are benign in their influence and will displace the normal strains from dental plaque. Interest in this area has focused upon the construction of mutants of *S. mutans* lacking lactate dehydrogenase, since lack of this crucial enzyme means that they produce less lactic acid and are, therefore, less likely to promote dental caries. Hillman *et al.* (2000) have carried out a series of genetic manipulations to knock out the lactate dehydrogenase gene, at the same time introducing a gene from another bacterium encoding alcohol dehydrogenase in order to overcome the otherwise toxic effects of NAD–NADH imbalance. In order to give this mutant a competitive advantage in colonizing plaque, they also introduced the genes for production of a bacteriocin (an inhibitory peptide) that has a wide spectrum of activity against other plaque bacteria. The two basic premises of this approach have a firm experimental basis, as lactate dehydrogenase mutants are less cariogenic in rats and there is support for the colonization ability of bacteriocin-producing strains from observations in humans and monkeys.

Replacement therapy experiments are not restricted to lactate dehydrogenase mutants. Other researchers have tried a very different approach, introducing a gene for production of the enzyme urease into *S. mutans*, so that it can generate alkali and so neutralize acid accumulation in plaque. Recognizing the importance of sucrose-derived glucans in plaque cohesion, Japanese researchers introduced genes for a dextranase gene and for an enzyme that makes cycloisomaltoligosaccharides (inhibitors of GTF) into the plaque bacterium *S. gordonii*.

A number of these replacement strategies have been tested in animal models, and there were reports in 2002 that research on replacement therapy with the lactate dehydrogenase mutant was shortly to move to experiments with human volunteers. As in trials of other anti-caries agents, such trials are likely to be initially in adults. The success of the strategy could be monitored by following the ability of the mutant strain to become established in plaque and by measuring the capacity of plaque from the volunteers to produce acid when exposed to sugars. Only later can investigations with a caries-prone group (i.e. children) be undertaken. The main areas of uncertainty in the replacement therapy approach relate to the unpredictable ecological consequence of the release of a genetically modified organisms, and in many ways the questions are the same as those relating to any GM organisms—will the mutant be stable and will it exchange DNA with the normal microflora? How will the overall balance of the bacterial population be affected? While every care can be taken in the construction of the mutant, it is impossible to predict the answers to these questions at the moment. Finally, it is necessary to recognize the widespread public unease about GM products, so even a product with many potential advantages might prove unacceptable.

Inhibition of mutans streptococci

Current means of preventing plaque-related dental diseases are largely non-specific, relying upon mechanical removal of dental plaque or upon the use of antibacterial agents or detergents which act on a range of bacteria (Russell 1994). Although in some instances the preventive effect may be due to a differential action upon particular organisms, such selectivity has usually only been recognized *after* an agent has empirically been found to be efficacious. An example is the realization that mutans streptococci show exceptional sensitivity to chlorhexidine and that following a course of treatment, they may take several months to recover to their initial level, whereas other, non-cariogenic species recover much sooner. Even non-specific anti-plaque agents can thus have a beneficial effect in destabilising the plaque microflora so that mutans streptococci, poor colonizers at the best of times, are reduced to such a level that they do not readily rise to a sufficiently high proportion of the plaque population to pose a threat.

Chlorhexidine

Chlorhexidine is the most effective antibacterial agent that has found wide application in dentistry, particularly in the treatment of gingivitis and as an adjunct to periodontal therapy. Oral rinsing or topical application of chlorhexidine causes a rapid drop in the viability of plaque bacteria, and its effect on mutans streptococci has been well studied. Numbers of mutans streptococci can be reduced to undetectable levels, yet will gradually return to the original levels over a period of several months, with the occlusal surfaces of molar teeth (the most caries-prone sites) being the first to be recolonized. It is thus apparent that regular or continuous application of chlorhexidine would be necessary to achieve long-term suppression, unless chlorhexidine treatment is being used as a short-term measure to reduce mother–child transmission or being combined with some other treatment. Chlorhexidine varnishes have the potential to have a long-term effect, and there have been mixed reports of their efficacy in reducing salivary levels of mutans streptococci. Only a few papers have described research that looked both at the microbiological marker and at the effect on caries, and again mixed results have been obtained. It seems that this variable experience is due to practical difficulties in achieving and maintaining adequate coverage of teeth with the varnish. The concept has been demonstrated to be valid, but

translating research results into a robust procedure that can be applied in practice with good reliability is proving difficult (Forgie *et al.* 2000).

Xylitol

The value of non-sugar sweeteners in caries prevention is addressed in Chapter 10. Xylitol was introduced as a non-sugar sweetener on the basis of the fact that it is not metabolized by bacteria such as *S. mutans*. This on its own is clearly advantageous, but an added bonus is that xylitol has an antibacterial effect. This is because the xylitol molecule, a sugar alcohol, is structurally similar to fructose. It is thus transported by the phosphotransferase systems responsible for uptake of fructose, and is phosphorylated as it crosses the membrane. However, in the absence of enzymes to take it further along metabolic pathways, xylitol phosphate accumulates inside the bacterium where it exerts a toxic effect. Some will be dephosphorylated in a 'futile cycle' that is a drain on energy and therefore slows growth. The overall effect is a selective antibacterial effect on bacteria that can transport xylitol but not utilize it (Tanzer 1995). The effect on mutans streptococci has been best documented, though other plaque bacteria (particularly streptococci and lactobacilli) are also subject to the effect. Regular consumption of xylitol has been demonstrated to result in a reduction of numbers of *S. mutans*, and also have a caries protective effect (Soderling *et al.* 2001) Most of the studies have delivered xylitol as a constituent of chewing gum, and some authors have found that gum containing sorbitol is just as effective, raising the question as to whether the benefits come from the sugar substitute or from the beneficial effects of stimulating salivary flow. Of course, the increased buffering by saliva will prevent plaque pH remaining at a low value and so indirectly is likely to result in a reduction in numbers of *S. mutans* by stopping selective conditions from developing.

Blocking of adhesion

Considerable research has been carried out on identifying adhesins on the surfaces of plaque bacteria and characterizing the receptor molecules to which they bind. These receptors may either be host macromolecules adsorbed to the tooth surface in salivary pellicle or components of the surfaces of other bacteria. Characterization of the binding reaction opens up possibilities for interfering with the binding either by the use of soluble analogues of the receptor or by treating with excess free adhesin. There has been one preliminary report of using an excess of a receptor to block attachment: *Actinomyces* type 2 fimbriae recognize salivary molecules containing β-linked GalNAc and it has been reported that, in volunteers who had rinsed their mouths with GalNacβ1-3Galα1-O-ethyl, there was a reduction in the total number of *Actinomyces* as well as a reduction in total plaque mass. Laboratory studies have also shown the possibility of the alternative approach of using an excess of adhesin, and a short peptide of 20 amino acids corresponding to the binding region of *S. mutans* antigen

Experimental approaches to control *S. mutans*

- Replacement Therapy with non-acid producing mutant
- Reduce numbers with bacteriocide such as chlorhexidine
- Xylitol interferes with metabolism
- Block adhesion with receptor analogues

I/II has been tested in experiments where it was applied to the teeth of volunteers (Kelly *et al.* 1999). The levels of *S. mutans* had previously been reduced to undetectable levels by chlorhexidine treatment, and the topical application of peptide was repeated every other day for 2 weeks. All control subjects became recolonized to the original level over the next 3 to 4 months but of the four test subjects who received the peptide, only one became recolonized within the time period. Under these experimental conditions, which were similar to those used to test passive application of antibody (see below) it appears that there may be a crucial stage at which interference with the attachment of *S. mutans* to receptors can have a long-term beneficial effect in decreasing its ability to become established as a major plaque organism. There clearly remains much to be done in resolving such aspects as the best formulation of the peptide for easy delivery to the tooth site and the frequency of application needed for a sustained effect. Nevertheless, the results reinforce the validity of an approach that aims to stop *S. mutans* gaining a foothold, rather than attempting to reduce already high levels.

Inhibition of specific enzyme reactions

Using metabolic inhibitors that block particular reactions unique to the target species is, in theory, a promising approach to therapy. Although a number of specific functions in oral bacteria can be proposed as potential targets for inhibitors, greatest attention has been paid to the glucosyltransferases (GTF). Beneficial effects might be expected from either preventing the formation of glucans or digesting them once formed. Known inhibitors of GTF include structural analogues of sucrose which compete for the active site and are likely to be relatively specific for enzymes which have sucrose as a substrate. Examples of such competitive inhibitors are 6-amino derivatives of sucrose, acarbose, 6-deoxy-sucrose, deoxynojirimycin, and ribocitrin. Other agents which have been shown to inhibit GTF include natural products such as polyphenols found in tea, cocoa, or fruits, and a number of small molecules including Zn^{2+} ions, Tris, pyridine, and amino sugars. Amongst the wide range of substances tested, none has yet been identified that can be regarded as being both a potent inhibitor and highly specific for GTF. These are properties that are desirable if a substance is to suppress GTF sufficiently and to have a beneficial effect while having no adverse side effects by inhibiting other enzymes.

Caries vaccines

Antibodies to the oral streptococci can be detected in saliva from an early age, though the pattern of response to different antigens shows great variability. Despite numerous studies, however, no convincing evidence has emerged that this immune response controls the developing microflora. This remains one of the great puzzles, not just for the oral cavity but for other permanently colonized mucosal sites—how is the balance between commensal bacteria and host response maintained in equilibrium? On the other hand, there is now substantial evidence that a strongly enhanced response induced by immunization or by passive application of antibody can influence their ability to colonize and/or cause disease (Koga *et al.* 2002).

Research into a dental caries vaccine has been carried out in many laboratories around the world in the last thirty years or more, and there is convincing evidence that it is possible to achieve a high level of protection against caries in experimental animals by the use of vaccines which rely upon intact *S. mutans* as immunogen. In common with the trend in the development of other human vaccines, considerable effort has been expended on defining the protective components of *S. mutans*, in the expectation that a purified subunit vaccine would induce a more consistent immune response, and would be less likely than whole bacteria to cause any adverse side-reactions. Although a range of cellular components have been investigated, most progress has been made with GTF preparations and cell wall proteins. There is good evidence that a GTF-based vaccine can protect rats against caries caused by *S. sobrinus*, with most of the protective effects being limited to smooth surface lesions. On smooth surfaces, GTF-mediated glucan formation is likely to be of major importance for adhesion of *S. sobrinus,* which can explain the success of GTF vaccines in this experimental model. However, experiments in which macaque monkeys were immunized with GTF from *S. mutans* showed no protective effect. It is thus necessary to examine carefully the relevance of the two animal models to human disease. The rat has tooth morphology and a pattern of decay different from the human and is not naturally colonized by *S. mutans*. In monkeys, as in humans, the main points of attack are in occlusal fissures and interproximal sites, with *S. mutans* being the principal organism associated with disease progression; protection against smooth surface attack is therefore of relatively little importance. Furthermore, many caries vaccine experiments using rats have employed *S. sobrinus* as the challenge organism; and it must be remembered that *S. sobrinus* is commonly found in less than one-third of the human population and its contribution to caries in humans is unclear. Monkey experiments may offer a more suitable disease model but

Dental caries vaccine

- Rats, mice, and monkeys have been protected against caries by immunization with whole bacteria or pure proteins derived from *S. mutans*
- No adverse effects of immunization have been reported
- Difficulties remain over the introduction of a clinical trial of an injectable caries vaccine
- Research has demonstrated the feasibility of alternative approaches using recombinant vaccines, orally administered vaccines, or passive immunization

present considerable problems in terms of husbandry and cost with consequentially small experimental groups. Therefore, although it may be desirable to test any proposed vaccine on non-human primates, rats are likely to be more convenient for preliminary experiments so long as caution is exercised in extrapolation of results to humans.

Barriers to introduction of a caries vaccine

The first promising results with caries vaccine trials in non-human primates were obtained in the 1970s. Two wall-associated proteins of *S. mutans* were tested as vaccines. One, referred to as Antigen A and administered as an intra-muscular injection, was reported to protect both rats and monkeys against caries and was then taken through the subsequent stages of testing for toxicity in animals and human adult volunteers. The other, the major surface adhesin known as Antigen I/II, also confers protection in rats or monkeys. Despite promising test results, neither protein has advanced to the stage of human clinical trials and it may be useful to consider some of the reasons. Questions can always be raised about the validity of animal data (*e.g.* tooth structure in rats, small size of experimental groups of monkeys, ecological consequences for other plaque bacteria), but proposals to introduce a novel vaccine against a human disease also introduce a whole range of ethical and politico-economic issues that extend far beyond laboratory findings. These apply to any novel vaccine but demand particularly close attention when the proposal is to vaccinate against caries. Principal among these is the question of risk–benefit because, for a non-life threatening disease which is regarded as a minor (and avoidable) affliction in medical terms, no adverse reactions can be tolerated. Particular concern has been raised with regard to streptococcal vaccines, because of the known phenomenon of antigenic cross-reaction between streptococcal proteins and heart tissue. While such cross-reaction between *S. mutans* proteins and heart tissue has been described, the nature of the phenomenon and its potential for causing pathological changes remains incompletely explained and, though it now appears that no hazard exists, it is difficult to allay all fears.

It should be noted that the introduction of *any* novel vaccine is fraught with difficulties, not least because of concern that any mishaps (or newspaper scare stories) can have a disastrous effect on public attitudes and participation in immunization schemes even for unrelated but well-established vaccines such as those for pertussis, polio, and diphtheria. The safety requirements for a vaccine against a disease that is not life-threatening must be very stringent, not just because of the risk–benefit equation for protection against caries, but because of concerns that public confidence in mass-vaccination campaigns could be damaged. The vulnerability of such campaigns to adverse publicity has been vividly illustrated by the experience with whooping cough vaccine in the 1980s and, more recently, measles, mumps, rubella (MMR) vaccine. In both cases public concern over one particular vaccine had a knock-on effect on uptake of other vaccines. As a consequence, many children went unprotected

and the result was a resurgence in incidence of disease in subsequent years.

Serious consideration was given, around 1985, to the initiation of trials in humans of vaccines utilising *S. mutans* wall-associated proteins in the UK and other countries. Some questions about the extent of the available experimental data remained to be answered, but the overriding concern was related to the place of a caries vaccine in national vaccine policies. This, together with a perception that other anti-caries measures were adequate, was a decisive factor in the decision not to proceed with research leading to trials of an injectable vaccine at that time. The decision altered perceptions of what sort of caries vaccine might be acceptable, but the fact remains that experimental evidence shows that an immunological approach to caries control is valid, and the principle of immune intervention to control caries remains highly attractive. Research has continued along a number of lines to find the best antigen and the best way of inducing an immune response.

Novel antigens

Traditionally, the walls of Gram-positive bacteria have been represented as being fairly simple in structure (compared to the walls of Gram-negatives), but an increasing number of surface proteins are now being recognized and the recent determination of the entire genome sequence of *S. mutans* has provided new avenues for exploration. There is no doubt that further knowledge of the surfaces of plaque bacteria will present new potential targets for immune agents. There is also increasing emphasis on defining specific antigenic epitopes within each antigen, and of defining the type of immune response that they would induce.

Novel immunization strategies

An alternative to an injectable vaccine is one which is administered orally, with the added attraction that stimulation of the gut mucosal immune response may also be manifested in the oral mucosa, giving an increased level of secretory IgA antibody in the oral cavity. An intranasal route of immunization has also been explored in mice and recently, humans. Strategies being investigated as a means of achieving a protective secretory immune response include the fusion of antigens to cholera toxin B subunit, the incorporation of antigens into liposomes and the cloning and expression of antigens in avirulent *Salmonella*. An understanding of the structure and function of possible protective antigens has led a number of research groups to use fusion proteins that are constructed of fragments of GTF incorporating the active site and/or glucan-binding domain together with the binding region of antigen I/II, in order to get a dual protective response against two major antigens. Once an immunogen has been selected, the stages of research involve first, the demonstration of the induction of an immune response, then an effect on *S. mutans*, and finally an influence on the development of caries. A number of laboratories around the world, principally in the USA and Japan, are involved in this work and have reported success in experiments with rats or mice. A major challenge is to develop immunization regimes that lead to a sustained high level of antibody secretion.

Passive immunization

A different approach to that of inducing an immune response by vaccination is to apply ready-formed antibodies topically. Using monoclonal antibodies directed against Antigen I/II, Ma *et al.* (1998) have reported that they have been able to control reimplantation of *S. mutans* on cleaned tooth surfaces in monkeys and in human volunteers. Monoclonal antibodies are, however, extremely expensive to produce at present; so alternative cheap sources of antibody for passive immunization have been sought. The yolk of eggs from immunized hens contains substantial amounts of immunoglobulin; and two groups of workers have reported that antibody from this source, when incorporated into a sucrose-containing diet, reduces the level of caries in rats infected with *S. mutans*. Another ready source of antibody is colostrum (the first milk yield after birth) from immunized cows, and this also has proved promising in rat experiments. In trials with human volunteers, using a bovine antibody mouth-rinse, however, there was no effect on the total numbers of *S. mutans* but a shift in the type of *S. mutans* occurred, with a small-colony type replacing a type with large colonies. This highlights a potential difficulty with procedures based on specific antibodies, which may be *too* specific. If a variant of *S. mutans*, which has different epitopes from that originally used to raise the antibody is present in the oral cavity, then it will evade immunological clearance. It is thus essential that to be effective, the protective antibodies must be directed against antigens which show no variation and are universally conserved throughout all the range of *S. mutans* types which are naturally present in the population. From another point of view, when selecting an *S. mutans* antigen as a target for preventive strategies, the possibility of cross-reactions with other oral streptococci must be borne in mind, as inhibition of harmless species could be counter-productive.

Microbiological prediction of caries

The discussion relates to methods to prevent caries. If we cannot prevent the disease, can we at least predict the risk of its occurrence and take steps to minimise the impact on identified high-risk individuals? In 1975, it was first reported that by measuring the numbers of mutans streptococci in saliva it was possible to identify high risk individuals. The results indicated that over 10^6 colony-forming units per ml of saliva was a strong predictor of risk of subsequent caries. For any predictive test to be of practical value, it is essential to know its sensitivity and specificity, the proportion of true and false positive and negative results, and whether it has general applicability to a range of different population groups. The consensus now is that, except in young children, microbiological tests on their own do not have sufficient reliability to pick out high-risk individuals for a population group

(Powell 1998). Microbiological data can, however, be valuable in more complex risk assessment schemes where other influences such as past caries experience, salivary properties, and diet are also factored in. The commercial chairside tests designed to culture mutans streptococci from saliva also have a use in patient education and motivation, as well as providing an objective way of monitoring compliance with dietary advice. While some of us may be delighted by being shown that we harbour all these germs in our mouths, the revulsion of others can be a strong motivating factor. And so we come full circle back to van Leeuwenhoek!

Conclusions

- Dental caries is a bacterial disease, modified by environmental factors such as diet and conditions in the mouth.
- Many of the preventive strategies already available to dentists work because they influence the bacterial challenge to the susceptible tooth surface. For example, fissure sealants make habitats unavailable, chewing gum stimulates saliva flow and affects pH levels in plaque, chlorhexidine disrupts the balance between bacterial species.
- Research into the microbiology of caries has shown that *S. mutans* is the major, but not the only, species associated with caries.
- Understanding of the acquisition of *S. mutans* has provided the opportunity to prevent or delay initial infection while our knowledge of the environmental conditions that favour increase in *S. mutans* in plaque can be applied in patient management.
- The application of modern molecular biology techniques to the study of *S. mutans* has presented a range of novel approaches to prevention of dental caries.

References

Caufield, P.W., Cutter, R.J., and Dasanayake, A.P. (1993). Initial acquisition of mutans streptococci by infants: evidence for a discrete window of infectivity. *Journal of Dental Research*, **72**, 37–45.

Colby, S.M. and Russell, R.R.B. (1997). Sugar metabolism by mutans streptococci. *Journal of Applied Microbiology*, **83**, 80S–88S.

Forgie, A.H., Paterson, M., Pine, C.M., Pitts, N.B., and Nujent, J.J. (2000). A randomised controlled trial of the caries-preventive efficacy of a chlorhexidine-containing varnish in high-caries-risk adolescents. *Caries Research*, **34**, 432–439.

Hillman, J.D., Brooks, T.A., Michalek, S., Harmon, C.C., Snoep, J.L., and van der Weijden, C.C. (2000). Construction and characterization of an effector strain of *Streptococcus mutans* for replacement therapy of dental caries. *Infection and Immunity*, **68**, 543–549.

Jenkinson, H.F. and Demuth, D.R.(1997). Structure, function and immunogenicity of streptococcal antigen I/II polypeptides. *Molecular Microbiology*, **23**, 183–190.

Kelly, C.G., Younson, J.S., Hikmat, B.Y., Todryk, S.M., Czisch, M., Haris, P.I., Flindall, I.R., Newby, C., Mallet, A.I., Ma, J.K.C., and Lehner, T. (1999). A synthetic peptide adhesion epitope as a novel antimicrobial agent. *Nature Biotechnology*, **17**, 42–47.

Kleinberg, I. (2002). A mixed-bacterial ecological approach to understanding the role of the oral bacteria in dental caries causation: an alternative to *Streptococcus mutans* and the specific-plaque hypothesis. *Critical Reviews in Oral Biology and Medicine,* **13**, 108–125.

Koga, T., Oho, T., Shimazaki. Y., and Nakano, Y. (2002). Immunization against dental caries. *Vaccine*, **20**, 2027–2044.

Kohler, B. and Andreen, I. (1994). Influence of caries-preventive measures in mothers on cariogenic bacteria and caries experience in their children. *Archives of Oral Biology,* **39**, 907–911.

Loesche, W.J. (1986). Role of *Streptococcus mutans* in human dental decay. *Microbiology Reviews*, **50**, 353–380.

Ma, J.K.C., Hikmat, B.Y., Wycoff, K., Vine, N.D., Chargelegue, D., Yu, L., Hein, M.B., and Lehner, T. (1998). Characterization of a recombinant plant monoclonal secretory antibody and preventive immunotherapy in humans. *Nature Medicine*, **4**, 601–606.

Marsh, P.D. (1994). Microbial ecology of dental plaque and its significance in health and disease. *Advances in Dental Research*, **8**, 263–271.

Powell, L.V. (1998). Caries prediction: a review of the literature. *Community Dentistry and Oral Epidemiology*, **26**, 336–371.

Russell, R.R.B. (1994). Control of specific plaque bacteria. *Advances in Dental Research,* **8**, 285–290.

Soderling, E., Isokangas, P., Pienihakkinen, K., Tenovuo, J., and Alanen, P. (2001). Influence of maternal xylitol consumption on mother–child transmission of mutans streptococci: 6-year follow-up. *Caries Research*, **35**, 173–177.

Tanzer, J.M. (1995). Xylitol chewing gum and dental caries. *International Dental Journal*, **45** (Suppl. 1), 65–76.

Thorild, I., Lindau-Jonson, B., and Twetman, S. (2002). Prevalence of salivary *Streptococcus mutans* in mothers and in their preschool children. *International Journal of Paediatric Dentistry*, **12**, 2–7.

van Ruyven F.O., Lingstrom P., van Houte J., and Kent R. (2000). Relationship among mutans streptococci, "low-pH" bacteria, and iodophilic polysaccharide-producing bacteria in dental plaque and early enamel caries in humans. *Journal of Dental Research*, **79**, 778–784.

5

Managing caries in enamel

Managing caries in enamel

Edwina Kidd and June Nunn

Introduction—what is caries?

It is important to understand what caries is, to follow the logic of its suggested management. Dental caries is a process which may take place on any tooth surface in the oral cavity where a microbial biofilm (dental plaque) is allowed to develop over a period of time.

Formation of the biofilm is a natural physiological process (see Chapter 4). It is important to remember that the biofilm is not a haphazard collection of micro-organisms, but a community with a collective physiology, which can solve the specific physico-chemical problems posed by the environment at the site. The bacteria in the biofilm are always metabolically active, causing minute fluctuations in pH. These may cause a net loss of mineral from the tooth when the pH is dropping. This is called demineralization. Alternatively, there may be a net gain of mineral when the pH is increasing. This is called remineralization. The cumulative result of these de- and remineralization processes may be a net loss of mineral and a carious lesion that can be seen. Alternatively, the changes may be so slight that a carious lesion never becomes apparent (Fig. 5.1).

From this description it becomes obvious that the carious process is a ubiquitous, natural process. The formation of the

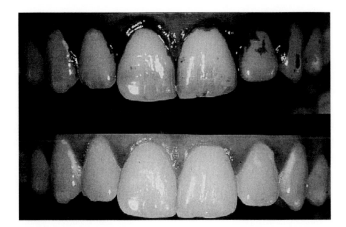

Figure 5.1 The upper anterior teeth of a young adult. In the upper picture, a disclosing agent reveals the plaque, while in the lower picture, the plaque has been removed. White spot lesions are visible on the canines, but not on other tooth surfaces, although plaque is present. (See Plate 1.)

biofilm and its metabolic activity cannot be prevented, but disease progression can be controlled so that a clinically visible enamel lesion never forms.

Logically, management depends on appreciating that the de- and remineralization processes can be modified. For instance, if the biofilm is partially or totally removed, mineral loss may be stopped or even reversed towards mineral gain.

Factors which influence the magnitude of the pH fluctuations are also very important and many of these can be influenced. For instance, the composition and thickness of the microbial deposits, the diet, the fluoride ion concentration, and the salivary secretion rate. These biological factors can in turn be influenced by various sociological parameters such as a person's behaviour, attitudes, their knowledge and beliefs and their affluence or poverty.

The carious process and the carious lesion

Carious lesions can form on any tooth surface exposed to the mouth; thus they can form on enamel, cementum, or dentine. This chapter will concern the enamel lesion; but the reader should appreciate that the principles of management of the process are the same, irrespective of the tooth tissue involved.

It is perhaps unfortunate that the word 'caries' is used to denote both the carious process that occurs in the biofilm at the tooth or cavity surface and the carious lesion that forms within the tooth tissue as a result of the process. The carious lesion can be thought of as a reflection of the carious process. The metabolic activity in the biofilm (the process) cannot be seen; it is the reflection, or consequence, of this process that the dentist can see. Thus the dentist is working on a reflection of reality and this may cause confusion as to where the 'action' is. Please stand in front of the mirror and look at your reflection. Do you like what you see? If you do not what might you do? Maybe you could get some new clothes, lose some weight, change your hairstyle, or even see a plastic surgeon. You are, of course, sensibly concentrating on the real you and it probably would not occur to you to pick up a brick and smash the mirror! Now please go into the clinic. All the dentists who are filling holes in teeth are, in a way, smashing the mirror; unless they have *also* concentrated on teaching the patient to control the metabolic activity in the biofilm.

The concept of activity

Thus far the carious process has been presented as an ubiquitous, natural phenomenon at the crystal level. The process is spread over time but it does not have to progress. Lesions, at any stage of their activity, can be arrested by improved plaque control, sensible dietary changes, and judicious use of fluoride. While examining patients, you may detect enamel carious lesions and it is possible to get a very good idea of their depth of penetration into the tissues. However, it is just as important to decide whether these lesions are active and progressing or already arrested. This judgement is essential for logical management because active lesions require active management whereas arrested lesions do not.

This makes it sound as if these decisions about activity are easy to make—like telling black from white. Unfortunately, this is not the case; because, we are dealing with a continuum of changes and the shades of grey are also relevant. Thus an active lesion may be rapidly or slowly progressing and parts of a lesion may be active while other areas are arrested.

Caries activity

- The caries process may or may not be progressive
- Lesions may be active
- Lesions may be arrested—by diet, oral hygiene, and use of fluorides

The validity and reliability of diagnostic decisions

It thus appears that diagnostic decisions are made in conditions of uncertainty. Will the dentist always be correct in the diagnosis of the presence of a lesion and its activity? We now come to a very important point about diagnosis—it should always be considered in terms of its validity and reliability. Validity means whether the diagnosis reflects the true condition. Reliability concerns whether the result would be reproducible either by the same dentist on a different occasion or by a different dentist.

It is now appropriate to consider the consequence of errors of diagnosis of activity. Suppose a dentist judges an enamel lesion to be active when it is in fact arrested. The consequences of the error will be that the dentist will institute preventive non-operative treatment and this was not required. Supposing, on the other hand, the dentist judges a lesion to be inactive, and does not institute preventive treatment, when in fact the lesion is active. Now the progression of the lesion is likely to continue unchecked. The first of these two errors is called a false positive, the second a false negative.

If you were the patient, bearing in mind some errors will always be made, which error would you prefer—to be treated unnecessarily or not be treated when action was required? Please consider this from the point of view of an enamel carious lesion and then alter your perspective so that 'treatment' now implies some irreversible action e.g. tooth extraction or a filling. Your perspective might change depending on the consequences of false positive and false

negative diagnosis in terms of treatment. You might also like to consider the same scenario from the point of view of the dentist, rather than the patient. This is a particularly thought-provoking exercise, where one decision reaps more reward, financially, than another. Maybe this even pertains to your student clinic where, perhaps, points are awarded for restorative treatments, but credits are not given for preventive care. We digress into ethics!

It is fortunate that dentists see patients on recall. Thus, a diagnostic decision can be re-evaluated on a subsequent occasion. Since patients are so intimately concerned with the management of the carious process, they must certainly be informed of the diagnosis; and should participate in discussion of treatment options. After all, the teeth belong to the patient, but the responsibility of the professional is to give advice based on the best evidence.

Caries risk assessment

The previous sections concentrated on individual lesions, but these lesions are clustered in individuals. It is important to assess an individual patient's susceptibility to carious lesion formation and progression. This is an important part of contemporary practice for the following reasons:

- it makes economic sense to target preventive treatments at the appropriate risk group.

- dental care neither begins nor ends with a single course of treatment, but is ongoing. When a course of dental treatment is complete, the dentist and the patient decide when it would be wise to check that all is well. This recall interval is based partly on an assessment of the risk of disease progression.

- patients should be made aware of their risk status. This knowledge encourages them to keep appropriate recall appointments and to become involved in their own preventive care and, if they pay for this, may help them budget for dental bills.

Factors relevant to assessment of caries risk

The factors relevant to caries risk are outlined in Table 5.1 and discussed subsequently.

Social history

Many studies have shown that dental caries is now concentrated in socially deprived people; and other diseases, such as some cancers and coronary artery disease, are similarly concentrated. The following features of the social history may also be present in high-risk patients:

- Caries in siblings may be high.
- The patient possesses little knowledge of dental disease.
- Dental attendance is irregular and dental aspirations low.
- The patient's use of snacks is high.

Medical history

Medically compromised and disabled people may be at a high risk of and from caries. Users of long-term medicines can be a

Table 5.1 Factors relevant to caries risk

HIGH RISK	LOW RISK
Social History	
Socially deprived	Middle class
High caries in siblings	Low caries in siblings
Low knowledge of dental disease	Dentally aware
Irregular attender	Regular attender
Ready availability of snacks	Work does not allow regular snacks
Low dental aspirations	High dental aspirations
Medical History	
Medically compromised	No medical problem
Disabled	No physical problem
Xerostomia	Normal salivary flow
Long term cariogenic medicine	No long-term medication
Dietary Habits	
Frequent sugar intake	Infrequent sugar intake
Use of Fluoride	
Non-fluoride area	Fluoridation area
No fluoride supplements	Fluoride supplements used
No fluoride toothpaste	Fluoride toothpaste used
Plaque Control	
Infrequent ineffective cleaning	Frequent effective cleaning
Poor manual control	Good manual control
Saliva	
Low flow rate	Normal flow rate
Low buffering capacity	High buffering capacity
High S. mutans and Lactobacillus counts	Low S. mutans and Lactobacillus counts
Clinical Evidence	
New lesions	No new lesions
Premature extractions	No extractions for caries
Anterior caries or restorations	Sound anterior teeth
Multiple restorations	No or few restorations
History of repeated restorations	Restorations inserted years ago
No fissure sealants	Fissure sealed
Multiband orthodontics	No appliances
Partial dentures	

xerostomia. Patients with rheumatoid arthritis may also have Sjögren's syndrome, which affects the salivary and lacrimal glands, leading to a dry mouth and dry eyes. Finally, many medicaments, such as antidepressants, antipsychotics, tranquilizers, antihypertensives, and diuretics, cause dry mouth. When a practitioner is in doubt as to whether a patient's medication is likely to cause a dry mouth, a formulary that notes such complications should be consulted. One further group of patients who may have a dry mouth is that with eating disorders. Hyposalivation, combined with dietary chaos, can cause dental problems.

The medical history is one of the factors in a caries risk assessment that can change. A vigilant dental practitioner ideally detects this change and informs the patient appropriately before too much damage is done.

Plaque control

Dental plaque is the most important risk factor for dental caries, because caries is the result of metabolic activities in this biofilm, and unless it is present, caries does not occur, regardless of any other factors. All patients with poor plaque control do not inevitably develop caries, but oral hygiene with a fluoride toothpaste is the bedrock of caries control in all patients. If, for any reason, oral hygiene becomes difficult, perhaps because of handicap, age, or illness, caries risk increases. Thus, patients who clean their teeth infrequently and ineffectively or have poor manual control may be at high risk. The ability to clean the mouth effectively may also change with time. Family dentists and hygienists are in an ideal position to detect this change.

Dietary habits

High sugar intake can be a caries risk factor. As with all factors, it is not possible to state unequivocally that all patients who have a high sugar intake develop dental decay, and some dentists interpret this as negating the value of dietary analysis and advice. It is unusual, however, to find a patient with multiple active carious lesions who does not have a high sugar intake. Dietary habits can also change with time, particularly with lifestyle change, such as starting work, retirement, and bereavement; again, a vigilant practitioner ideally notices such changes.

Use of fluoride

Fluoride delays the progression of dental caries; thus patients who do not use a fluoride-containing toothpaste may be at risk. Numerous studies have shown water fluoridation is beneficial in caries prevention, particularly in areas of deprivation (see Chapter 3).

Saliva

Many features of saliva affect the risk of developing caries. Xerostomia has already been discussed as a predisposing factor. Numerous research studies have also suggested that salivary counts of mutans streptococci and lactobacilli are predictors of caries risk. This huge volume of work appears to show that low counts often predict low risk well on an individual patient basis, but the opposite is not necessarily true.

problem, if the medicines are sugars-based. Today, many sugars-free medicines are available, but dentists should always check the sugars content of any medications their patients take frequently.

Perhaps the most relevant factor in a medical history is a dry mouth. Patients who have had radiotherapy in the region of the salivary glands for a head and neck malignancy suffer from

Clinical evidence

Clinical evidence has been shown to be the best predictor of caries risk. Thus, patients with the following characteristics are at high risk:

- Multiple new lesions
- History of premature extractions for caries
- Multiple restorations
- Anterior caries or restorations
- History of requiring frequent replacement restorations

Much of this information can be elicited from a new patient by a careful history. The clinical and radiographic examination of clean, dry teeth is of great importance and reveals whether lesions are present and whether they are likely to be active or arrested.

A practitioner who knows his or her patients can hone this initial assessment to near perfection and detect a change in risk status before too much damage has been done. In some patients, placing an appliance, such as a partial denture or an orthodontic appliance, in the mouth can change risk status such that caries develops. The reason for this is that the appliance favours plaque stagnation.

Summary

An experienced practitioner is able to assess caries risk in less time than it takes to read through the previous account of the process. Research confirms logic and has shown that a practitioners' best guess is a good assessor of risk status.

Site predilection for the caries process

- Any surface where the microbial biofilm remains undisturbed
- Partially erupted teeth
- Depth of the fissure system
- Approximally, below the contact point

Histopathological features of enamel caries

Enamel reactions during eruption

When a tooth erupts into the oral cavity, the enamel is fully mineralized. Normal and sound enamel consists of crystals of hydroxyapetite so tightly packed that the enamel has a glass-like appearance. It is translucent and the dentine shines through to give a yellow-white colour to the tooth.

The enamel crystals are arranged in rod (prism) and interrod enamel. Between the crystals are minute spaces filled with water and organic material. These spaces form a fine network of diffusion pathways or pores in the enamel.

The outermost enamel is rather porous with the openings of the striae of Retzius on the surface and these perikymata grooves act as larger diffusion pathways. The numerous pits of the Tomes

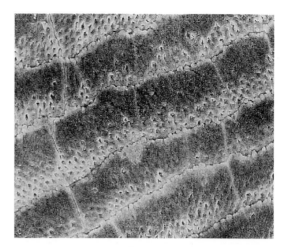

Figure 5.2 An SEM picture of a newly erupted enamel surface after removal of the pellicle. The perkymata and Tomes process pits can be seen. Originally published in *Textbook of Clinical Carology* (Munksgaard) 1994 and reproduced with permission. (See Plate 2.)

processes can be seen as well as a number of developmental defects, called focal holes (Fig. 5.2). In vivo, all these features are filled with protein.

Once the enamel erupts into the oral cavity, it is covered by the metabolically active biofilm and is continually modified by the alternating de- and remineralizations of the carious process.

Eruption is an important time. The tooth emerges gradually over a number of months. The partly erupted tooth does not participate in mastication and it is difficult to clean. For these reasons, microbial accumulation is enhanced, and during this time there are many episodes of de- and remineralization. This is the carious process at a sub-clinical level.

The deeper parts of the fissure system are particularly protected from removal of the biofilm and visible signs of caries may develop where bacterial deposits remain for the longest period of time.

A similar situation exists approximally because bacteria are protected beneath the contact point and along the gingival margin, where plaque control may also be poor.

From this description it is obvious that there is no such thing as a 'caries susceptible site' but there are sites where microbial deposits are likely to remain undisturbed. These areas, although not unique chemically, may well develop clinically visible lesions. It is interesting to know that it was G.V. Black who first pointed this out in 1908, so we are not dealing with new knowledge here!

Ultra structural changes in enamel related to the biofilm

An elegant series of *in vivo* experiments followed the development of the initial lesion formed under an undisturbed biofilm. These conditions were created by cementing bands onto teeth, which were subsequently extracted for orthodontic purposes. The bands

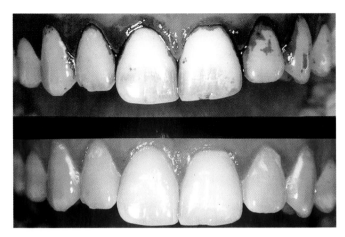

Plate 1 The upper anterior teeth of a young adult. In the upper picture a disclosing agent reveals the plaque while in the lower picture the plaque has been removed. White spot lesions are visible on the canines but not on other tooth surfaces although plaque is present. (Figure 5.1, p. 79.)

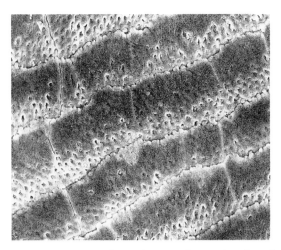

Plate 2 An SEM picture of a newly erupted enamel surface after removal of the pellicle. The perkymata and Tomes process pits can be seen. Originally published in *Textbook of Clinical Carology* (Munksgaard) 1994 and reproduced with permission. (Figure 5.2, p. 82.)

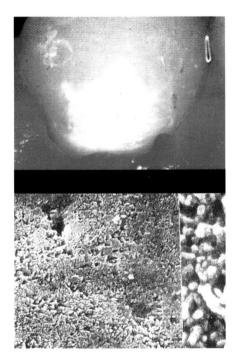

Plate 3 A clinical and SEM picture of a white spot lesion formed under an orthodontic band after 4 weeks of plaque stagnation. Clinically the lesion is opaque with a matt surface. Ultrastructurally there is dissolution of the perikymata overlappings and dissolution of the surface enamel. Originally published in *Textbook of Clinical Carology* (Munksgaard) 1994 and reproduced with permission. (Figure 5.3, p. 83.)

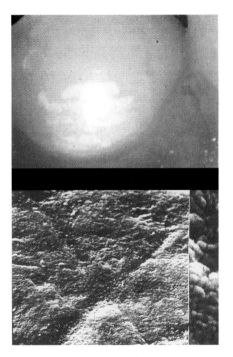

Plate 4 A clinical and SEM picture of a white spot lesion formed under an orthodontic band after removal of the biofilm. The lesion surface is now shiny and hard as a result of abrasion or polishing of the partly dissolved surface of the active lesion. Originally published in *Textbook of Clinical Carology* (Munksgaard) 1994 and reproduced with permission. (Figure 5.4, p. 83.)

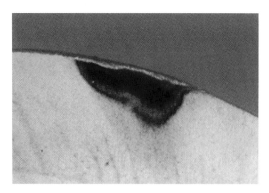

Plate 5 Longitudinal ground section through a small white spot lesion in enamel examined in water with polarized light. The body of the lesion shows as an area of positive birefringence beneath a relatively intact, negatively birefringent surface zone. (Figure 5.5, p. 84.)

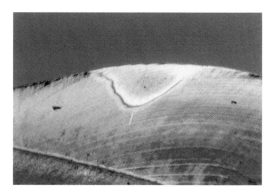

Plate 6 Longitudinal ground section through a small white spot lesion in enamel examined in quinoline with polarized light. The translucent zone is at the advancing front of the lesion and the dark zone is superficial to this. The striae of Retzius are well marked within the body of the lesion. (Figure 5.6, p. 84.)

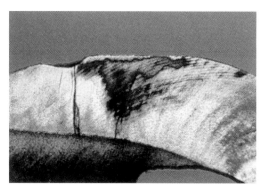

Plate 7 Longitudinal ground section of a natural carious enamel lesion in a tooth extracted from a patient aged 70 years, examined in water in polarized light. This lesion was arrested and similar in appearance to the lesion in Figure 5.20. Well-mineralized laminations are obvious within the body of the lesion, particularly on its occlusal aspect. (Figure 5.7, p. 85.)

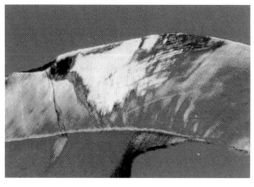

Plate 8 The same section as in Figure 5.7 (Plate 7) examined in quinoline with polarized light. Wide, well-developed dark zones are obvious at the advancing front of the lesion, within the lesion, and at the surface of the lesion. (Figure 5.8, p. 85.)

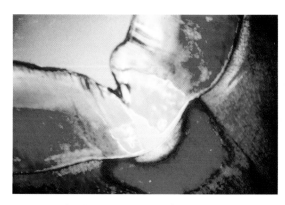

Plate 9 Longitudinal ground section of a natural occlusal carious lesion examined in quinoline in polarized light. The lesion forms in three directions, guided by prism direction assuming the shape of a cone with its base towards the enamel-dentine junction. The undermining shape of this lesion is purely a function of anatomy. (Figure 5.9, p. 85.)

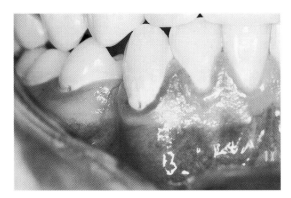

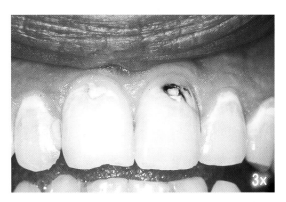

Plate 10 Active smooth surface cervical lesions. These are mat and visible on a wet tooth surface. Cavities can be seen on some lesions. These lesions can be arrested by plaque control alone. (Figure 5.11, p. 86.)

Plate 11 Arrested smooth surface cervical lesions. Notice the healthy gingival margins indicating good plaque removal. The lesions are shiny and are slightly brown from exogenous stains picked up from the mouth. (Figure 5.12, p. 86.)

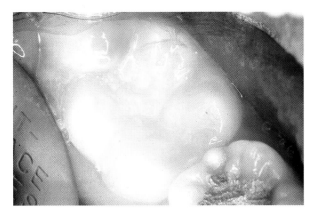

Plate 12 This erupting molar appears caries free but it is not. Figure by courtesy of *Dental Update*. (Figure 5.13, p. 87.)

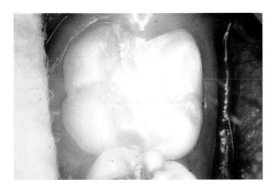

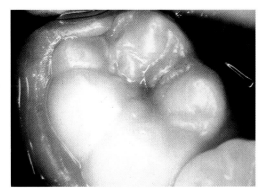

Plate 13 The surface has now been disclosed, brushed to remove all stained plaque, and thoroughly dried. A white spot lesion is now obvious at the entrance to the fissures. Figure by courtesy of *Dental Update*. (Figure 5.14, p. 87.)

Plate 14 The grey discolouration of this occlusal surface is caused by demineralized, discoloured dentine shining through relatively intact enamel. This lesion was visible in dentine on bitewing radiograph. Figure by courtesy of *Dental Update*. (Figure 5.15, p. 87.)

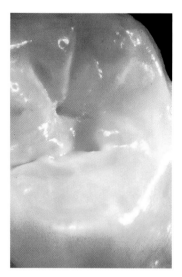

Plate 15 There is a microcavity in the white spot lesion in this occlusal surface. It looks like a slightly widened fissure or a small hole left by a woodworm. Histologically this lesion is well into dentine and it may be visible in dentine on a bitewing radiograph. Figure by courtesy of *Dental Update*. (Figure 5.16, p. 88.)

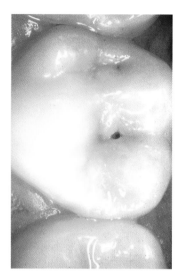

Plate 16 A cavitated lesion exposing dentine. This lesion is visible in dentine on a bitewing radiograph. Figure by courtesy of *Dental Update*. (Figure 5.18, p. 88.)

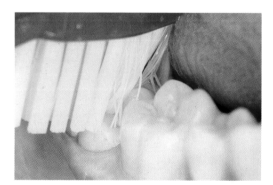

Plate 17 Cleaning a partly erupted tooth with a toothbrush. The parent should stand behind the child and bring the brush in at right angles to the arch. Figure by courtesy of *Dental Update*. (Figure 5.22, p. 90.)

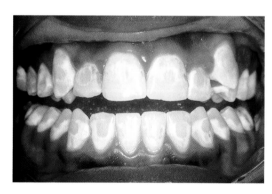

Plate 18 An orthodontic nightmare! Multiple white spot lesions have formed on tooth surfaces around the orthodontic brackets. Both plaque control and diet were unfavourable. (Figure 5.24, p. 91.)

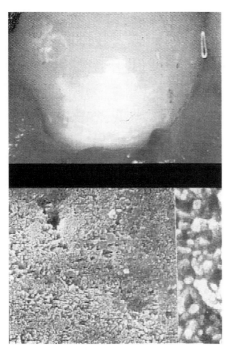

Figure 5.3 A clinical and SEM picture of a white spot lesion formed under an orthodontic band after 4 weeks of plaque stagnation. Clinically, the lesion is opaque with a matt surface. Ultrastructurally, there is dissolution of the perikymata overlappings and dissolution of the surface enamel. Originally published in *Textbook of Clinical Cariology* (Munksgaard) 1994 and reproduced with permission. (See Plate 3.)

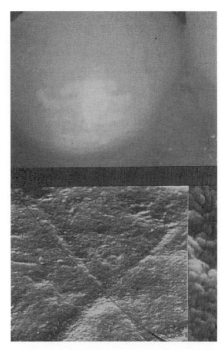

Figure 5.4 A clinical and SEM picture of a white spot lesion formed under an orthodontic band after removal of the biofilm. The lesion surface is now shiny and hard as a result of abrasion or polishing of the partly dissolved surface of the active lesion. Originally published in *Textbook of Clinical Cariology* (Munksgaard) 1994 and reproduced with permission. (See Plate 4.)

prevented mechanical disturbance of the plaque. After varying periods of time, the bands were removed and replicas of the surfaces taken for scanning electron microscopy. The teeth were then left uncovered and mechanical plaque control was resumed, further replicas showing how the surface reacted after biofilm removal.

After one week of undisturbed biofilm formation, no changes in the enamel were seen clinically, even after careful air-drying. However, at the ultrastructural level, there were signs of direct dissolution of the outer enamel surface. This was seen as an enlargement of the intercrystalline spaces due to partial dissolution of the individual crystal peripheries.

After two weeks with completely undisturbed plaque, the enamel changes were visible clinically after air-drying. The 'white spot' lesion was now visible. After three and four weeks, these changes could be seen without air-drying, the lesion being opaque with a matt surface. Ultrastructurally, there was complete dissolution of the thin perikymata overlappings, marked dissolution corresponding to developmental irregularities such as Tomes' processes, pits and focal holes, and continued enlargement of the intercrystalline spaces (Fig. 5.3).

Thus, the surface participates in the enamel reaction from the very beginning of lesion formation by direct dissolution of the outermost microsurface and enlargement of intercrystalline diffusion pathways. This direct surface erosion is most likely partly responsible for the matt surface of the active lesion.

When the orthodontic bands were removed, allowing disturbance of the biofilm, the white appearance diminished and the surface became hard and shiny again. Ultrastructural studies showed wear of the external microsurface (Fig. 5.4). Thus the return to a shiny, hard surface was a result of abrasion or polishing of the partly dissolved surface of the active lesion. This important series of experiments shows the precise relationship of the lesion to the biofilm, and shows that regular disturbance of the biofilm will arrest the lesion by removing the acid-producing organisms.

The white spot lesion

The same series of experiments also extracted teeth at varying times to allow detailed examination of sections in polarized light. After only one week of undisturbed biofilm formation, this examination showed a slight increase in enamel porosity and the tissue beneath the porous outer microsurface was more porous than the microsurface itself. This so-called subsurface demineralization became more obvious at weeks two, three, and four and the classical histological zones of the white spot lesion in polarized light could be identified. These zones are the surface zone and body of the lesion, best seen after imbibition of sections in water (Fig. 5.5) and the dark zone and primary translucent zone seen after imbibition of sections is quinoline (Fig. 5.6).

Several models have been proposed to explain the relative protection of the outer 10–30 microns of enamel against further

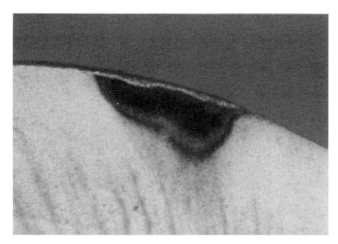

Figure 5.5 Longitudinal ground section through a small white spot lesion in enamel examined in water with polarized light. The body of the lesion shows as an area of positive birefringence beneath a relatively intact, negatively birefringent surface zone. (See Plate 5.)

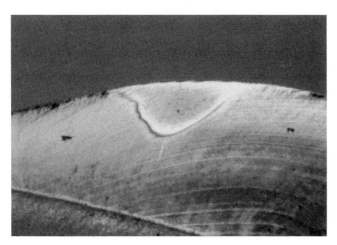

Figure 5.6 Longitudinal ground section through a small white spot lesion in enamel examined in quinoline with polarized light. The translucent zone is at the advancing front of the lesion and the dark zone is superficial to this. The striae of Retzius are well marked within the body of the lesion. (See Plate 6.)

dissolution. A physico-chemical explanation seems important. Dissolution is caused by an undersaturation with respect to enamel apatite and a formation of fluorapatite in the enamel surface caused by a supersaturation with respect to fluorapatite. A protective role of salivary proline-rich proteins and other salivary inhibitors, such as statherin, has also been emphasized. These inhibit demineralization and prevent crystal growth. They are macromolecules and cannot penetrate the deeper parts of the enamel, thus their stabilizing role is limited to the surface enamel. It is also possible that the outer enamel is special in terms of its ultrastructure and chemical composition.

Removal of the orthodontic bands and resumption of tooth cleaning resulted in reduced porosity of the deeper parts of

lesions. A gradual return of enamel fluids to supersaturation with respect to apatites causes a shift in equilibrium of minerals at the sites of demineralization. Arrested lesions showed a widening of the dark zones indicating this reprecipitation. However, although the surface of the lesion may become hard and shiny and the white spot becomes less obvious, some interior opacity remains because some sub-surface porosity is still present. It should be noted that these arrested lesions are actually more resistant to a subsequent acid attack than sound enamel.

The shape of the white spot lesion is determined by the distribution of the biofilm and the direction of the enamel prisms. Thus, on an approximal surface, the lesion formed beneath the biofilm is a kidney-shaped area between the contact facet and the gingival margin. Within the enamel, spread of dissolution takes place along the enamel prisms. In section, the smooth surface lesion is conical (Figs 5.5 and 5.6). This conical shape is the result of systematic variations in dissolution along the enamel prisms. The oldest or most active part of the lesion is located along the central traverse. The conically shaped lesion represents a range of increasing stages of lesion progression beginning with dissolution at the ultrastructural level at the edge of the lesion. This emphasizes that the lesion is driven by, and reflects, the specific environmental conditions in the overlying biofilm. Figures 5.7 and 5.8 show histological sections through an arrested carious lesion, similar to that shown clinically in Figure 5.19. Arrested lesions are characterized by multiple dark zones, when examined in quinoline indicating re-deposition of mineral.

Caries on an occlusal surface is also a localized phenomenon in the deepest part of the groove–fossa system, where the bacterial accumulations receive the best protection against functional wear. The lesion forms in three dimensions, again guided by prism direction. The lesion thus assumes the shape of a cone with its base towards the enamel dentine junction (Fig. 5.9). It appears that the active biofilm is above the entrance to the narrow fissures and grooves. Ultrastructural studies show that the deepest part of the fissures usually harbour non-vital bacteria or calculus. This has important clinical implications explaining why occlusal lesion formation can be prevented on erupting molar teeth by removal of the biofilm with a fluoride toothpaste.

Using porosity in diagnosis

The porosity of the subsurface lesion can be turned to some advantage by the clinician. First it explains why the white spot lesion looks white and why a dentist, looking at a clean tooth surface can, using vision and a three-in-one syringe, determine the depth of penetration of the lesion. The lesion that is only visible on a dry tooth surface is probably in the outer enamel; whereas, a lesion visible on a wet tooth surface has penetrated most of the way through the enamel and maybe into the dentine.

This relates to the relative refractive indices of enamel, water, and air. Enamel has a refractive index of 1.62. In the sub-surface lesion, the pores are filled with a watery medium of refractive index 1.33. The difference in refractive index between water and the enamel

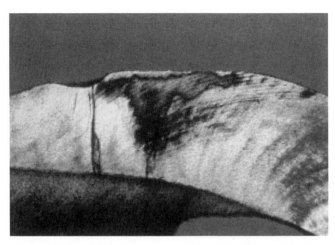

Figure 5.7 Longitudinal ground section of a natural carious enamel lesion in a tooth extracted from a patient aged 70 years, examined in water in polarized light. This lesion was arrested and similar in appearance to the lesion in Figure 5.19. Well mineralized laminations are obvious within the body of the lesion, particularly on its occlusal aspect. (See Plate 7.)

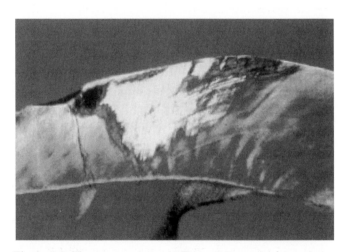

Figure 5.8 The same section as in Figure 5.7 examined in quinoline with polarized light. Wide, well developed, dark zones are obvious at the advancing front of the lesion, within the lesion, and at the surface of the lesion. (See Plate 8.)

affects the light scattering and makes the lesion look opaque. If the surface is now dried, air, refractive index 1.0, replaces the water. The difference in refractive index between the air and the enamel is now greater than that between the water and the enamel. This means, the lesion becomes more obvious or an earlier lesion can be detected.

Porosity is the basis of many techniques that detect carious lesions; for instance, radiography, and two quantitative techniques, quantitative light-induced fluorescence and electrical resistance. These techniques allow quantitation of the degree of porosity. When used once they will detect demineralization, but

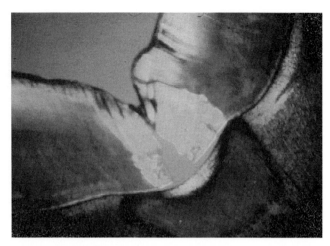

Figure 5.9 Longitudinal ground section of a natural occlusal carious lesion examined in quinoline in polarized light. The lesion forms in three directions, guided by prism direction, assuming the shape of a cone with its base towards the enamel–dentine junction. The undermining shape of this lesion is purely a function of anatomy. (See Plate 9.)

when used on a longitudinal basis, they potentially allow the dentist to follow lesion progression or arrest.

Before concluding the section on sub-surface porosity, a word of caution is, however, appropriate. The dentist must be careful when using a sharp probe. It is very useful to gently draw the point across the lesion to detect a matt surface indicating an active lesion. It is, however, most unwise to jab the sharp probe into the lesion to see whether it is 'sticky'. The probe is likely to cause a cavity and this will encourage biofilm stagnation and lesion progression.

Shape of the carious lesion

- Determined by distribution of the biofilm
- Guided by the direction of enamel prisms
- On approximal surfaces; kidney shaped between contact facet and gingival margin
- On occlusal surfaces: cone-shaped

Diagnosis of enamel caries

It is important to recognize active enamel caries at the stage of the white spot lesion so that preventive treatment has a chance to arrest lesion progression.

Prerequisites for early diagnosis

Caries diagnosis requires

- good lighting
- clean teeth
- a three-in-one syringe so that teeth can be viewed both wet and dry

- sharp eyes with vision aided by magnification. This is particularly necessary for older dentists who are unlikely to be able to see as well as they did in their youth.

- Reproducible bitewing radiographs

The white spot lesion, although caused by plaque, is also obscured by it. A logical way to proceed is for the dentist to examine the teeth both before and after removal of plaque. Many experienced practitioners choose to carry out their examination immediately after the patient has seen the hygienist.

The three-in-one syringe is invaluable in the diagnosis of the depth of penetration of the white spot lesion. A white spot lesion that is visible only when the enamel has been thoroughly dried has penetrated about halfway through the enamel. A white or brown spot lesion that is visible on a wet tooth surface has penetrated all the way through the enamel, and the demineralization may be in the dentine. Demineralization may be in dentine before cavitation occurs, but the lesion can still be arrested if plaque control can be established.

Finally, good bitewing radiographs are essential for the diagnosis of approximal lesions where a contact point is present. A film holder and beam aiming device should always be used to ensure the correct angulation of the beam and as an aid in reproducing the same geometry in any subsequent radiograph (Fig. 5.10). Where a lesion is to be monitored for progression or arrest, this reproducibility of view is essential; otherwise, an apparent change in the lesion may simply be an artifact of geometry.

Diagnosis of active and arrested lesions on individual tooth surfaces

Free smooth surfaces

Vision is the salient diagnostic tool. Uncavitated, active lesions are close to the gingival margin and have a matt surface (Fig. 5.11).

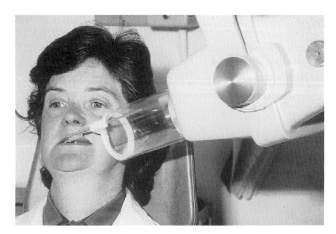

Figure 5.10 A bitewing radiograph is being taken. The film is in a film holder and a rod comes out of the mouth at right angles to the film. The cone of the X-ray machine is lined up with a circular attachment to this rod. This ensures a reproducible set up with the X-ray beam passing at right angles to the film.

Inactive lesions may be further from the gingival margin, white or brown in colour with a shiny surface (Fig. 5.12).

Occlusal surfaces

Visual examination and examination of the bitewing radiograph are both important. The active, uncavitated lesion is white, often with a matt surface (Figs 5.13 and 5.14). The corresponding inactive lesion may be brown. These enamel lesions are not visible on a bitewing radiograph. The enamel lesion that is only visible on a dry tooth surface is the outer enamel lesion. The lesion visible on a wet surface is all the way through enamel and may be into dentine. Cavitated lesions may present as microcavities with or without a greyish discoloration of the enamel (Figs 5.15 and 5.16). The microcavity is easily missed on visual examination, unless the surface is perfectly clean and dry. Careful examination of bitewing radiographs is important and serves as a useful safety net to avoid

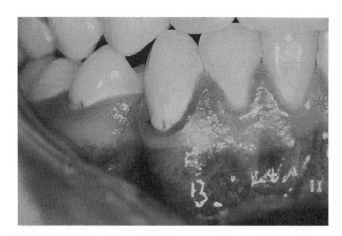

Figure 5.11 Active smooth surface cervical lesions. These are matt and visible on a wet tooth surface. Cavities can be seen on some lesions. These lesions can be arrested by plaque control alone. (See Plate 10.)

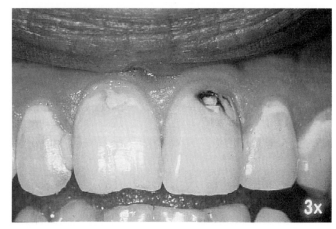

Figure 5.12 Arrested smooth surface cervical lesions. Notice the healthy gingival margins indicating good plaque removal. The lesions are shiny and are slightly brown from exogenous stains picked up from the mouth. (See Plate 11.)

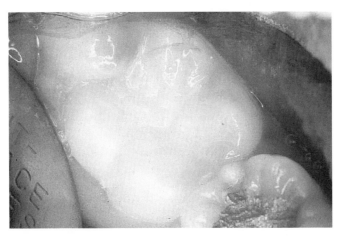

Figure 5.13 This erupting molar appears caries free but it is not. Figure by courtesy of *Dental Update*. (See Plate 12.)

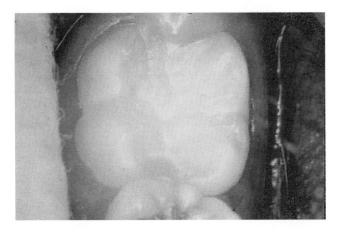

Figure 5.14 The surface has now been disclosed, brushed to remove all stained plaque and thoroughly dried. A white spot lesion is now obvious at the entrance to the fissures. Figure by courtesy of *Dental Update*. (See Plate 13.)

Radiographic interpretation: important points

- An approximal enamel surface that appears to be caries-free may have a lesion whose porosity is not sufficient to show on a radiograph

- A lesion in the enamel on a bitewing radiograph is histologically in the dentine. The lesion is unlikely to be cavitated

- It is not possible to judge the activity of the lesion from a single bitewing radiograph. It is also not possible to know whether a lesion is cavitated from its appearance on radiograph

- A series of radiographs, perhaps taken at yearly intervals, is required to judge lesion progression or arrest. It is essential to use film holders and beam aiming devices so that the views are reproducible. Slight alterations in the beam angle will affect the radiographic view

- Fibreoptic transillumination is not helpful in detecting an approximal enamel lesion, but can be used to detect lesions in dentine

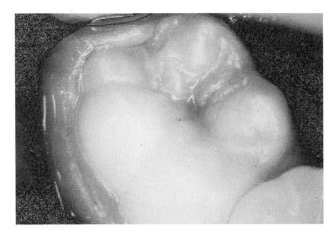

Figure 5.15 The grey discolouration of this occlusal surface is caused by demineralized, discoloured dentine shining through relatively intact enamel. This lesion was visible in dentine on bitewing radiograph. Figure by courtesy of *Dental Update*. (See Plate 14.)

missing microcavities. A lesion that has been missed on visual examination but found on radiograph has been called hidden caries (Fig. 5.17). More advanced lesions may present as cavities exposing dentine (Fig. 5.18). Cavitated lesions are usually visible in dentine on a bitewing radiograph. Cavitated occlusal lesions, whether microcavities or cavities down to dentine, are usually active because the patient cannot clean plaque out of the cavity.

Approximal surfaces

Sometimes an enamel lesion is visible because the adjacent tooth has been extracted. This is often an arrested lesion (Fig. 5.19). Its surface is shiny and the lesion is brown because it has picked up stain from the mouth. However, usually an adjacent tooth precludes a direct visual examination and now the bitewing radiograph is the salient diagnostic tool (Fig. 5.20).

A number of points should be made about interpreting the radiograph.

A defining moment clinically

It is important to discuss whether progression into dentine or cavitation are defining moments clinically as far as lesion management is concerned. It has already been stated that the driving force for lesion progression is the metabolic activity in the biofilm. In the uncavitated lesion, this biofilm is on the tooth surface, while in the cavity the biomass plugs the hole. As far as management is concerned what matters is whether the patient can access and remove the biofilm. Dentine involvement per se is irrelevant. On a smooth cervical surface, a toothbrush can remove plaque from a cavity (Fig. 5.11). On an approximal surface even the most fastidious of flossers cannot arrest a lesion by plaque control alone because the floss will not enter the cavity. This is where operative dentistry is essential to restore the integrity of the tooth surface, so that the patient can clean.

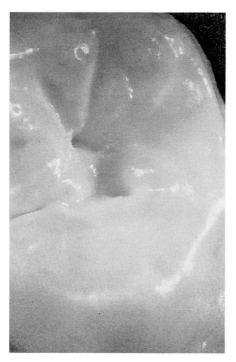

Figure 5.16 There is a microcavity in the white spot lesion in this occlusal surface. It looks like a slightly widened fissure or a small hole left by a woodworm. Histologically, this lesion is well into dentine and it may be visible in dentine on a bitewing radiograph. Figure by courtesy of *Dental Update*. (See Plate 15.)

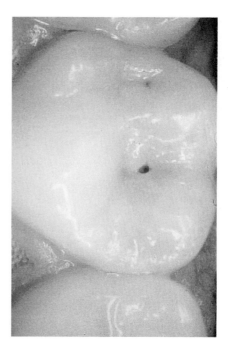

Figure 5.18 A cavitated lesion exposing dentine. This lesion is visible in dentine on a bitewing radiograph. Figure by courtesy of *Dental Update*. (See Plate 16.)

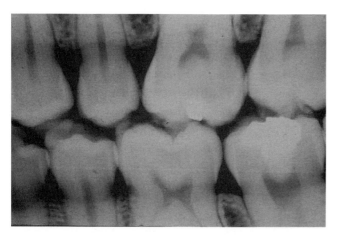

Figure 5.17 A bitewing radiograph showing occlusal caries in dentine in the lower first molar. Note the enamel lesion is not visible on the radiograph.

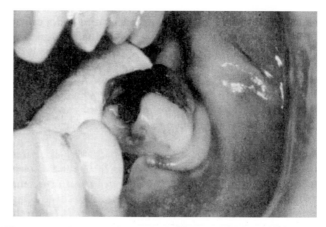

Figure 5.19 An arrested smooth-surface approximal lesion on the mesial surface of the lower second molar. This lesion probably stopped progressing after extraction of the first molar.

Caries management

The management of active caries always requires preventive treatment, and in cases in which cavities preclude plaque control, operative treatment is also needed. Figure 5.21 provides a caries control checklist that practitioners and other members of the dental team may find useful. The term preventive treatment is used because this implies active intervention by the dental team that is skilful, time-consuming, and worthy of payment. It is not an 'observe' or a 'wait and watch' approach.

All patients should be put into a caries risk category, either high or low with all others designated as medium risk.

Patient involvement

The carious process can be arrested by meticulous plaque control, dietary modification, judicious use of fluoride, and salivary

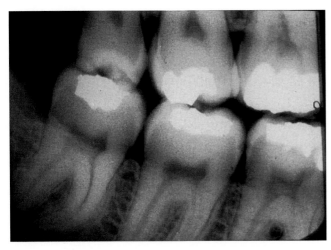

Figure 5.20 A bitewing radiograph showing carious lesions in enamel on the distal surface of the first molar and the mesial surface of the second molar. Histologically, these lesions will be in dentine but they are probably not cavitated.

stimulation. Each of these approaches requires the active cooperation of the patient. The patient is in control of his or her own dental destiny because it is the patient, not the dentist, who influences the carious process. For this reason, it is absolutely essential to involve the patient from the outset, and the patient must acknowledge the problem and have some sense of control over it.

One of the best ways to ensure active patient cooperation is to turn the patient into his or her own personal dentist, so that the patient can perform a check-up every day. The dentist should give the patient a mirror and show the patient his or her own carious lesions. The dentist should show the patient the white spot and a red and swollen gingival margin that bleeds on probing. Disclosing solution should be applied to demonstrate the plaque in that specific position. The dentist should explain how plaque causes caries and show the patient his or her own radiographs. The dentist should explain that the patient is looking at decay and that the cause must be found so that the process can be arrested. It should be explained that only the patient can carry out this part of the treatment. The ability of the patient to understand his or her essential role in disease control greatly influences the prognosis.

Above all, the dentist must begin to determine the patient's wishes with respect to the caries problem. What effort is the patient prepared to make in caries control? Fillings have an important role to play in restoring cavities and thus facilitating the patient's plaque control, but they are only part of the treatment. Direct questioning on attitudes may not be helpful, however, because a patient may tend to answer a question in a way that, 'pleases' the dentist. It can take a long time before the patient's attitudes are revealed. These attitudes are important in assessing prognosis and in logical and realistic treatment planning.

Communication
Involve the patient; they are in control.

High caries risk patients will have multiple active lesions.

Show the patient the lesions, clinically and on radiographs.

Why is this patient high risk?
Is it: Plaque control?
Fluoride use or lack of it?
Diet?
Are these factors alterable?
Low salivary flow?

Preventive Treatment
Plaque control:
    Mechanical: Disclose
                     Show the patient
                     See them in action
                     Recall and reassess

    Professional:

Fluoride: Check toothpaste
                 Mouthwash
                 Varnish

Diet: Use diet sheet
                 Negotiate goals
                 Record these
                 Reassess

Salivary flow: Is it low?
                 What lubricants does patient use?
                 Use of chewing gum
                 Use of artificial saliva

Fissure sealing
                 To aid plaque control

Figure 5.21 A caries control checklist.

Why the patient is a caries risk

The dentist needs to determine the relative importance of the various caries-promoting factors for the individual patient. Unless the practitioner and the patient can work together to find the cause of the problem, relevant solutions cannot be found. The involved patient begins to understand the relevance of the partnership approach and often enters into the detective work of determining the cause with admirable gusto.

The following should always be checked for their relative importance in the high-risk patient:

- *Plaque control*: A disclosing agent should be used so that the patient can see the relationship between plaque and carious lesions.

- *Diet*: All patients designated as high risk should keep a diet sheet.
- *Fluoride history*: The fluoride content of the water, toothpaste, and any mouthwash the patient uses should be checked.
- *Salivary flow*: Both stimulated and unstimulated salivary flow should be measured.

Some risk factors such as plaque control, diet, and fluoride use are amenable to alteration by the patient. Other risk factors, such as a dry mouth, are less amenable to alteration. For instance, a patient with Sjögren's syndrome may always be at high risk and may always have to make strenuous preventive efforts.

A dental practitioner is also unlikely to be able to modify or alleviate social deprivation in a particular patient, but may be able to observe social factors change over time, sometimes for better and sometimes for worse.

Mechanical plaque control

Regular disturbance of the biofilm with a toothpaste containing fluoride will prevent the formation of visible lesions and will arrest lesions that have already formed.

The dentist should check whether the patient's toothpaste contains fluoride. It is suggested that small children should use the adult, family paste but a small pea-sized portion of toothpaste should be used. Small children cannot spit and will, therefore, swallow the paste and this precaution will avoid fluorosis.

The dentist should show the patient, and the parent in the case of a child, the white spot lesions and then disclose the teeth. This will demonstrate the relationship of the biofilm to the lesion. Now watch the patient in action with a toothbrush to remove the plaque, helping improve technique where necessary.

The patient should be encouraged to feel the shiny, plaque-free surface with their tongue with the aim of achieving this feel at home. The dentist should note whether the patient *can* remove plaque. If the patient *can* but *does not*, the problem is motivation not manual dexterity.

With children, particular attention should be paid to the occlusal surface of erupting teeth. The erupting tooth is below the line of the arch and will be missed by the brush unless it is brought in at right angles to the arch (Fig. 5.22). It should be noted that an occlusal surface is most susceptible to plaque stagnation during eruption and teeth can take months or years to erupt. There is huge individual variation in eruption times. Molars take longer to erupt than premolars but within a specific tooth type there is great variation from person to person. The prevention programme must, therefore, be tailored to the needs of the individual. The patient and parent should be seen on regular recall until they are able to attend with the surface plaque-free after home cleaning. If this is consistently not achieved consideration should be given to fissure sealing the surface with a resin to block the groove–fossa system thus aiding plaque control.

Where a bitewing radiograph shows an approximal lesion in the outer enamel, the patient, or the parent in the case of a child, should be shown how to use dental floss.

Professional prophylaxis

In caries-active patients who do not master plaque control, and/or in patients with severely decreased salivary secretion, it may be necessary to support the patient with professional tooth cleaning. The procedure is described in Fig. 5.23.

Use of fluoride

The dentist should check that the patient is using a fluoride toothpaste. Some products formulated for sensitive teeth and some herbal toothpastes do not contain fluoride. The paste should be used twice daily and cleared from the mouth by spitting out only, rather than vigorously rinsing.

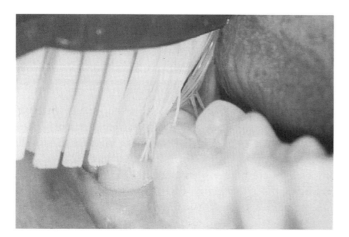

Figure 5.22 Cleaning a partly erupted tooth with a toothbrush. The parent should stand behind the child and bring the brush in at right angles to the arch. (By courtesy of *Dental Update*.) (See Plate 17.)

PROFESSIONAL TOOTH CLEANING.

1. Disclose plaque and give oral hygiene instruction.

2. Remove remaining plaque with fluoride-containing polishing paste. A pointed bristle brush should be used in the handpiece to clean plaque from the fissures and a soft, rubber cup for free smooth surface. Proximally the paste is applied with floss or an international brush depending on the local anatomical conditions.

3. Disclose again and check all plaque has been removed.

4. Apply topical fluoride (2% NaF or Duraphat varnish)

5. Control visits. The interval between appointments should be every 2–3 weeks initially but may be extended as cooperation is improved and the patient reaches satisfactory levels of plaque control.

Figure 5.23 Professional prophylaxis.

A reasonable aim for this patient would be to try to confine sugar to mealtimes.

Salivary flow

Salivary flow should be measured because a feeling of a dry mouth may be subjective rather than actual.

When the salivary glands are capable of secreting, chewing gum stimulates salivary flow. A chewing gum with an artificial sweetener (sorbitol or xylitol) should be chosen in preference to a sugar-containing gum. Of the two artificial sweeteners, xylitol seems the better as this product may suppress counts of some acidogenic microorganisms.

Sometimes patients with a dry mouth suck sweets or sip sweet drinks to alleviate the problem. This is obviously very unwise in patients who are already at high risk to caries because they are short of saliva.

Patients with very dry mouths may benefit from artificial salivas. These may be based on carboxymethyl cellulose with added calcium, phosphate, and fluoride ions. A product is also available based on porcine mucin but this would obviously be unacceptable to some religions.

Fissure sealing

An additional preventive tool to halt caries progression is fissure sealing. If the patient or parent cannot totally prevent the establishment of the biofilm in pits and fissures of the erupting or erupted teeth, then we need to look at alternative means of protecting these vulnerable sites. Occluding the pit or fissure mechanically is one such means.

Fissure sealants are materials that are chemico-mechanically retained within the pit or fissure, and thus prevent the ingress of biofilm. Provided the sealant material is retained in its entirety and that there is no marginal leakage, such vulnerable sites remain free of caries.

Size of the problem

We know from epidemiological studies that the molar pits and fissures are those most likely to become carious. Occlusal caries has been shown to account for 83% of the total caries burden in children between 5 and 17 years of age. There is good evidence from national epidemiological data on both children and adults to indicate that the predilection for caries to develop on these specific sites continues through from the time of eruption into early adult life.

Since the advent of acid etching of enamel as described by Buonocore in the 1950s, we have had increasingly reliable means of retaining resin material in pits and fissures. Despite this, the provision of sealants, especially in young adults, remains low. Clinicians have concerns about the possibility of sealing in caries, since the detection of white spots lesions is difficult. One study in the Netherlands has demonstrated lesions into dentine detected radiographically, below sealed surfaces. For the most part, on the evidence available, sealing in early or incipient lesions does not appear to lead to caries progression. This premise has

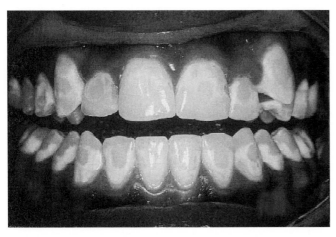

Figure 5.24 An orthodontic nightmare! Multiple white spot lesions have formed on tooth surfaces around the orthodontic brackets. Both plaque control and diet were unfavourable. (See Plate 18.)

A fluoride mouthrinse (0.05% sodium fluoride) used every day is a useful fluoride supplement in a high-risk patient, although the cost of the product may preclude its use by some patients. These rinses should not be used in children under 6 who cannot rinse and spit as there is a risk of fluorosis if the solution is swallowed. Fluoride mouthrinses are a sensible precaution in children wearing fixed orthodontic appliances. These appliances make plaque control more difficult and very unsightly white spot lesions can form around the brackets if oral hygiene is poor and diet unfavourable (Fig. 5.24). Both children and patients with dry mouths favour minimally astringent products.

Surgery application of fluoride varnish is a useful preventive measure, and particularly valuable in those unlikely to comply with a daily mouthwash regime. The method of application is given in Figure 5.23.

Dietary advice

Dietary advice should be based on a diet sheet. Figure 5.25 shows one day in a diet sheet kept by a young man with many approximal lesions in outer enamel on bitewing radiograph. The occlusal fissures of molar teeth were already filled.

The sugar attacks have been highlighted, and the number of individual attacks has been written at the top. This gives the dentist the opportunity to explain the Stephen curve and the importance of decreasing the frequency of sugar intake. The dentist should try to get the patient to suggest changes. This approach helps the patient to set realistic goals and enables the dentist to see whether the relationship between diet and caries has been understood by the patient. The dentist should check that the main meals are adequate, and a list of foods that are safe for teeth may be helpful here. The negotiated dietary change should be recorded on paper, so that the patient can take this away and ponder at leisure. The dentist should record the goals agreed in the notes so that specific enquiry can be made at the next visit.

	THURSDAY (10)		FRIDAY		SATURDAY	
	Time	Item	Time	Item	Time	Item
Before Breakfast	7:15	Milk shake 1 pint of ice cream Semi-skimmed milk.				
Breakfast	8.30	Black Coffee 2 packets of sugar.				
MORNING	10.00 12.00	Coffee/sugar 2 cheese rolls Coffee/sugar Twix candy bar				
Mid-day Meal	12.30	2 cheese rolls Piece of cake Mint Apple				
AFTERNOON	15.30 17.00	Coffee/sugar Tea/sugar 5 biscuits				
Evening Meal	19.30	Pizza Ribena Ice cream				
EVENING	21.30 22.30	Glass of Coke Glass of Coke				

Figure 5.25 One day out of a diet sheet. The sugar attacks have been underlined and the number of individual attacks (10) has been written at the top.

been tested clinically. In some trials, teeth scheduled for orthodontic extractions where there was clinical evidence of active caries, have been sealed prior to extraction. Histological examination of these teeth after extraction indicated cessation of the caries process. Other trials have taken enamel biopsies and tested for microbial activity before sealant placement and after extraction of these teeth. Results show a marked decrease in microbial activity.

Points to remember

- Occlusal caries accounts for 83% of the caries burden of 5–17-year-olds in the UK

- 1993 Child Dental Health Survey: Adolescents with sealants: 34% in England, 31% in Wales, 52% in Scotland, 47% in Northern Ireland

- After 10 years of age, mean number of carious teeth significantly lower for adolescents with sealants

- 1998 Adult Dental Health Survey: 5% of all adults had sealants, 23% of 16–24-year-olds

Indications for sealants

As in earlier discussions in this chapter, sealant placement needs to be considered in the context of risk factors, both for the individual patient and for individual teeth. It is vital that sealants are placed where there are sound clinical indications for doing so,

supported by appropriate radiographs, in this case bitewings, and with consideration for the medical, dental, and social history of the patient. The British Society of Paediatric Dentistry lays down criteria for sealant placement, and their guidelines are currently in use in the UK.

As far as patient selection is concerned, the essential elements of those guidelines are that sealants are advised where a child or a young person is compromised in some way, and in whom the development of caries and/or its treatment is a risk. This is the main category of patients in whom sealants for the primary dentition may be advisable. The other categories of patients for whom sealants are advised are those who have experience of caries in primary teeth.

If the risk factors outlined above are identified in a patient, then it is prudent to seal all susceptible sites on permanent teeth, as soon after eruption as is practicable. Where caries has affected one or more permanent molar teeth, the remaining sound pits and fissure should be sealed.

Procedure to adopt for the application of sealants

- Decide patient's risk category: medical, dietary, oral hygiene

- Decide patient's dental risk category (low = less than 2 other lesions in the mouth)

- Determine if patient has pits and fissures that anatomically predispose to development of stagnation areas

Efficiency and effectiveness of fissure sealants

Whether a method is efficient or effective, that is, does it do the job for least cost and does it achieve the stated objective, is a matter of real concern to clinicians.

Similarly, clinicians need to be confident that sealants will be retained and that caries of the partial or non-sealed surface, which may go undetected, will not result.

The first longitudinal study to report on the use of fissure sealants employed a self-curing resin that was applied only once and not topped-up at any time subsequently. After 15 years, 28% of the sealants were totally retained and 35% were partially retained. Significantly, more of the sealed teeth remained caries free: 68% as compared with 17% in the non-sealant group. A similar trial in Sweden took the opportunity to repair the sealants on first molars when the second molars were sealed. Data from this trial indicated that after 20 years, 87% of the surfaces were either fully or partially sealed and only 13% had active caries or had been restored.

Reasons given by clinicians against the use of sealants

- Not effective—sealant material lost
- Danger of sealing in dental caries
- Not efficient—seal more teeth than would ever become carious
- Acid etchant leaves the remainder of the surface vulnerable

This retrospective analysis of data from the public dental health programme in Sweden would suggest that the systematic placement of sealants to the occlusal surfaces of permanent molar teeth, soon after eruption, is a cost-effective public health measure.

While effectiveness is not, therefore, in dispute, cost-efficiency of sealants is a concern of clinicians and is another reason why this preventive measure is not in more widespread use. Certainly, the indiscriminate application of sealants to every pit and fissure, of every tooth in all patients is not a cost-efficient approach. As with other measures, sealants need to be targeted at those teeth and individuals that are at high risk of, and from, the development of dental caries.

Another feature in the argument surrounding cost is who applies the sealant. In many countries where there are auxiliary programmes, fissure sealants become more cost-efficient, particularly, when carefully targeted.

Implicit in both arguments on efficiency and effectiveness, is the issue of maintenance. Regular reviews and top-ups of lost or partially retained sealants are important. In Sweden, longitudinal studies over 20 years have shown that maintained sealants produce a long-lasting caries preventive effect. Sadly, a Scottish prospective study to investigate a system for assessing the quality of sealants, showed over half of them to be inadequate in terms of coverage or caries prevention. This serves to emphasize the importance of maintenance.

Comprehensive preventive care

Fissure sealing should not be viewed in isolation from other preventive measures such as dietary counselling, oral hygiene instruction, and topical fluoride agents. Studies show that applying fissure sealants in combination with fluorides and, in some cases, chlorhexidine, is superior in terms of protection against caries than using these modalities alone.

Materials

The most successful materials as fissure sealants, in terms of retention and thus caries prevention, are the bis-GMA resins. These have been in use since the 1970s and have not been superseded, although newer materials enjoy a vogue until longevity studies indicate that they do not compare well with the conventional resins. There has been concern in recent years over the potential oestrogenicity of resin-based sealant materials. Bis-GMA is synthesized from Bisphenol A (BPA) and, theoretically, residual BPA could mimic the role of natural steroid hormones. This risk is negligible and should not detract from the very positive health gain for a targeted sealant programme.

Materials used as fissure sealants: Early materials (1904–1950)

- Silver nitrate
- Zinc phosphate/amalgam ('Prophylactic odontotomy')
- Black copper cement

Newer materials (1966–present day)

- Cyanoacrylate resins
- Urethane resins
- bis-GMA resins
- Glass ionomer cements
- Resin-modified glass ionomer cements

In Australia, glass ionomer cements (GICs) are used as sealant material in the School Dental Service. These materials are as effective as resin-based materials in preventing caries. However, in Sweden, the evidence on cost-effectiveness is less clear: placement of the material is more efficient if the clinician is assisted; but, it takes longer to place than resin-based materials and this adds to the cost of the procedure.

Glass ionomer cements have the advantage that they release fluorides; resin-modified GICs theoretically, from in-vitro, laboratory-based studies release more fluoride into the adjacent enamel and thus have the potential to prevent caries in these sites compared with fluoride-containing resin-based material. The latter also suffer the disadvantage that fluoride-release may compromise the integrity of the material and its retention must, therefore, be in some doubt.

One distinct advantage of GICs is that the material can be placed on the occlusal surface of partially erupted teeth that are notoriously difficult to isolate, and thus seal well, using conventional resin materials. Even if only partially-retained, while in-situ they act as a fluoride reservoir and there is evidence to show that material may be retained well into the depth of the fissure explaining the caries protection often afforded despite apparent loss.

The conventional resin-based materials may be either filled or unfilled, and light- or self-polymerizing. Extensive trials have been conducted on these alternates, and there is no good evidence to suggest that one is more superior in terms of retention and caries prevention than another. A filled resin will have more bulk and thus may require some finishing if excess is applied, although this is true of unfilled resins. The filled resin will have more wear resistance. However, more viscous materials may not penetrate into the space created by acid etching to ensure that there is a good marginal seal.

The choice of material and thus the mode of polymerization is more a matter for personal choice, since there is no significant difference in retention rates between the different modalities. Visible light curing of resins or modified GICs for that matter, gives the clinician more control over the setting of the material. While clinicians working in most of the developed countries will have ready access to curing lights, the same is not true in developing countries where self-polymerizing materials may be preferable.

Variations in the type of materials that may be used as sealants

- Filled or unfilled resins
- Chemical or light-cured resins
- Tinted clear or opaque resins
- Resins, GICs or resin-modified GICs
- Fluoride-releasing or fluoride-free

Application considerations

A vexed question in relation to the preparation for sealant placement is the need for professional prophylaxis prior to enamel conditioning. The consensus is that this is not necessary unless there is gross debris on the surface, since acid etching will clear the surface to be sealed. When prophylaxis is used, some materials appear to increase retention rates, at least *in-vitro*. For example, sodium bicarbonate or fluoride-containing toothpaste, as compared with pumice. This confirms the currently held view that there is no contraindication to use of topical fluorides prior to sealant placement.

As well as alternative materials, many different approaches to the application of sealants have been advocated. For example, the use of lasers and air abrasion in comparison with conventional acid etching of the enamel prior to sealant application, or even laser curing of the resin. While the *in-vitro* studies on these alternatives are sometimes promising, there is no good scientific evidence to date to support the incorporation of these into clinical guidelines and they must, as yet, remain novel approaches that require further evaluation.

Other issues such as methods of isolation (cotton-wool roll and saliva ejector versus rubber dam isolation), liquid or gel etchants and tinted, clear, or opaque sealant resins have not given statistically different results in terms of superior sealant retention where one approach has been adopted in preference to another.

Issues to consider in the application of sealants

- Is prophylaxis required?
- Which isolation method to use?
- Whether to use gel or liquid etchant?
- What material to use?
- Which curing system to consider?

Management of caries into enamel and dentine

In the section on diagnosis of active and arrested lesions, we describe the clinical and radiographic diagnosis of occlusal caries. The early lesion can be arrested by mechanical plaque control (see Section: Mechanical plaque control), but if good plaque control is consistently not achieved, a fissure sealant should be placed. However, where decalcification is noted and the patient is in a high-risk category as described above, it is deemed sensible to investigate the fissure with the smallest round bur. Provided the lesion is contained within enamel, the defect can be made good with an acid-etch retained composite, supplemented by a compatible sealant material. It must be borne in mind, however, that a significant proportion of these sites will be minimally affected, indeed will have no radiolucency on bitewing radiographs and should perhaps be considered for sealant application alone.

Once a cavity is present on an occlusal surface, arrest by plaque control alone is not normally possible. At this stage the lesion is

Clinical presentation and procedures to adopt

• Caries-free surface • No other carious lesions • No medical risk/disability • Good dietary and plaque control • No lesions seen on bitewing radiographs	• No sealants but monitor for risk change
• Demineralized pit/fissure • Less than two other lesions in the mouth • Questionable diet/plaque control • No dentine involvements on Bitewing radiiographs	• Fissure sealant and monitor
• Demineralized pit/fissure • More than two other lesions in the mouth • Questionable diet/plaque control • No dentine involvement on BW radiographs	• Either fissure seal or • Enamel biopsy and replace with composite to defect and sealant to remainder of occlusal fissure pit/fissure system
• Cavitated pit/fissure • Dentine involvement on bitewing radiographs	• Sealant restoration

usually visible in dentine on a radiograph and now operative intervention is required. The preferred method of restoration is a 'sealant restoration'.

In this technique, the cavity is enlarged with a small bur to access the soft, infected dentine, which is now removed with slow round burs and excavators. The cavity is restored with adhesive filling materials (composite bonded to enamel and dentine or GIC to replace the dentine, topped off with composite resin to replace the enamel). A fissure sealant is now used to protect the remaining fissure system.

In the short term, the longevity of such restorations, as judged by complete sealant retention and no caries, would appear to be good. This is not always the case in the long term. However, a significant proportion of material is usually partially or fully retained, caries prevalence is low, and these restorations efficiently conserve tooth tissue. It is, of course, beholden on the clinician to review and maintain such restorations. Little or no disease implies more, not less, vigilance.

Conclusions

This chapter details the contemporary views on the early carious lesions in enamel, from the time of eruption to the establishment of a biofilm. An understanding of the process, at the histopathological level, is vital to understanding the potential for interruption of the continuum and thus prevention of progression of dental disease. The dynamic nature of the process, of de- and remineralisation, is explored as is the rationale for the current apporach to diagnosis.

There are a multitude of factors to take into account when considering an individual's risk for the development of dental caries and part of the chapter has looked at the most significant, for example, medical and social background, diet and fluoride exposure. The remainder of the chapter is devoted to consideration of the management of caries in enamel through evidence-based strategies: for example, patient and individual oral hygiene factors, the role of fluorides and that of fissure sealants, but in a pragmatic way.

References

Carvalho, J.C., Thylstrup, A., and Ekstrand, K. (1992). Results after 3 years non-operative occlusal caries treatment of erupting permanent first molars. *Community Dentistry Oral Epidemiology*, **20**, 187–92.

Disney J.A., Graves R.C., Stamm, J.W., *et al.* (1992). The University of North Carolina Risks Assessment Study: further developments in caries risk prediction. *Community Dentistry Oral Epidermiology*, **20**, 64–75.

Ekstrand, K.R., Ricketts, D.N.J., and Kidd, E.A.M. (2001). Occlusal caries: pathology, diagnosis and logical management. *Dental Update*, **28**, 380–87.

Fejerskov, O., and Manji, F. (1990). Reactor paper: risk assessment in dental caries. In: *Risk Assessment in Dentistry*. J.D., Bader, (ed). Chapel Hill,N.C.: University of North Carolina Dental Ecology. pp. 215–217.

Fejerskov, O. (1997). Concepts of dental caries and their consequences for understanding the disease. *Community Dentistry Oral Epidemiology*, **25**, 5–12.

Holmen, L., Thylstrup, A., Øgaard, B., and Kragh, F.A. (1985). Scanning electron microscopic study of progressive stages of enamel caries in vivo. *Caries Research*, **19**, 355–67.

Holmen, L., Thylstrup, A., Øgaard, B., and Kragh, F.A. (1985). A polarized light microscropic study of progressive stages of enamel caries in vivo. *Caries Research*, **19**, 348–54.

Holmen, L., Thylstrup, A., and Årtun, J. (1987). Surface changes during the arrest of active enamel carious lesions in vivo. A scanning electron microscope study. *Acta Odontologica Scandinavia*, **45**, 383–90.

Holmen, L., Thylstrup, A., and Årtun, J. (1987). Clinical and histological features observed during arrestment of active enamel carious lesions in vivo. *Caries Research*, **21**, 546–54.

Further reading

Fejerskov, O., and Kidd, E.A.M. (eds). Dental Caries (in press). Blackwell, Oxford.

British Society of Paediatric Dentistry: fissure sealants in paediatric dentistry; a policy document. *Int. J. Paed. Dent.* 2000, **10**, 174–7.

British Society of Paediatric Dentistry. UK National Clinical Guidelines in Paediatric Dentistry: Management of the stained fissure in the first permanent molar. *Int. J. Paed. Dent.* 2000, **10**, 79–83.

6

Prevention of pulpal and periapical disease

Prevention of pulpal and periapical disease

John Whitworth

Introduction

Apical periodontitis is a term to describe inflammatory conditions of the periodontal tissues that are caused by irritants in the pulp canal system. While the majority of these lesions develop around root apices, apical periodontitis can occur laterally or in furcal regions, associated with any natural or pathological communication between the pulp space and the periodontium.

Apical periodontitis and the pulpitis from which it usually develops are serious conditions at an individual and population level and should not be trivialized in an age of improved dental health. They remain a prominent cause of pain and loss of oral function in all countries with a high prevalence of dental caries, dental trauma, and operative dentistry; and their treatment is costly of time, financial resource, and dental tissue. Untreated, they may progress to life-threatening sepsis, and even symptom-free, chronic lesions carry the risk of acute flare-up or systemic interaction.

This chapter will review the aetiology and epidemiology of apical periodontitis, before considering how dentists can prevent pulp and periapical breakdown in practice. All of these preventive measures are defined by the European Society of Endodontology (1994) as endodontic treatment; procedures designed to maintain the health of all or part of the pulp, or to preserve periapical health when a pulp has died.

Apical periodontitis

- Pulpitis and apical periodontitis are prevalent in all countries with a high experience of caries, dental trauma, and operative treatment
- They are responsible for significant personal suffering; and can progress to serious, life-threatening sepsis
- The operative treatment of pulpitis and apical periodontitis is costly of time, financial resource, and tooth tissue
- Prevention is beneficial at a personal and community level, and endodontic procedures are available to maintain the health of all, or part of the pulp or to preserve periapical health when the pulp has died

Aetiology of apical periodontitis

Apical periodontitis usually affects teeth containing necrotic pulp tissue, and traditional texts made links between non-vital pulp tissue, 'stagnant' body fluids, and periapical inflammation. Such hollow tube theories regarded necrotic pulp canals as spaces into which tissue fluids from the periapex would flow and mingle with dead tissue to form an irritant cocktail, whose subsequent percolation back through the apical foramen would trigger periapical breakdown. The first suggestion that agents other than damaged host tissues may be involved in periapical irritation in fact came much earlier than that, when Miller (1890) discovered micro-organism in necrotic pulps. Sampling, culture, and identification techniques were then rather crude, and it was many decades before scientific and microbiological methods were able to establish a clearer cause and effect relationship between microbial infection and disease in the pulp and periapex.

Some key and surprisingly recent milestones include:

- the discovery by Kakehashi et al. in 1965 that in germ-free animals, pulp tissue could tolerate wide exposure to the mouth for many months without adverse effects. Pulp tissue remained healthy and reparative calcific barriers were commonly laid down despite the impaction of hair and foodstuffs into the open wounds. By contrast, the pulps of normal animals whose mouths contained micro-organisms predictably died after exposure to the mouth, with the development of periapical inflammation and bone loss;

- the careful microbiological studies of Sundqvist (1976) on human teeth devitalized by trauma, which revealed that teeth with necrotic, infected pulp canal contents developed apical periodontitis, while teeth with necrotic pulps but no cultivable microflora remained in periapical health; and

- the primate study of Moller et al. (1981) in which pulps were mechanically devitalized, either under aseptic conditions or allowing infected saliva to enter. Only the animals in which micro-organisms had been allowed to enter developed apical periodontitis. Teeth with sterile necrotic pulps had no detectable periapical lesions.

Numerous clinical and laboratory studies have been built on these foundations, and few would now challenge the overwhelming body of evidence linking pulp break down and the development of apical periodontitis with microbial infection. It is clear that dead pulp tissue and 'stagnant' tissue fluids in the pulp canal space are not sufficiently irritant in themselves to provoke a response in the periapical tissues that would initiate or sustain apical periodontitis. They may, however, provide a warm, nutritious and defenceless niche for microbial infection to become established, and it is the introduction of this non-host antigenic material which is the key to the development of pathological changes in the periapex. A graphic example is provided by the clinical scenario in which a pulp loses vitality following a traumatic incident that catastrophically disrupts its apical blood supply. Although the tooth may darken and become unresponsive to thermal and electrical pulp testing, the patient reports no adverse symptoms; and radiographs provide no evidence of periapical inflammation. Suddenly, often years later, and after the most minor incident or dental intervention, the tooth becomes exquisitely painful to bite on and classic signs of periapical inflammation appear. The explanation is that the defenceless, sterile, necrotic pulp tissue became infected, perhaps by a single microbial cell, which gained access through an exposed dentinal tubule or incomplete enamel/dentine crack. Exponential growth rapidly converted well-tolerated, sterile canal contents into a highly irritant body of material, capable of eliciting a significant inflammatory response.

There are of course exceptions, including giant cell foreign body reactions to materials such as vegetable matter, talcum powder, or endodontic paper points, which gain access to the periapex through the open canal system, and occasional neoplastic lesions presenting as inflammatory disease. Common lesions are, however, common and signs of periapical disease usually mean an infected, necrotic pulp space.

Periapical changes are triggered principally by the by-products of microbial metabolism and toxins such as lipopolysaccharides from the cell walls of dying Gram-negative micro-organisms. Diffusion into the periradicular tissues heralds defensive inflammatory and immune responses, whose damaging consequences include bone resorption. It is important to note that micro-organisms themselves rarely migrate from the root canal system, and that the periapical lesion is not the focus of disease, rather it is the response of host tissues to contain infection and prevent its potentially serious extension (Nair 1997). Simply removing periapical tissues by surgical means or prescribing antibiotics will not cause the lesion to heal, since its cause is contained in the avascular environment of the pulp space. Lesions can only be prevented by protecting pulps against infection or by treating infected pulp systems before changes can affect the periradicular tissues. Similarly, established lesions can only be expected to heal if endodontic infection is eliminated and prevented from recurring, either by extracting the offending tooth, or by completing root canal treatment which manages infection as well, in biological terms, as an extraction would.

Source and nature of the endodontic microflora

Endodontic infection is usually derived from the normal oral flora, which gains entry to the pulp space through carious lesions, pulpal exposure by trauma or operative dentistry, or through incomplete enamel/dentine cracks. Blood-borne spread of micro-organisms

from a distant site (anachoresis) is now considered unlikely as a cause of pulp canal infection.

While the oral flora represents a diverse, mixed flora of more than 500 cultivable species, the necrotic pulp canal is a specialized environment, selecting a narrower microflora. Bacteria are usually implicated, though yeasts are occasionally reported. Species which invade and colonize the dying pulp are predominantly aerobic, Gram-positive organisms, but in time, these give way to an increasingly anaerobic Gram-negative flora, typically comprising of 2 to 8 species in any canal. Mixed collections of microbial species have been shown to interact nutritionally, supporting each other in the growth and evolution of a mature microbial climax community (Sundqvist 1992). It is not known if there is such an entity as a healthy root canal flora, or if any infection of the pulp space represents a pathological entity. Periodontists have long debated specific and non-specific plaque hypotheses in the aetiology of marginal periodontitis. Less research is available to indicate whether a specific mass of any micro-organism or if specific species or combinations of species are necessary for apical periodontitis to develop. There is, however, some evidence that single-species infections are just as capable of producing periapical inflammation as mixed infections, though the latter are typically associated with larger lesions. This may reflect longer-established infections which have had greater time to develop in complexity and provoke reactive changes in the periapex, or the selection of especially virulent organisms as microbial communities evolve.

Specific species have, however, been associated with the development of symptoms, and while precise mechanisms have not been elucidated, it is likely that virulence factors, such as proteolytic enzymes, immunogenic capsular material, or ability to compromise host defence mechanisms may be responsible. The Gram-negative, anaerobic Prevotella, Porphyromonas, and Fusobacterium species have special associations in this regard.

For now, it must be considered that any microbial infection of the pulp space is unwelcome and capable of inducing pulp inflammation, breakdown, and the development of apical periodontitis. Dentists should work to avoid any exposure of the pulp space to the oral flora.

Endodontic microflora

- Pulpitis and apical periodontitis are microbial diseases, caused by members of the oral flora
- Pulpitis is prevented by denying micro-organisms entry to the pulp
- Apical periodontitis is prevented by preserving pulpal health or cleaning the pulp system before microbial toxins can affect the periapical tissues
- The special environment of the pulp canal supports mixed infections which are progressively anaerobic, Gram-negative, and nutritionally inter-related
- There is currently no such entity as a healthy pulp canal flora. Any microbial infection is considered undesirable and should be prevented

Epidemiology of apical periodontitis

Endodontics is one of the most technically exacting disciplines in dentistry. For this reason, much of the research and most of the standard texts have focused on mechanical aspects of clinical technique, rather than the biology and epidemiology of the disease being treated. This contrasts strongly with the related disciplines of cariology and periodontology, for which there are substantial published data on prevalence and treatment need.

Dental caries is understood to be the single most common cause of pulp death and apical periodontitis, but quite how much disease it causes is not known. Some understanding of scale is provided by countries with nationalized healthcare systems, such as the UK, in which it is known that more than 1 million root canal treatments are undertaken on permanent teeth each year, at a cost in excess of £40 million. This figure takes no account of the many teeth extracted in preference to being retained by root canal treatment, and similar numbers of teeth with non-vital pulps which are symptom-free, or episodically uncomfortable for which no treatment is sought. The cost of root canal treatment also takes no account of the price to be paid for coronal restoration of damaged, pulpless teeth, or of any remedial care required in the future for the management of treatment failure.

A number of studies have attempted to quantify pulp death and development of apical periodontitis in response to operative dental procedures. Many of these, such as the provision of crowns, must presumably have followed earlier episodes of dental disease and repair such as caries and cavity restoration. It seems evident that crown preparation is associated with increasing levels of endodontic breakdown as observation periods increase. Approximately, 2–4% of pulps may lose vitality within the first 5 years of crown cementation, a figure which rises to almost 20% at 20 to 25 year recall (Valderhaug *et al.* 1997). This has serious pathological and economic implications in populations with high life expectancy, and demands serious thought before embarking on aggressive courses of restorative treatment, even in patients entering middle age.

Service planning requires some knowledge of disease prevalence in the community to be served. Levels of apical periodontitis have seldom been investigated in caries screening studies, since radiographic exposures are needed. However, studies have been undertaken to quantify apical periodontitis as a distinct disease entity. All surveys from developed countries have revealed substantial normative treatment need, including the management of previously untreated periapical disease, and retreatment of lesions which failed to heal after initial care.

A comprehensive summary of prevalence data for apical periodontitis, largely based on Scandinavian and European studies was made by Eriksen in 1998. Table 6.1 shows that 33% of 20–30 year olds have at least one periapical lesion, a figure which rises to 62% for those over 60. It is striking to compare apical periodontitis (infected pulp canal space requiring complex intervention) with data for marginal periodontitis (1 CPITN score of 4, denoting the need for complex intervention). Arguably, apical periodontitis is far more prevalent in Western societies than advanced forms of periodontal disease, with implications in terms of resource allocation for its conservative treatment, risks of acute flare-up or the need for extraction.

The risk of acute flare-up in chronic apical periodontitis has been estimated as 5% per year, in other words, 50% over a 10 year period. Of greater concern to some is the silent damage which may result from untreated or inadequately treated periapical disease. In a homeopathic age, when many accept that unquantifiably small amounts of agents are able to exert beneficial or deleterious effects on the body, and links are being made between chronic inflammatory conditions and systemic malaise, many find the prospect of harbouring asymptomatic, chronic infectious lesions as undesirable as the spectre of an acute episode. There is, however, no clear evidence at the present time to support or refute such systemic links (Murray and Saunders 2000).

The quality of endodontic treatment has been the subject of numerous investigations in a range of countries and healthcare systems. Evaluations are usually based on a radiographic judgement of the technical standard of treatment, using criteria associated with success, which are published by European and American Endodontic associations. Almost all have concluded that standards of service delivery in practice are disappointing, and likely to result in high levels of treatment failure and persistent periapical disease. Table 6.2 summarizes quality evaluations from a range of countries.

Table 6.1 Prevalence of serious marginal periodontitis and apical periodontitis in Europe

Disease	Age group (years)				
	20–30	30–40	40–50	50–60	60+
Apical periodontitis	33	40	48	57	62
Marginal periodontitis	0	14	20	25	26

(Courtesy Blackwell Sciences)

Table 6.2 Endodontic treatments considered technically satisfactory and likely to prevent or heal apical periodontitis in various countries

Country	Year	% cases considered technically satisfactory
Sweden	1990	30
Switzerland	1991	27
Netherlands	1993	50
USA	1995	42
Germany	1997	14
England & Wales	1998	10
Belgium	2000	43

The clear message from all of this is that pulp infection, breakdown, and the development of apical periodontitis is better prevented than allowed to develop. Prevention begins by understanding how pulps can be protected from injury and infection, and by working with natural defences to preserve pulpal health.

Epidemiology and complications

- Apical periodontitis is probably more prevalent than advanced forms of marginal periodontitis in Western communities
- The technical quality of endodontic treatment prescribed to treat apical periodontitis is disappointing in most countries
- The risk of acute exacerbation is approximately 50% over a 10 year period, but the behaviour of individual lesions is unpredictable
- Concerns are growing about possible links between chronic apical periodontitis and systemic malaise
- Apical periodontitis is better prevented than allowed to develop and require difficult, costly treatment

Natural defences against the oral environment

Enamel

In pristine health, the dental pulp is protected from injury by dentine, enamel, and a sound investing periodontium. The majority of threats to pulpal health come through the crown after loss or damage to enamel. Enamel, which is 2.5 mm thick over cusp tips and has the hardness of mild steel, acts as a simple physical barrier against the oral environment. Chemically, it is composed of 96% mineral with 4% organic matter, but no cells. Its capacity to remineralize after acidic challenge is well-documented, but it is incapable of new growth after fracture or loss. For this reason, suspicious, early enamel lesions are no longer probed as there is a risk of converting an area of sub-surface demineralization capable of physiological repair into an area of cavitation which cannot be restored without operative intervention. Similarly, conservative dentists now favour minimally invasive, enamel-preserving resin-bonded restorations rather than enamel and dentine sacrificing alternatives.

Preservation of enamel is important, and no dentist should forget their primary role in preventing and limiting enamel-destroying caries, trauma, and tooth wear; or think the restorative treatments they provide are better than undamaged tissue. Any thickness of enamel protects the underlying tissues, and few pulps die and become infected in the presence of intact enamel.

Dentine/pulp complex

Breach of protective enamel coverage opens dentine to the mouth and places the pulp at risk. The consequences depend on the extent of tissue injury, the nature of any insults which come to bear, and the underlying condition of the pulp. These can range from minor dentine sensitivity to pulp necrosis and serious spreading infection. Dentine and pulp are anatomically and functionally linked

and should be considered together as a *dentine–pulp complex*. Dentine encases and provides physical protection for the body of the pulp and the cytoplasmic processes of its peripheral odontoblasts, which extend deep into its tubular structure. The pulp, in turn, provides tissue fluid which hydrates dentine, and may provide some degree of toughness. Movement of dentine/pulp fluid is also responsible for dentine sensitivity following enamel loss. Rapid fluid movement under drying, thermal, or osmotic stimulation, excites sensory nerve endings in the body of the pulp, to warn of tissue injury. Pulp nerves are also believed to be involved in mechanoreceptive feedback to the masticatory system, which may limit chewing forces and potentially damaging flexural overload of teeth (Randlow and Glanz 1986). The absence of such protection, in addition to the tissue loss often associated with pulpless teeth probably explains their vulnerability to fracture.

The defensive capacity of the pulp is greatly compromised if it loses its dentine coverage and is exposed directly to the mouth. Similarly, dentine offers the body little or no defence against microbial infection without the help of a functioning pulp. Exposed dentine should, therefore, be treated with respect as a living tissue, and efforts made to limit further loss and prevent its assault by chemical, physical, and microbial agents, which may inflame and threaten survival of the pulp.

Physical protection

Insulation

Soft tissues are damaged by heat, which can disrupt blood flow and denature protein components. Dentine is a good thermal insulator, and is capable of protecting the pulp from damaging temperature changes provided that 1–2 mm thickness of tissue remains. If it is thinned to 1 mm or less, as may happen in a heavy crown preparation, its defensive capacity is seriously compromised, and the cellular components of the pulp may be at risk of damage.

Restriction of diffusion

Exposed dentine surfaces are porous. Fluid-filled tubules communicate from the external surface to the pulp, providing avenues for externally applied agents to injure pulp tissue. Tubules are narrower and more widely spaced in peripheral than circumpulpal dentine, with some 15000 tubules mm^{-2} of dentine at the amelo-dentinal junction as opposed to 65000 tubules mm^{-2} at the pulp chamber roof (Fig. 6.1). Deeper layers of dentine are thus more porous than superficial layers, and the relative risks of deep tissue injury are apparent.

When chemical and microbial irritants are applied to dentine, they may be diluted by the constant outward flow of tissue fluid from the pulp through opened dentinal tubules. In addition to simple dilution, dentinal fluid has buffering, and possibly even humoral immune activity, to limit the penetration of irritants. The nature of tubular fluid appears to change after dental injury. Within hours of cutting dentine for a cavity or crown, disruption of the odontoblast layer allows plasma proteins including albumin, fibrinogen, and IgG derived from the pulp vasculature, to

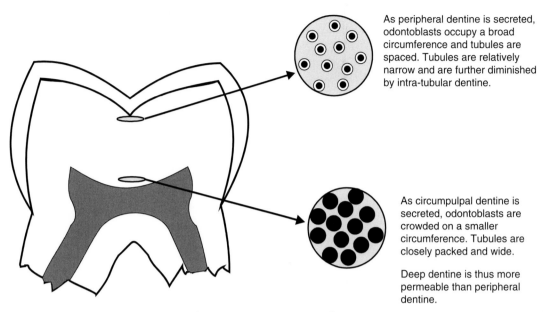

As peripheral dentine is secreted, odontoblasts occupy a broad circumference and tubules are spaced. Tubules are relatively narrow and are further diminished by intra-tubular dentine.

As circumpulpal dentine is secreted, odontoblasts are crowded on a smaller circumference. Tubules are closely packed and wide.

Deep dentine is thus more permeable than peripheral dentine.

Figure 6.1 The increased porosity of deep dentine

concentrate in dentinal tubules, increase the viscosity of tubular fluid and reduce dentine permeability to external agents. The duration of these changes is not known.

Dilution mechanisms are again dependent on dentine thickness. One millimetre of remaining dentine reduces the effects of toxic material to 10% of the original level, while 2 mm of dentine prevents any toxic action on the pulp.

Longer-term irritation, for example, associated with a slowly advancing carious lesion or tooth wear stimulates hard tissue deposition. Peri(intra)-tubular dentine is laid down within dentinal tubules to narrow their lumena and reduce the area of an exposed dentine surface which is porous. Opened dentinal tubules are invariably sealed off further at their pulpal extent by tertiary 'irritation' dentine, whose tubular structure is more sparse and haphazard, and discontinuous with that of primary or physiological secondary dentine. These changes generally seal off tubular communications with the pulp, and little, if any, dentine sensitivity or pulp inflammation is noted in cases of long-standing, non-progressive dentine exposure.

Whenever dentine surfaces are cut with burs or hand instruments, a smear layer is generated, consisting of fine dentine particles and variable amounts of salivary components and micro-organisms. This material is typically pushed 1–5 microns into dentinal tubules to form 'smear plugs', which can reduce dentine permeability by as much as 78%. While this cannot strictly be considered a natural process, it is a helpful accident of nature that hard tissue preparation results in tissue changes, which may be protective.

All of these processes work to spare the soft-tissue of the pulp from major irritation and injury. In teeth with vital pulps, bacteria may enter dentine, but they do not enter the pulp in significant numbers unless caries advances to within 0.5 mm of the

chamber, invades irritation dentine, or there is direct exposure of pulp tissue to the mouth (Reeves and Stanley 1966).

Inflammation

Like other soft connective tissues in the body, the pulp responds to irritation by mounting an inflammatory response. Inflammation can be observed in the pulp whenever dentinal tubules are opened, but the consequences are not necessarily serious. Inflammatory responses are helpful in killing occasional micro-organisms which stray into the pulp, and in creating inflammatory exudates to dilute other irritant agents applied to dentine. While it is true that the pulp occupies a rigid, *non-compliant* space which does not swell to decompress inflamed tissue, it should not be thought that pulp tissue is helpless in the face of insult. Earlier concepts of the intra-pulpal pressure rising during inflammation to overcome the perfusion pressure of the arterioles feeding it were disproved by Van Hassel in 1971. Such responses would lead to avascular necrosis or infarction, which is not a common cause of pulp death. Despite the rigid case, pulp is a surprisingly compliant tissue, provided internally by a rich concentration of proteoglycans in its ground substance, which are compressible and physically cushion tissue in areas adjacent to regions of inflammation and locally increased pressure, protecting them from damage. Unusual arterio-venous shunts are also represented in the pulp, allowing the diversion of blood flow away from areas of increased pressure, preventing vascular stasis and avascular necrosis. Immunological processes are also active in the pulp. These can have beneficial as well as damaging effects on pulp cells.

Inflammatory responses represent the final layer of defence against the entry of micro-organisms from the oral cavity and pulpal breakdown. When the pulp is overcome, inflammatory changes may confine microbial infection to the periphery of the pulp, subjacent to the area of microbial entry, before changes

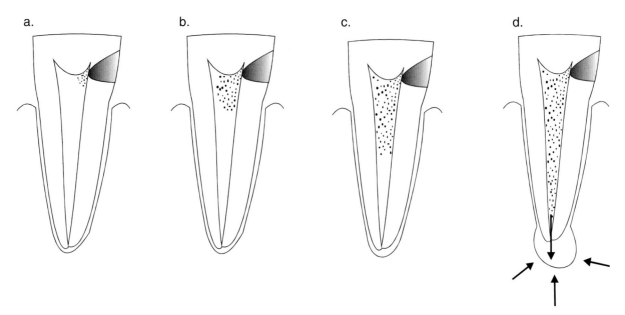

Figure 6.2 Progressive break down of the pulp. Pulp death is not immediate and total. Inflammatory changes spread from a peripheral point of infection (a), spreading first centrally (b), and then apically (c), until the entire pulp is overwhelmed (d). The fight to protect against microbial invasion then moves to the periapex. Progressive break down allows the successful application of amputation (pulpotomy) techniques which excise infected tissue and preserve the healthy tissue beneath.

progress centrally and then apically as defences are overwhelmed (Fig. 6.2). This resilience of pulp tissue provides an opportunity in specially defined circumstances to preserve part of the pulp in health after amputation of diseased, microbially contaminated tissue (see section 'Preserving injured pulps').

Apical periodontium

Inflammation

When infected pulps break down, toxic microbial metabolites diffuse through apical, lateral and furcal portals of communication to inflame the associated periodontal tissues. It is important to understand that the area of periradicular inflammation does not represent the focus of infection. Inflammatory changes are simply the means by which the body seeks to provide another layer of defence against

tissue invasion, and spread of microbial irritants throughout alveolar bone and beyond. The cause of the lesion remains the infected root canal system with few micro-organisms migrating beyond its confines. Effective treatment of established apical periodontitis must, therefore, be targeted at the infected pulp canal contents, not the reactive changes in the periradicular tissues themselves.

Preventing pulp injury in operative dentistry

Despite the best efforts of primary prevention, few people maintain pristine dental health throughout life. Most experience some degree of tissue damage by dental caries, tooth wear or trauma and require the application of restorative materials, usually after mechanical or chemical hard tissue preparation.

Local anaesthetics

Highly perfused tissues are often well placed to survive injury and heal quickly. Most dental local anaesthetic solutions contain a vasoconstrictor, which is added to enhance the depth and duration of pain control, and to limit bleeding in certain operative procedures. One adverse consequence is that they can have a profound effect on pulp blood flow, dependent on the agent and route of administration. Periodontal ligament infiltration of lidocaine with 1:100 000 epinephrine, for example, reduces pulpal blood flow by 75% within 5 minutes, returning to normal only after 75 minutes. Local infiltration of a similar solution containing 1:80 000 epinephrine reduces pulp blood flow by 30% for more than one hour, whilst even inferior alveolar block with the same

Natural defences against apical periodontitis

- Teeth possess sophisticated layers of defence to protect themselves from the oral flora

- Few pulps become infected and die in the presence of intact enamel

- Exposed dentine and pulp work together as a complex to reduce dentine permeability in the face of externally applied irritants

- The pulp is a resilient organ in the absence of microbial invasion. This resilience opens opportunities to preserve part of the pulp in health even after microbial injury

- No dentist should forget their primary role in preventing and limiting damage to dental hard tissues, or think the restorative treatments they provide are better than undamaged tissue

solution reduces canine blood flow by 43%. Taken in isolation, these effects probably present no great threat to pulp tissue, which can tolerate ischaemia for more than one hour by switching to anaerobic metabolism. However, reduction of blood flow, in combination with an especially aggressive, over-heating preparation may theoretically compromise a tissue with relatively low circulation and heat-redistributing capacity, causing tissue injury and even rupture of the peripheral vasculature with bleeding into the pulp chamber and dentine. A pulp with reduced perfusion may also generate less tissue fluid, and the protective outflow of dentinal fluid may be curtailed.

These observations are not a call for the use of vasoconstrictor-free local anaesthetics during lengthy operative procedures on sensitive dental tissues. They do, however, raise awareness that all aspects of dental care can conspire to injure the pulp, and that operative interventions should be justified, as minimal as possible, and conducted with care.

Hard tissue preparation

Managing dentine caries and preparing teeth for crowns requires hard tissue removal. While tissue loss is inevitable, the manner in which it is removed may be open to debate, and there is general agreement that healthy tissue should be preserved as far as possible.

Area of preparation

Dental tubules affected by caries are often narrowed by intra-(peri)tubular dentine, and walled off at their pulpal extent by reactive tertiary dentine. Excavation of caries just to the lateral limit of the lesion is unlikely to open fresh tubules, which are relatively easy pathways of irritants to the pulp. The days of cavity 'extension for prevention' have now passed in favour of more conservative approaches in which attempts are made to simply remove caries and unsupported tissue, and meet the basic physical needs of the bulk restorative material. Even so, it is not always easy to identify precisely, the extent of affected tissue; and iatrogenic damage is easy, especially with high speed rotary tools. Efforts have been made to identify affected tissue by the use of dyes, but most have resulted in over-estimation of the extent of caries. Alternative, and possibly more conservative, methods of caries removal include the use of lasers, and the application of microabrasion, in which cavities are effectively sand-blasted free of diseased tissue. The caries-dissolving agent Carisolv (MediTeam, Göteborg, Sweden) offers a more conservative, therapeutic approach to caries removal, which is kind to pulp tissue (Young and Bongenhielm 2001). Crown preparation rarely involves the removal of diseased tissue, and the large area of previously unopened tubules which are exposed to the mouth by crown preparation can be particularly damaging.

Depth of preparation

Depth of preparation is significant in relation to the porosity of deep dentine and the reduced capacity of thinned dentine to provide thermal protection and dilution of irritants. In addition, preparation into deep dentine risks transecting odontoblast processes close to the cell-body, which inevitably results in odontoblast death. Provided that the pulp remains healthy, lost cells will be replaced by new odontoblast-like cells, but the dead tract which immediately results is an open pathway for microbial invasion of the pulp.

In summary, there is sound scientific rationale that dictates hard-tissue preparation should be as minimal as possible to eradicate disease and allow adequate properties of the chosen restorative material.

Heat generation

Hard tissue preparation generates frictional heat. This is a special issue if dentine is prepared with large burs travelling at high angular velocity, with heavy pressure and without water cooling. Most deep dentine preparation is currently undertaken with high-speed burs—applied with light, intermittent touch—and with focused water spray from more than one direction. This, added to relatively minimal dentine preparation wherever possible, means that severe thermal pulp damage is avoided in most cavity and crown preparations.

Dessication

Further injury can come from the injudicious use of the air syringe during the examination and preparation of dentine surfaces. Streams of air are able to force fluid flow through capillary-like dentinal tubules, which can pluck odontoblasts from the pulp, lodging them in dentinal tubules, where they rapidly break down. Dentine surfaces should not be fully dried unless essential for restorative purposes. The advent of hydrophilic bonding resins and impression materials make this a rare necessity.

Dental materials and the pulp

It is logical to consider whether restorative dental materials applied to dental tissues can harm the pulp. Concerns have traditionally focused on acids and monomers, which were believed to diffuse through freshly cut dentine surfaces to inflame and kill pulps. It is not long since the use of base and lining materials was the norm in cavity restoration to act as protective and insulating barriers to safeguard the dentine–pulp complex.

Evidence has gradually been amassed from germ-free animal studies and from surface-sealing studies (Fig. 6.3) that dental materials are generally non-toxic to the dental pulp, and can be placed in direct contact with pulp tissue without provoking serious inflammation and pulp necrosis. In most circumstances, reparative hard-tissue barriers are laid down in response to such traditionally *tissue damaging* materials as monomer-containing composite resins and acidic zinc phosphate cement (Cox and Hafez 2001).

The key issue is whether micro-organisms are present in the cavity or not, either remaining after cavity preparation, or entering the cavity by microleakage at the restoration margins.

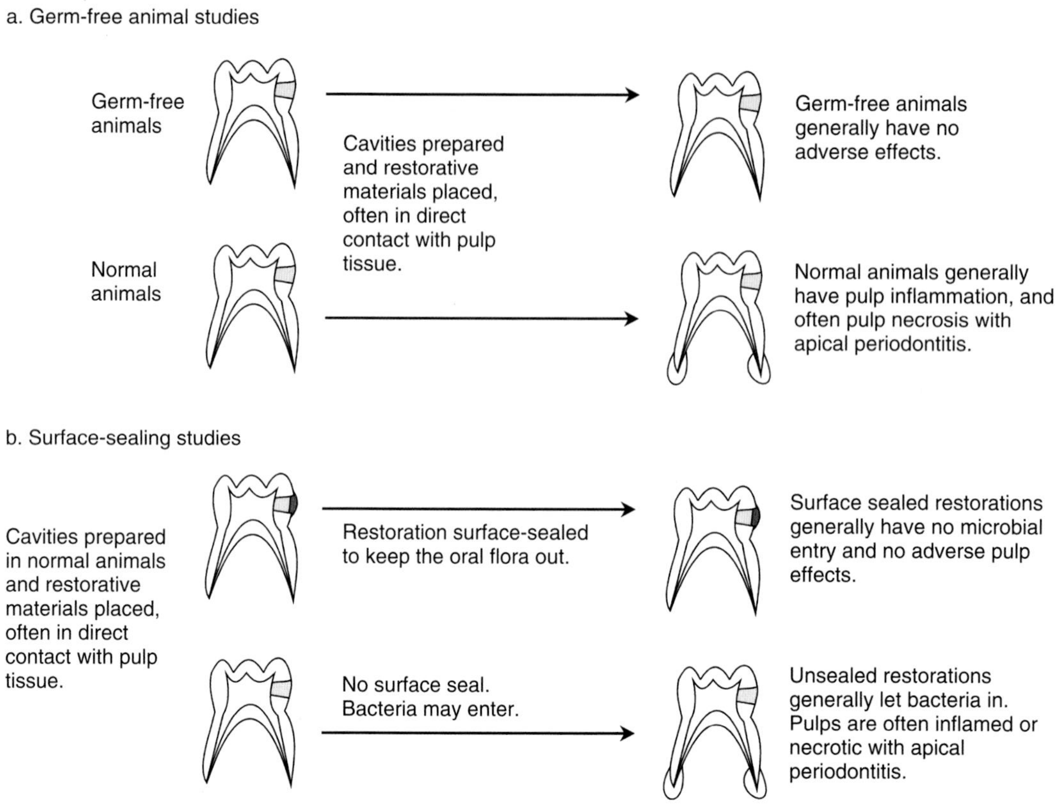

a. Germ-free animal studies

Germ-free animals

Normal animals

Cavities prepared and restorative materials placed, often in direct contact with pulp tissue.

Germ-free animals generally have no adverse effects.

Normal animals generally have pulp inflammation, and often pulp necrosis with apical periodontitis.

b. Surface-sealing studies

Cavities prepared in normal animals and restorative materials placed, often in direct contact with pulp tissue.

Restoration surface-sealed to keep the oral flora out.

Surface sealed restorations generally have no microbial entry and no adverse pulp effects.

No surface seal. Bacteria may enter.

Unsealed restorations generally let bacteria in. Pulps are often inflamed or necrotic with apical periodontitis.

Figure 6.3 Germ-free animal and surface-sealing studies to test the irritancy of dental materials. (a) Germ-free animal studies (b) Surface-sealing studies.

Against this background, the physical properties of dental materials and their ability to create and maintain marginal seal against the oral environment are critical to success. Probably as important is the skill and thoroughness of the dentist in creating a blood and saliva-free environment for material adaptation and in ensuring proper marginal adaptation of restorations. The relevant features of dental materials in terms of pulp health are discussed below.

Ability to bond to or seal interfaces with dental hard tissues

Materials providing a long-term fluid and bacteria-tight interface with dental tissues are likely to be well-tolerated by the pulp. Marginal sealing is a property associated with hydrophilic resin bonding systems and glass–ionomer cements, although their long-term sealing ability is less certain. Amalgam restorations do not form chemical bonds with dentine, and the relative corrosion resistance of contemporary non-gamma 2, high-copper amalgams may compromise their ability to form tight margins by material corrosion. Cavity varnishes, or increasingly, priming and sealing amalgam cavities with resin bonding agents, may represent a wise precaution before restoration with non-sealing materials. Poor adaptation is particularly associated with provisional crown and bridgework, in which vast areas of freshly cut dentine are potentially at risk. The potential merit of resin-sealing all

preparations before temporization has been discussed, though without clear consensus.

Dimensional stability during setting

Laboratory studies have shown that many contemporary dental materials form strong bonds with dental hard tissues. Many of these studies take little account of the realities of material behaviour and handling in the clinical setting. Most materials contract to some degree during setting, and the degree to which this impacts on performance can be greatly influenced by the manner in which the material is applied and the configuration of the cavity preparation. In many circumstances composite resins, which are expected to bond well, may develop shrinkage forces which overcome bond strengths with cavity walls, bringing about marginal failure and opportunity for leakage from the moment the restoration is placed. Curing contraction is usually compensated by later hygroscopic expansion of polymeric materials in contact with saliva. This may improve marginal adaptation, but will not re-establish broken adhesive bonds.

For composite resins, the risks of polymerization-induced marginal breakdown are controlled by incremental build-up and curing of material the lamellar build-up of restorations with flowable material which is able to move to compensate for shrinkage in the deepest layers before building stiffer materials more superficially; and by directing curing light in the knowledge that the material will cure towards it.

Glass ionomer cements enjoy greater dimensional stability and reduced risk of polymerization-induced marginal breakdown. Dental amalgams form no bonds with cavity margins, but may expand slightly on setting to enhance marginal adaptation.

Coefficient of thermal expansion

The mouth is a harsh environment, with many, irregular cycles of thermal exchange every day. Thermal flux brings about volumetric change, and materials which do not have coefficients of thermal expansion comparable with dental tissues may undergo marginal breakdown with time. Most composite resins demonstrate marginal breakdown and percolation of oral fluids beneath the restoration with time. Whether the prior sealing of dentine by the bonding agent spares the pulp from injury is not known. Again, problems of this sort are less pronounced with glass ionomer cements.

Amalgam restorations have markedly different expansion behaviour to tooth tissues, but have probably been able to compensate for such changes by dynamic corrosive events at the restoration/tooth interface.

The properties of all dental materials must be considered in relation to pulp health. Evidence on basic biocompatibility is certainly important, since the development of materials toxic to host tissues cannot be supported. The physical properties of materials, including clinical methods of securing and preserving long-term marginal seal are just as important if the restoration is to do its ultimate job of protecting the pulp as well as intact enamel would.

Operative dentistry and prevention

- Operative dental treatment can compromise the natural defences of teeth, and make them more vulnerable to microbial invasion
- Tooth preparation should always be justified and as minimal in area and depth as possible
- The dentine/pulp complex should be treated as a sensitive, living tissue, avoiding overheating, and overdrying, and taking steps to seal it from contamination by the oral flora
- Dental restorative materials have little direct pulpal toxicity. Entry of micro-organisms at cavity/restoration interfaces is the key cause of postoperative pulp inflammation and breakdown
- The physical properties of restorative materials and careful manipulation to enhance long-term marginal seal are more important for pulp survival than their chemical composition

Preserving injured pulps

The situations in which pulps are in acute danger and in which dentists can actively intervene to preserve health are in the management of:

- deep caries and
- pulp exposure by accidental or iatrogenic trauma.

Dental caries is still the commonest cause of pulpal injury. The clinical management of dental caries emphasizes complete excision of carious dentine to eliminate infection and prevent disease progression. The prepared cavity is then sealed—fluid and bacteria-tight—to prevent new infection or the reactivation of any micro-organisms that were inadvertently left.

Indirect pulp capping

Occasionally, a particularly deep carious lesion in a vital, symptom-free tooth presents the clinician with a dilemma. Should the lesion be fully excised in the knowledge that the pulp will become directly exposed to the mouth, or should some diseased dentine be left in order to avoid direct pulp exposure?

Complete excision of caries from the periphery of the cavity is not negotiable, and this must be meticulously completed before attempting to manage diseased tissue on the pulpal walls. A clean working environment should also be secured, ideally with a well-sealing rubber dam, but at least with appropriate suction and cotton-wool isolation. Conventional teaching is then based on the view that the advancing front of a carious lesion contains demineralized but sterile dentine, which can be safely left in the depths of the cavity preparation. It is currently impossible to judge with accuracy when this condition has been reached, and practice is highly variable and subjective. When a comfortable degree of excavation has been achieved, the dentine/pulp complex is treated with a wound dressing described as an 'indirect pulp cap', usually a setting calcium hydroxide cement, before restoring the cavity against the oral environment. The purpose of the calcium hydroxide cement is to create a bactericidal, high pH environment, in which the pulp can lay down further dentine to wall itself off from further injury. It has been claimed that calcium hydroxide actively promotes the deposition of reparative dentine, but there is no evidence that it has any special powers in this regard, other than to secure a clean arena for the pulp to get on with its natural activity in the face of irritation. There are no clear data on the success of such procedures, though all experienced dentists have witnessed recurrent caries and pulp involvement under restorations.

Stepwise excavation

Without objective criteria and any assurance that remaining caries will have arrested, some dentists advocate a stepwise excavation procedure to allow more thorough caries removal. Here, soft dentine in the depths of the preparation is treated with a calcium hydroxide cement, but the cavity is sealed temporarily. Two months later, by which time it is hoped that the pulp will have laid down reactive dentine and retreated from the carious front, the cavity is re-entered for complete caries removal.

Since the degree of initial diseased tissue removal and the critical mass for activity is unknown, and since it is known that most restorations leak, stepwise excavation appears rational, and the limited number of studies would confirm this both in primary and permanent teeth.

Novel approaches are required to deal with this clinical problem, and work continues on materials which may be better placed to induce hard-tissue deposition and to sterilize and harden any cariously affected dentine. One example is an anti-microbial resin polymer, which can impregnate softened dentine in a comparable manner to wood hardeners used to treat areas of timber decay. Another involves the fumigation of cavity preparations with bactericidal ozone. Such approaches may open new management options in the years to come.

Direct pulp capping

Despite careful excavation, pulps are frequently exposed to the mouth during cavity preparation. They are also commonly exposed in complicated coronal tooth fractures. The key determinants of outcome are the underlying condition of the dental pulp and the ability of the dentist to prevent tissue infection. The condition of the pulp may occasionally be easy to assess by the history of symptoms or by the outcome of sensitivity tests before treatment. However, the histological status of the pulp bears little relation to reported symptoms, and conventional pulp testing, even if it was done before local anaesthesia and cavity preparation, is extremely crude.

When dental caries has extended into the pulp in a true carious exposure, the pulp is infected with micro-organisms, and has little chance of survival, even if there are no presenting symptoms. Similarly, a traumatic exposure left open to the mouth for 24 hours is contaminated with micro-organisms, and has little chance of survival if the cavity is simply restored.

The best prognosis is for traumatic pulpal exposures, treated as soon as possible after the event. The tooth should be isolated with a well-sealing rubber dam, the pulp wound cleaned, and haemostasis secured with sodium hypochlorite solution. Haemostasis is critical for the success of any direct pulp capping procedure. Failure to achieve adequate haemostasis probably reflects greater-than-anticipated pulpal inflammation, and a consequently poor prognosis. Classically, the pulp wound is then covered with setting calcium hydroxide cement to further disinfect the exposed pulp and encourage the deposition of a reparative dentine bridge. However, there is convincing evidence that bridges induced by calcium hydroxide are incomplete and porous and do not provide long-term pulp protection, especially if restorations leak at a later stage (Cox et al. 1996). In recent years, considerable interest has focused on dentine-bonded composites as materials able to secure the clean, well-sealed environment for more predictable and complete pulpal repair. These approaches are now accepted and widely practiced, though long-term outcomes are not known. Calcium hydroxide no longer holds a position of glory as a unique pulp regenerative agent, and the realization that it is the conditions created by the restorative material that allow healing to take place has opened the search for alternative approaches. A variety of materials, including glass ionomer cements, and the exceptionally well sealing and biocompatible Mineral Trioxide Aggregate (Maillefer/Dentsply, Ballaigues,

Switzerland) have their advocates. Radical new bioactive approaches, such as the application of human growth factors for induced dentine bridge formation are also under widespread investigation. It is, however, important to emphasize once again that the underlying condition of the pulp is critical to success. Even bioactive molecular approaches will be ineffective in the case of a dying pulp.

Pulp amputation

Simple pulp capping of carious and long-standing (>24 hours) traumatic exposures cannot be recommended. In immature teeth, where the pulp has not yet completed its task of root formation, and where root canal treatment would be difficult, advantage can be taken of the pulp's great healing ability. In these situations, pulp amputation is advocated, in which an attempt is made to excise all of the affected tissue and leave the sterile, healthy radicular pulp to complete tooth development.

Working under aseptic conditions, the infected coronal 2–3 mm of pulp tissue are removed under sterile saline irrigation with a high speed diamond bur. An indication of the underlying pulp condition is provided by the degree of bleeding from the wound. Bleeding should be slight and readily controlled in healthy tissue, and sodium hypochlorite may be washed over the wound for further disinfection. No attempt should be made to mask the condition of the pulp by attaining haemostasis with an astringent. If haemostasis is not achieved, then further tissue should be removed. The same range of wound dressings may again be applied; traditionalists favouring calcium hydroxide cements, while others favour resins, MTA, or biological approaches. In any event, the tooth should be restored tightly and kept under review. This approach was initially adopted by Cvek in 1978 for the management of traumatic pulp exposures, and his long-term successes were in excess of 80%. However, the utility of the approach is reinforced by recent studies showing high levels of success in the management of carious pulp exposures in young permanent molars (Nosrat and Nosrat 1998).

The benefits of excising infected tissue are well recognized by paediatric dentists, who have shunned simple pulp capping as a high-risk procedure for the preservation of exposed primary pulps. Apical periodontitis in the young carries the same dangers of pain and sepsis, but has added dimensions in terms of damage to subjacent permanent teeth, risks associated with emergency tooth extraction and orthodontic consequences following unplanned tooth loss. Maintenance of healthy pulp tissue is therefore important, and coronal pulpotomy is the accepted norm for the deeply carious primary molar. This is ideally done under rubber dam with a sharp excavator or bur, taking care to free the coronal chamber of soft tissue and cut back to healthy radicular pulp stumps. A wound dressing is then applied to the radicular pulp, before restoring the tooth bacteria and fluid-tight. Clinical research has focused strongly on the choice of medicament and its impact on success. In reality, outcome again is probably more dependent on the condition of the radicular pulp tissue and the ability to eliminate and exclude infection than on the precise composition of chemicals applied. In carefully selected cases, it has been shown that approximately 80% of cariously exposed primary molars will be preserved without evidence of apical periodontitis, whether the pulp stumps are treated with formocresol or calcium hydroxide (Waterhouse *et al.* 2000). Attempts have begun to assess the condition of pulp tissue more objectively by measuring inflammatory mediators in blood from cut surfaces, and relating this to clinical outcome. High levels of PGE_2 have been associated with higher levels of pulp break down and apical periodontitis, regardless of the wound dressing (Waterhouse *et al.* 2002). Efforts to apply astringents such as ferric sulphate to control bleeding may appear logical, but may not help the clinical outcome. Bleeding, which is difficult to control may indicate that the tissue is in an irreversible state of inflammation and will break down whatever medicament is subsequently applied.

This is an exciting area for adult and paediatric dentistry, and one in which molecular biology will make great inroads to support diagnosis and treatment in the decades to come.

Injured pulps

- Pulps which have become infected after carious or traumatic exposure can be preserved
- Clinical outcome depends on the underlying condition of the pulp, and the ability to eliminate and prevent recurrence of infection
- Cutting pulp to eliminate infected tissue is acceptable to prevent total pulp breakdown in primary and permanent teeth
- Better methods are needed to assess the condition of the exposed pulp
- Molecular biology is likely to deliver novel diagnostic and therapeutic tools in the years ahead

Prevention of apical periodontitis after pulpal breakdown

Classical signs of irreversible pulp inflammation include spontaneous pain, and prolonged pain on thermal stimulation. In the early stages of pulp breakdown, pulpal infection can be quite superficial (Fig. 6.2), and there are frequently no signs of periapical involvement. As degeneration proceeds, deeper areas of the pulp and adjacent dentine become infected and changes extend to the apical periodontium. The best prognosis for conventional root canal treatment occurs when a pulp canal system is managed before there is extensive infection and apical periodontitis develops. Measures which assist in the elimination of infection and the prevention of its recurrence are central to long-term periapical health.

Creating a clean environment

Rubber dam isolation of the working field is mandatory, not just to protect patients from the dangers of dropped instruments, but to control against the influx of micro-organisms, and allow the use of strong disinfectants. It is not sufficient for the dam to be in place; it must seal. All caries and plaque should also be thoroughly removed before any attempt is made to enter the pulp chamber.

Entering the system

It is essential that the pulp system is fully unroofed to open the coronal entrances of all canals for entry. Standard textbooks show classical cavity outlines for all teeth and once the chamber is found, blunt-ended endodontic access burs allow the chamber to be quickly and safely unroofed to its full extent. Knowledge of pulp anatomy is essential for predictable care, including common anatomical variants which, unentered, will harbour infected pulp tissue and give rise to apical periodontitis. The benefits of magnification and supplementary light cannot be over-estimated in endodontics, and the operating microscope has revealed infinite anatomical variation in canal systems. However, commonly missed anatomy continues to be the lingual canals of lower incisors and canines and the mesiopalatal canal of upper molars.

The opened chamber should be filled from the outset with an antimicrobial and tissue solvent irrigant, of which sodium hypochlorite remains the gold standard.

Removal of tissue

Bulk removal of a vital pulp is still most efficiently achieved with barbed broaches, which are available in a range of diameters for even fine and curved canals. It is important to remove large portions of vital tissue before commencing canal preparation, since files can compact soft tissue in the canal, where it will form an obstruction to full instrumentation and become necrotic under bacterial infection to cause apical periodontitis.

Determining the level of the wound

Root canal treatment involves the removal of pulp tissue, the preparation of the canal to a pre-determined level, and the installation of a sealing root filling, which will serve as a wound dressing against the cut soft tissue surface.

The length of preparation, and therefore, the level of the soft tissue wound is the working length. It is important that the level determined does not leave a pulp stump which cannot be sustained by any residual apical perfusion. Equally, the wound should not be placed out into the periapical tissues, which to this point have not been involved in a disease process. In reality, it is very difficult to determine from radiographs exactly where preparation extends to in relation to the apical foramen, and great hope is placed in new-generation electronic apex locators which certainly appear to make the process more accurate.

Reassuringly, it has been shown that if pulp tissue is completely removed under strictly aseptic conditions, periapical health will be maintained by root fillings extended to within 2 mm of radiographic root end (Friedman 1998). Preservation of working length is important, but length is frequently lost during the preparation of curved canals by the generation of obstructions. These are generally blockages caused by dentine chippings and due to inadequate irrigation, or ledges (steps) created on canal walls by inflexible instruments. The advent of rotational cutting and flexible nickel–titanium alloys for instrument manufacture has almost completely eliminated the occurrence of these procedural errors, allowing predictable and rapid canal preparation to length.

The purpose of canal instrumentation is to enlarge major root canals concentrically, ridding them of pulp tissue and infected dentine, and allowing entry of further irrigant to the deep parts of the canal system. After a 40 year period of instrument standardization, enlarging tools are now available in a range of tapers and designs, offering canal preparations which are large apically and minimally flared, small apically and greatly flared, and anything in between. There is currently no consensus on which approach or preparation system delivers the most predictable results in vital or non-vital cases. What is clear is that any of the currently available nickel–titanium systems will allow better control and reduction in procedural errors during the shaping of root canals (Gluskin *et al.* 2001).

Single or multiple-visit care

The advent of rapid canal preparation techniques make it technically possible for most dentists to complete root canal treatments at a single visit. Clinical research evidence has suggested that a single session of instrumentation and disinfection is inadequate to properly clean infected cases, and so the application of an antimicrobial intra-canal dressing has been advocated for cases of apical periodontitis.

The situation is different for cases without apical periodontitis where there is little infection in the deeper parts of the canal system. For these cases, there is consensus that single visit treatment is preferred, provided that this does not lead to compromise in mechanical instrumentation and use of antimicrobial and tissue-solvent irrigant. Thirty minutes of canal contact with frequently exchanged, 2% sodium hypochlorite solution is generally considered adequate for disinfection and cleansing.

Preserving the clean environment

After mechanical instrumentation, sites treated for periodontal disease are installed on a maintenance programme for periodic plaque control. Endodontic sites cannot be repeatedly re-entered for plaque control, so the environment must be preserved by other means. The pulp canal space is, therefore, obliterated with inert, non-toxic filling materials which aim to deny the entry of nutrients through apical, lateral, or coronal portals to micro-organisms left after treatment, and prevent the entry of new infection from the mouth. Gutta percha and sealer remain the commonest materials for this purpose, and can be adapted to the canal interior by cold compaction or after softening with solvents or heat. Thermoplastic obturation techniques are more likely to drive materials into secondary anatomy, and have been hailed as better and more complete filling techniques than cold methods. However, no system has been shown to preserve periapical health better than cold lateral condensation, which remains the most widely taught and practiced filling technique worldwide.

Regrettably, *in vitro* studies have shown that all root fillings leak and that all are vulnerable to marginal percolation by fluids and micro-organisms from the mouth if they are not protected by a well-sealing coronal restoration.

Carefully conducted root canal treatment is successful in preventing apical periodontitis in 83–100% of cases. By contrast, treatment of established apical periodontitis is successful in only 46–93% of cases. Clearly, these figures, taken from a range of clinical studies, present diverse pictures of success, but the message is clear—prevention is better than cure.

Prevention of apical periodontitis

- It is easier to prevent apical periodontitis than to heal it once it is established
- Effective prevention in the irreversibly pulpitic tooth involves meticulous removal of micro-organisms and substrate from the pulp system, and sealing it against new infection
- Infection control should underpin every action at every stage of root canal treatment
- Contemporary devices such as magnification, electronic apex location, nickel–titanium instrumentation, and thermoplastic obturation may enhance infection control. They should not, however, take precedence over infection control basics, such as a well-sealing rubber dam and the use of sodium hypochlorite for irrigation

Preventing apical periodontitis after root canal treatment

The root canal treated tooth has none of the complex physical and responsive barriers to protect the apical periodontium from the oral flora. It has also been shown that coronally unsealed root fillings are traversed by non-motile micro-organisms within 4–40 days. Root canal treated posterior teeth are also at risk of cuspal fracture, which may involve the roots and result in treatment failure. It is, therefore, critical to restore root canal treated teeth as soon as possible after the root filling is completed. In molars, this can be as simple as a cuspal coverage amalgam or composite restoration, extended 2–3 mm into all root canals, and often supplemented by a resin bonding agent (Nayyar *et al.* 1980).

Root canal treated premolars and anterior teeth are especially vulnerable if they are restored with provisional post crowns, which are notoriously ill-fitting and allow large-scale leakage. If early restoration is not possible, these teeth should ideally be sealed with a coronal restoration and overlaid with a removable partial denture. Alternatively, coronal seal can be secured with a direct post cemented into the newly filled canal, and a plastic core material. Fibre posts and composite cores present a particularly exciting immediate restoration, supported now by long-term clinical evidence (Ferrari *et al.* 2000), and easily retrieved for canal re-entry if required.

The placement of intracanal posts is not without its risks, notably root perforation during post channel preparation, and compromise of the apical root filling by over extension. Iatrogenic communications between the canal system and periodontium are usually associated with the development of apical periodontitis as micro-organisms from the mouth gain entry to the canal and wound. Apically, at least 4 mm of root filling material must remain after post channel preparation to safeguard periapical health. Both of these errors can be prevented by first melting out root filling material to the desired level before shaping the post-channel with appropriate twist drills. Better still, intracanal posts should be avoided wherever they are not essential to retain the coronal restoration.

Finally, pulpless teeth are incapable of sensation and will not alert the host to caries or other damage which may expose the root filling to the oral microflora. Root filled teeth should, therefore, be examined with extreme care during clinical review; and periodically radiographed to control for coronal caries, or the development of apical periodontitis.

Root canal treated teeth

- Root canal treated teeth can fail for non-endodontic reasons associated with new infection or reactivation of old infection
- They are also vulnerable to fracture and caries
- Root canal treated teeth should be restored quickly against the oral flora, incorporating features to prevent tooth fracture, and should be reviewed with radiographs to ensure periapical health and the absence of silent caries

Conclusions

- Pulpitis and apical periodontitis are microbial diseases caused by members of the oral microflora. They are common disorders in all developed countries and are responsible for substantial pain and suffering, and if inadequately treated, can progress to serious, disseminating sepsis.

- Teeth and their supporting structures contain sophisticated defences against entry of the oral microflora. Dentists should understand these defences, and be aware that the restorative solutions they provide for dental disorders are no match for intact dental tissue.

- The dentine/pulp complex is able to survive considerable insult, and approaches are available to safeguard the health of all or part of the pulp if it is injured. Molecular biology is likely to offer new solutions for the preservation and regeneration of pulp tissues, which have not been overwhelmed by microbial insult.

- Apical periodontitis can be prevented from developing if irreversible pulp injury is managed quickly and well by root canal treatment. Clinical procedures should be based on sound principles of infection control.

- The root canal treated tooth is vulnerable to periapical break down, if it is not adequately protected. Root filled teeth should be restored quickly with well-sealing coronal restorations, taking care not to compromise the root filling or create new portals of communication with the periradicular tissues.

References

Cox, C.F., and Hafez, A.A. (2001). Biocomposition and reaction of pulp tissues to restorative treatments. *Dental Clinics of North America*, 45, 31–48.

Cox, C.F., Subay, R.K., Ostro, E., Suzuki, S., and Suzuki, S.H. (1996). Tunnel defects in dentine bridges: their formation following direct pulp capping. *Operative Dentistry*, 21, 4–11.

Cvek, M. (1978). A clinical report on partial pulpotomy and capping with calcium hydroxide in permanent incisors with complicated crown fracture. *Journal of Endodontics*, 4, 232–237.

Eriksen, H.M. (1998). Epidemiology of apical periodontitis. In *Essential Endodontology: Prevention and Treatment of Apical Periodontitis*, Chapter 8 (ed. Orstavik, D. and Pitt Ford, T.R.), pp. 179–191. Blackwell Science: Oxford.

European Society of Endodontology (1994). Consensus report of the European Society of Endodontology on quality guidelines for endodontic treatment. *International Endodontic Journal*, 27, 115–124.

Ferrari, M., Vichi, A., Manochi, F., and Mason, P.N. (2000). Retrospective study of the clinical performance of fiber posts. *American Journal of Dentistry* 13(Special issue), 9B–13B.

Friedman, S. (1998). Treatment outcome and prognosis of endodontic therapy. In *Essential Endodontology: Prevention and Treatment of Apical Periodontitis*, Chapter 15, (ed. Orstavik, D. and Pitt Ford, T.R.), pp. 367–401. Blackwell Science: Oxford.

Gluskin, A.H., Brown, D.C., and Buchanan, L.S. (2001). A reconstructed computerised tomographic comparison of NiTi rotary GT files versus traditional instruments in canals shaped by novice operators. *International Endodontic Journal* 34, 476–484.

Kakehashi, S., Stanley, H., and Fitzgerald, R. (1965). The effect of surgical exposures of dental pulps in germ-free and conventional laboratory rats. *Oral Surgery, Oral Medicine, Oral Pathology* 20, 340–349.

Moller, A.J.R., Fabricius, L., Dahlen, G., Ohman, A.E., and Heyden, G. (1981). Influence on periapical tissues of indigenous oral bacteria and necrotic pulp tissue in monkeys. *Scandinavian Journal of Dental Research* 89, 475–484.

Murray, C.A., and Saunders, W.P. (2000). Root canal treatment and general health, a review of the literature. *International Endodontic Journal* 33, 1–18.

Nair, P.N.R. (1997). Apical periodontitis: a dynamic encounter between root canal infection and host response. *Periodontology 2000* 13, 121–148.

Nayyar, A., Walton, R.E., and Leonard, L.A. (1980). An amalgam coronal-radicular dowel and core technique for endodontically treated posterior teeth. *Journal of Prosthetic Dentistry* 43, 511–515.

Nosrat, I.V., and Nosrat, C.A. (1998). Reparative hard tissue formation following calcium hydroxide application after partial pulpotomy in cariously exposed pulps of permanent teeth. *International Endodontic Journal* 31, 221–226.

Randlow, K., and Glanz, P.O. (1986). On cantilever overloading of vital and non-vital teeth: an experimental clinical study. *Acta Odontological Scandinavica* 44, 271–277.

Reeves, R., and Stanley, H.R. (1966). The relationship between bacterial penetration and pulpal pathosis in carious teeth. *Oral Surgery* 22, 59–65.

Sundqvist, G. (1976). Bacteriological studies of necrotic dental pulps. Odontological dissertation number 7. University of Umea: Umea, Sweden.

Sundqvist, G. (1992). Associations between microbial species in dental root canal infections. *Oral Microbiology and Immunology* 7, 257–262.

Valderhaug, J., Jokstad, A., Ambjornsen, E., and Norheim, P.W. (1997). Assessment of periapical and clinical status of crowned teeth over 25 years. *Journal of Dentistry* 25, 97–105.

Van Hassel, H.J. (1971). Physiology of the human dental pulp. *Oral Surgery, Oral Medicine, Oral Pathology* 32, 126–134.

Waterhouse, P., Nunn, J., and Whitworth, J. (2000). An investigation of the relative efficacy of Buckley's Formocresol and calcium hydroxide in primary molar vital pulp therapy. *British Dental Journal* 188, 32–36.

Waterhouse, P.J., Nunn, J.H., and Whitworth, J.M. (2002). Prostaglandin E_2 and treatment outcome in pulp therapy of primary molars with carious exposures. *International Journal of Paediatric Dentistry* 16, 116–123.

Young, C., and Bongenhielm, U. (2001). A randomised, controlled and blinded histological and immunohistochemical investigation of Carisolv on pulp tissue. *Journal of Dentistry* 29, 275–281.

Further reading

Kim, S., Trowbridge, H., and Suda, H. (2002). Pulpal reactions to caries and dental procedures. In: Cohen, S., and Burns, R.C. (Eds.), *Pathways of the Pulp*, Chapter 15. (8th edn.) St Louis, Mosby. pp. 573–560.

Spangberg, L.S.W. (1998). Endodontic treatment of teeth without apical periodontitis. In: Orstavik, D., and Pitt-Ford, T.R. (Ed.) *Essential Endodontology: Prevention and Treatment of Apical Periodontitis*, Chapter 10. Blackwell Science: Oxford, pp. 211–241.

Pashley, D.H. (1996). Dynamics of the pulpo-dentine complex. *Critical Reviews in Oral Biology and Medicine* 7, 104–133.

Whitworth, J.M. (2002). *Rational root canal treatment in practice*. London, Quintessence Publishing Co. Ltd. pp. 1–131.

7

Tooth wear: aetiology, prevention, clinical implication

Tooth wear: aetiology, prevention, clinical implication

Linda Shaw

Introduction

Tooth wear is a relatively common problem and the source of many patient complaints. It is not a new phenomenon, but has received more attention in recent years. The type of tooth wear, its distribution, prevalence, and aetiology varies widely across populations and age ranges. However, the recent emphasis on tooth wear and its prevention is probably due to a combination of factors; we have an ageing population with increasing life expectancy, who remain dentate for longer, and who have greater expectations of dental care. At the other end of the age range, there is a cohort of young people who, possibly because of lifestyle factors, experience quite extensive tooth wear.

Definitions of tooth wear

Tooth wear is usually due to a combination of processes, the 'triumvirate' of abrasion, attrition, and erosion. It is unusual for wear to be solely attributed to one of these. Rather, tooth wear is due to all three processes with perhaps one of these predominating.

Abrasion is loss of tooth substance from the friction of a foreign body, often a toothbrush. There are case reports of many quite bizarre causes, including occupational hazards. *Attrition* is a loss of tooth substance due to tooth-to-tooth contact. It was very marked in predynastic Egyptians, prior to 3000 BC, and considered to be due to the sand content of the diet, and therefore, could be regarded as partly attrition and partly abrasion. Parafunctional activities such as nocturnal bruxism are probably a more common cause with the type of diet in the twenty-first century AD. *Erosion* is very different from these two physical types of tooth wear; it is the loss of tooth structure by chemical means, usually acidic, and not associated with mechanical or traumatic factors, or dental caries.

Although these three terms are well known and in common usage, there are other terms describing non-carious destructive processes involved in tooth wear, but these are much less well-known and not universally accepted. These are demastication and abfraction. *Demastication* is a term used for wearing away of tooth substance during mastication. This could be specifically applied to the type of wear shown by the ancient Egyptians, and would depend on the abrasivity of the food consumed. *Abfraction* has been defined as the wedge-shaped defect observed at the cemento-enamel junction. Axial forces on the tooth tend to concentrate stress in this region, and cause microfractures and tooth tissue loss. This is sometimes confused with cervical abrasion and requires further investigation to establish it as a separate entity.

Types of tooth wear

- *Abrasion*: wearing away of tooth substance through physical or mechanical processes with a foreign body
- *Attrition*: loss of tooth substance due to tooth-to-tooth contact
- *Erosion*: irreversible loss of dental hard tissue due to a chemical process not involving bacteria, and not directly associated with mechanical or traumatic factors or with dental caries
- *Demastication*: loss of tooth substance during mastication, influenced by the abrasivity of the food. This should be regarded as a combination of abrasion and attrition
- *Abfraction*: stress concentrations near to the gingival margins leading to microfractures. This probably increases the susceptibility to abrasion and erosion

Epidemiology of tooth wear

There has been subjective information published in the 1990s suggesting that tooth wear, particularly from erosion, has increased considerably. The scientific basis for this is somewhat uncertain. Undoubtedly, very different types of tooth tissue loss are observed in the older adult population than in children. It is, therefore, essential to consider them separately but to regard tooth wear as a continuum throughout life with very different aetiological factors at the ends of the age spectrum.

Prevalence in adults

The data available vary enormously, but a general estimate indicates that up to 97% of the adult population are affected; only about 7% exhibit what could be considered as pathological wear, which requires some form of management or treatment.

Although there are a few early case reports on tooth wear, the first large survey was published in 1972; this considered 10 000 extracted teeth in California. Other subsequently published surveys considered Roman and Anglo-Saxon skulls, and also found a high prevalence of tooth wear. However, none of these investigations could be considered as being representative of a population group.

The consistent finding from very disparate published studies is that tooth wear increases with age, and a certain amount is considered to be a normal 'physiologic' ageing process. An attempt has been made to determine 'threshold' levels, which are regarded as acceptable levels of wear for a given age. More recent studies using the Tooth Wear Index (TWI) of Smith and Knight have indicated that young adults are showing accelerated wear, which may pose a problem for the future.

Prevalence in children

There are more reliable data on the prevalence of tooth wear in the child and adolescent population. As with adults, there have been many case reports and several case–control studies, but there is now an increasing amount of information from well-conducted clinical trials and national surveys. One of the most important is the United Kingdom Child Dental Health Survey of 1993, in which a randomly selected sample of 17 061 children aged from 5 to 15 years was examined. It was found that 50 per cent of children aged 5 and 6 years had evidence of tooth wear, largely attributed to erosion, with almost 25 per cent having dentine involvement. Over half of palatal surfaces of primary upper incisors showed erosion in this age group. At eleven years of age, 2 per cent of children were found to have erosion in their permanent teeth.

An assessment of dental erosion was also included in the oral health examinations, which were part of the National Diet and Nutrition Surveys of pre-school children in 1992–93 and school age children in 1996. Again, these are very important epidemiological studies and involve large population sample sizes. They, too, confirmed the high levels of tooth wear, attributed predominantly to dental erosion, in children and young people.

These studies are cross-sectional investigations and do not give information about incidence, or the possible changing prevalence of tooth surface loss in children. However, inferences can be drawn as the National Child Dental Health Survey was based on data collected 2 years before the National Diet and Nutrition Survey data. The prevalence of any erosion in both primary and permanent dentitions was greater in the later study; for example, in 4–6 year olds 18% of the labial surfaces of upper primary incisors was affected in 1993, compared with 38% in 1995–96. The differences are less marked in the permanent dentition, but the trend to increasing levels of erosion is consistent.

Table 7.1 gives some of the data from the UK National Surveys, as well as two other epidemiological investigations from Birmingham and Liverpool. Although there are obvious differences in the measurement and calibration of erosion, the evidence from the epidemiological studies suggests that one-third of pre-school children and a half of teenagers have measurable tooth surface loss, which can largely be ascribed to dental erosion. This is not, as yet, the public health problem that dental caries continues to be, but vigilance is required to monitor whether the prevalence is increasing.

Prevalence of tooth wear

- One-third of pre-school children have significant tooth wear
- One-half of teenagers show tooth surface loss on incisor teeth that is largely due to erosion
- Approximately 7 per cent of adults exhibit 'pathological' wear, which requires some form of management or treatment
- There is some evidence that tooth wear due to erosion is increasing in the child and young adult population

Assessment

Measurement of tooth wear in general, and erosion, in particular, has been fraught with difficulties. There have been many systems used *in vitro* which plainly cannot be translated to the clinical environment. These include physical and chemical systems involving scanning electron microscopy, digital image analysis, profilometry, ultrasonography, 3-D-tomography, laser scanning, nuclear magnetic resonance imaging, micro-radiography, and hydroxyapatite dissolution. Many of these analytical systems are accurate and reproducible, but can only be used either *in vitro*, *in-situ*, or are extremely time-consuming and impracticable to apply clinically.

Table 7.1 Prevalence of dental erosion in children

	Age (in years)	% Children affected	% Labial surfaces of incisors affected
UK National Diet and Nutrition Survey (1994) [Hinds and Gregory 1994]	$1\frac{1}{2}$–$4\frac{1}{2}$	20	14
Millward, Shaw, and Smith (1994)	4–5	48	17
UK Child Dental Health Survey (1993)	4–6	52	18
	11–14		11
UK National Diet and Nutrition Survey (1996) [Walker *et al.* 2000]	4–6	–	38
Milosevic and Lennon (1994)	14	30	–

Table 7.2 Tooth wear index criteria

Code score	Surfaces	Criteria
0	B/L/O/I	No loss of surface characteristics
1	B/L/O/I	Loss of enamel surface characteristics
2	B/L/O/I	Loss of enamel, dentine exposed for less than one-third of surface Loss of enamel just exposing dentine
3	B/L/O	Dentine exposure for more than one-third of surface
	I	Substantial loss of dentine
4	B/L/O	Complete loss of enamel, or pulp exposure of secondary dentine
	I	Pulp exposure or exposure of secondary dentine

B = Buccal and Labial, L = Lingual and Palatal, O = Occlusal, I = Incisal.

Indices to measure tooth wear *in vivo* were first described in animal models, and were applicable to anaesthetized rats but not to conscious children. Many of the scales and indices subsequently suggested for human clinical studies have had diverse diagnostic criteria. The number and complexity of these indices demonstrates that it has been difficult to devise an ideal index for use in all clinical circumstances. There is no universally accepted, definitive index that is applicable to the diverse needs for research into the aetiology, prevention, management, and epidemiology of tooth wear, and monitoring of an individual patient. In adults, the TWI of Smith and Knight has probably achieved the greatest clinical acceptance; it measures tooth wear from all sources and does not differentiate between attrition, abrasion, and erosion. It is this index, with some modifications, that has been generally used in children. The main criteria are given in Table 7.2. The TWI has several advantages over other published indices; it has the ability to distinguish between 'normal' and 'abnormal' levels of tooth wear as acceptable levels of tooth wear have been published for all the differing age-groups; it is simple to use for individual or large population studies and satisfactory examiner reproducibility has been shown to be achievable.

In the UK a simple, qualitative index, largely using the criteria in the TWI but on index teeth, has been used in the national dental surveys. It should be noted that the calibration of the many examiners involved in these large surveys proved somewhat difficult. The data for the reproducibility of diagnosis indicated that the results should be interpreted with caution.

Aetiological factors

There is no doubt that the causes of tooth wear are multifactorial; the different types of tooth wear seldom exist as a single entity and the causes also are very seldom single or simple. It is a complex interaction of physical and chemical forces on a biological system. It is, therefore, somewhat arbitrary to consider each type of tooth wear individually, as though they were separate entities with distinct individual causative factors.

Assessment of tooth wear

- *In vitro in situ* systems use physical methods such as scanning electron microscopy, digital image analysis, profilometry, ultrasonography, 3-D-tomography, laser scanning, nuclear magnetic resonance imaging, and micro-radiography

- Chemical methods used *in vitro* include acid solubility studies, calcium and phosphorus dissolution and hydroxyapatite dissolution

- *In vivo* animal studies have been time consuming, subject to considerable error and not appropriate for translation to human clinical investigations

- The many published clinical indices suggest that it has been difficult to devise an ideal index for use in all clinical circumstances

- The Tooth Wear Index of Smith and Knight (1984) is a qualitative clinical index and has probably achieved the greatest general acceptance. It is intended for both epidemiological studies and individual patients for long-term monitoring of tooth wear

- Poor reproducibility of diagnosis of tooth wear in large surveys with many examiners indicate that the results of studies should be interpreted with caution

Abrasion

Most abrasion is located in the cervical area of teeth and associated with tooth brushing. Incorrect or over-vigorous brushing with an abrasive toothpaste is usually the prime aetiological factor. There has been a trend to the reduction in abrasivity of commercially available toothpastes. These are complex formulations and there needs to be a balance between oral health benefits and potential damage to teeth and soft tissues. It is not just the abrasive content of the toothpaste that is important; the abrasive type, particle size and surface, and the chemical effects of the other constituents will also affect the amount of abrasion. For example, most of the hydrated silica-based toothpastes have good cleaning values with a low to moderate dentine abrasivity. Obviously, other factors such as brushing force, bristle stiffness and particularly the frequency of and time spent on tooth brushing are very important in encouraging dental abrasion. There is strong evidence to show that abrasion increases enormously if the teeth are first exposed to an acidic erosive challenge, and then tooth brushing is undertaken shortly afterwards. Similarly, the tongue and other oral soft tissues may play a similar role.

There are many case reports of abrasion related to different foreign objects and substances repeatedly introduced into the mouth and contacting the teeth. These include such things as pipe-smoking, pen and pin chewing, and even bag-pipes!

Attrition

Wear caused by tooth-to-tooth contact during the normal function of eating should be minimal unless the diet is very abrasive such as that of the Ancient Egyptians. (This again shows the interrelation of factors.) However, there can be contact of the teeth for reasons other than eating; oral habits, such as parafunction, may contribute significantly to dental damage. Bruxism is considered to be one of the most significant parafunction activities of the stomatognathic system. It is usually defined as the habitual grinding, clenching, gritting, and gnashing of teeth during the day or night for non-functional purposes. Both conscious and subconscious grinding may occur, but the aetiology is not well understood. It has been shown to be related to several stress factors and occlusal discrepancies, although some of the published information relating to these factors is questionable.

It is uncertain whether occlusal interferences cause the bruxism which results in attrition, or whether the wear has resulted in the occlusal interferences. Wear facets are found on the occlusal surfaces of posterior teeth and the incisal edges of anterior teeth. These are flat and flush with the opposing tooth in contact. There is often an erosive element also to the tooth wear and then the opposing tooth surfaces do not contact each other evenly.

Evidence from Romano-British skulls and particularly from exhumed skulls, where there was an accurate recording of the age at death, suggests that attrition may have been more common in ancient populations. However, very few of them lived to the average life expectancy that we have in the twenty-first century. The patterns of wear on occlusal surfaces and assessment of islands of dentine and enamel are used for determining the age of individuals in forensic cases. It should be realized that this is likely to be relatively inaccurate due to the absence of reliable longitudinal data and variables such as diet, which may have played an important part in the development of wear.

Erosion

Not only is tooth wear a multifactorial condition but erosion itself has a mutifactorial aetiology. Figure 7.1 indicates some of the factors involved. Obviously, a susceptible tooth and time are required. There are factors within the individual, referred to as intrinsic factors, and external influences, referred to as extrinsic factors, which are all relevant. There appears to be a huge individual variation as far as susceptibility to erosion is concerned, with the actual anatomy of the mouth, salivary flow rates and buffering capacity, and mineralization of the tooth tissues all playing a part. For example in areas such as the lower incisor region, where there is pooling of saliva and relative protection by the tongue, the prevalence of erosion is lower.

Intrinsic sources of acid

All acids, whether from extrinsic or intrinsic sources, are capable of demineralizing tooth tissue and, therefore, of causing erosion. Intrinsic sources of acid are essentially gastric contents, which enter the mouth as a result of reflux and vomiting. There are also some occasional case reports of rumination—deliberately bringing food back into the mouth to re-chew—which has led to extensive erosion. Gastric reflux is much commoner than was once thought. Relatively, recent research has shown that, in the developed world, 7% of the adult population have gastro-oesophageal reflux on a daily basis and more than 30% every few days. The majority of this is asymptomatic, but there is a wide spectrum of disease and severity of reflux into the mouth. Sometimes the development of dental erosion is the first sign that reflux is occurring, and indicates that investigation of the gastro-oesophageal reflux may be required. General associated symptoms are heartburn, retro-sternal discomfort and dysphagia. People with neurological impairments such as cerebral palsy also have significantly higher levels of reflux. Some of the potential causes of reflux are shown in Table 7.3. Of particular significance is excessive alcohol intake as this is a potent cause of reflux, but alcoholic drinks in themselves may be an extrinsic acidic source.

Vomiting, either spontaneous or self induced, may be associated with a variety of medical problems. Some of the more common ones are given in Table 7.4. This phenomenon must continue over a long period to cause significant erosion, and again,

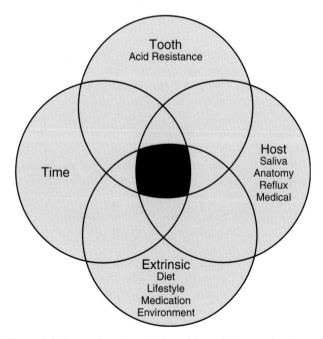

Figure 7.1 Interaction of multiple aetiological factors related to the development of dental erosion.

Table 7.3 Principal causes of gastro-oesophageal reflux

Increased gastric pressure	Obesity
	Ascites
Increased gastric volume	After heavy meals
	Obstruction
	Spasm
Sphincter incompetence	Hiatus hernia
	Diet
	Drugs, e.g. diazepam
	Neuromuscular, e.g. cerebral palsy
	Oesophagitis—alcohol

Table 7.4 Principal causes of vomiting

Psychosomatic	Stress-induced psychogenic vomiting
	Eating disorders
	Bulimia nervosa
	Anorexia nervosa
Metabolic and endocrine	Uraemia
	Diabetes
Gastro-intestinal disorders	Peptic ulcer, gastritis
	Obstruction
	Nervous system disorders
	Cerebral palsy
Drug induced	Primary, eg cytotoxics
	Secondary to gastric irritation e.g. alcohol, aspirin, non steroidal anti-inflammatory drugs
	Drug-induced xerostomia over an extended period may also influence erosion

Table 7.5 Erosion potential of some commonly available drinks

	pH	Titratable acidity	Erosion potential
Cola drinks	2.5	0.1	Medium
Carbonated orange	2.9	2.0	Medium
Grapefruit juice	3.2	9.3	High
Apple juice	3.3	4.5	High
White wine	3.7	2.2	Medium
Orange juice	3.8	4.5	High
Beer—bitter	3.9	0.6	Low
Lager	4.4	0.5	Low
Buxton sparkling water	5.1	0.1	Low
Perrier water	5.2	0.1	Low
Buxton still mineral water	8.1	-	-

there is a range in susceptibility. Current research shows an increasing prevalence of such conditions as bulimia and anorexia nervosa, both of which may be associated with self-induced vomiting.

Extrinsic sources of acid

There are many sources of acid from outside the body, which may affect the dental tissues. A series of case reports have related erosion to contact with fertilizers, dynamite, and various industrial processes using acids. Recently, an increased prevalence and severity of erosion has been shown in people with diverse work and leisure activities such as wine tasting and competitive swimming, which exposes the dentition to repeated contact with acids. However, it would be fair to say that these types of exposure are far less common than the extrinsic acid sources that are related to dietary intake. Dietary practices are changing from the traditional three meals per day to habits of 'grazing' and 'snacking'. There has been an enormous increase in soft drink consumption, and this is no longer confined to children but is being carried forward into adult life. A significant association has been shown between soft drink consumption and dental erosion, particularly, the bed-time consumption of fruit-based drinks. There are also acidic foods and practices that may be implicated such as high consumption of fruit, pickles, and sauces.

It is not only the pH of the food and drink that is important in the development of erosion, but also the titratable acidity. This is the amount of alkali that needs to be added to an acid to bring it up to a neutral pH. It, therefore, represents the amount of available acid, and is an indication of strength and erosive potential. Table 7.5 gives the pH and the titratable acidity of some commonly consumed drinks. Many proprietary brands of drinks have buffers added to them so that, although their pH remains low,

their titratable acidity is much reduced and they, therefore, have a reduced erosive potential.

Lifestyle influences

There has been a welcome emphasis in recent times on a healthy lifestyle, with a 'healthy' diet as just a part of it.

Encouragement to take regular exercise may also lead to increased consumption of acidic drinks; some of the sports drinks are not only acidic, but also contain a considerable amount of simple sugars. Both competitive swimmers and cyclists have been reported as having higher levels of dental erosion.

Conversely, there are unhealthy lifestyles that may be implicated in dental erosion. The use of the drug 'ecstasy' (3,4-methylenedioxy-methamphetamine) reduces salivary flow. The dry mouth combined with dehydration from vigorous exercise and excessive consumption of low pH drinks has also been linked to dental erosion.

Aetiology of tooth wear

- *Abrasion*: usually due to incorrect or over-vigorous brushing, but there are many unusual habits that are occasionally implicated

- *Attrition*: parafunctional activities, such as bruxism, are probably the most significant factors in the development of pathological tooth wear in contact areas

- *Erosion*: always multifactorial but one specific aetiological factor usually predominates
  - Intrinsic acid sources
    - Gastro-oesophageal reflux
    - Vomiting; spontaneous or self-induced
  - Extrinsic acid sources
    - Dietary, drinks etc.
    - Lifestyle influences

How can we prevent tooth wear?

Excessive tooth wear is still not a public dental health problem that dental caries and periodontal disease are. However, for a significant and increasing number of individuals, it is a serious oral condition, which can require very extensive and expensive treatment. It is vital that the existence of tooth wear is identified early and appropriate preventive measures put into place.

Abrasion

Prevention of abrasion is largely common sense. If the main aetiology is incorrect toothbrushing and/or the use of an overly abrasive toothpaste, then the technique and the paste can be changed. Other aetiological factors need to be identified and then appropriate advice given. This can occasionally be quite problematic if the cause of the abrasion is related to professional activities, such as in wind instrument players.

Abrasive foods are uncommon in developed countries, but may be significant factors in certain areas of the developing world. However, there are usually many health and social problems that may render tooth wear somewhat insignificant compared with these other public health concerns.

Attrition

If attrition related to parafunctional activity is found to be progressing to unacceptable levels, then prevention of further tooth surface loss must be considered. Although males consistently show more attrition than females, they experience far fewer symptoms of temporo-mandibular dysfunction or myofascial pain than females. The severity of attrition has not been shown to be strongly associated with the development of signs and symptoms. It has proved to be impossible to totally stop nocturnal bruxing activity; although drug therapy such as tricyclics will reduce REM (Rapid Eye Movement) sleep, which is when the majority of this activity takes place. The most realistic method of controlling attrition is not in the prevention of the parafunctional activity itself, but rather in the prevention of the damage it causes. An occlusal splint (mouthguard) can be constructed, which will prevent the tooth to tooth contact which results in attrition. For long term use, and to try to minimize the amount of bruxing activity, a hard occlusal guard to cover the maxillary teeth such as a 'Michigan Splint' is an option to consider. This, may require the use of a face-bow so that the models can be correctly articulated, and the occlusal surfaces constructed to a predetermined occlusal scheme.

There is no published evidence from clinical trials to show that alteration of the occlusion will eliminate bruxism, but it may have an effect on the site of the attrition. Occlusal management (adjustment) aims to direct the forces generated during bruxism through areas of the teeth and restorations that are best suited to accept them. This will, therefore, reduce mechanical failure, mobility, and wear.

Erosion

The first step in the prevention of erosion is making a diagnosis. Once suspicions have been raised, it is essential to record accurately the severity and extent. This will establish the clinical baseline so that any progression can be assessed, and the effects of preventive measures monitored. It may also be necessary to undertake these procedures in patients with marked abrasion and attrition.

- Record the clinical situation
  - For children, in the permanent dentition, and adults, take impressions for the production of good quality stone study casts.
  - Clinical photographs may be helpful.
  - Currently, the most useful diagnostic index is the Tooth Wear Index, but this is probably not sufficiently sensitive to detect small changes or to record erosion per se.
  - A silicone index can be prepared (see later).
- Try to determine the aetiological factors
  - Take an in-depth history to include a detailed dietary history, medical history, dental hygiene habits, and sensitive investigation about lifestyle factors.
  - A three-day diet history to include everything that passes the patient's lips is important. The periodicity of eating and toothbrushing is also important. Such habits as continuous sipping or 'frothing' of drinks should be noted. (Frothing is the habit of holding carbonated drinks in the mouth and sucking them in and out of the teeth to make froth. This tends to add the 'ultrasonic' effect of the bursting bubbles to the erosive effects of the acid. It also extends contact time.)
- Give appropriate dietary counselling
  - This can only be given after a thorough analysis of the diet and influencing factors. It must be tailored to the individual, bearing in mind the constraints that are operating on them. It needs to be given in a positive, individualized way to maximize compliance.
  - Limit acid foods and drinks to mealtimes.
  - Reduce frequency.
  - Avoid acidic substances last thing at night.
  - Finish meals with something alkaline such as a small piece of cheese or milk.
  - Avoid toothbrushing for at least an hour after acidic substances.
  - Check the formulations or constituents of any medication, mouthwashes, etc.
  - Chewing gum has been shown to stimulate salivary flow and increase buffering capacity, but may also cause increased gastric secretion. It should not be recommended

for children, probably below the age of 7 years, and is not suggested for those with a history of gastric reflux.

- Intrinsic acid sources
  - If there is any evidence or suspicion of gastric reflux, then referral to the general medical practitioner and onward to a gastro-enterologist or psychiatrist may be required. Medication may be helpful, but this obviously needs medical supervision.
  - If reflux or vomiting are occurring, then rinsing the mouth with water and sodium bicarbonate helps to neutralize the oral environment. People who have vomited often rush off to clean their teeth. This is quite the wrong thing to do and should be advised against. It has been shown that if teeth have been subjected to an acidic attack and are then brushed, up to five times as much enamel is removed. If reflux is occurring during sleep then an occlusal guard containing sodium bicarbonate can be used in adults or teenagers.
- Follow up
  - When the patient returns for a review, their compliance with all the advice given should be checked. Perhaps more importantly, the state of the dentition must be examined very carefully.
  - A localized silicone index should be taken of the original study casts in the area of most concern. This can be cut through with a sharp scalpel over the area (often the palatal aspect of the upper incisors). It is then transferred to be fit on to the patient. If there is any gap between the silicone index and the surface of the tooth, then there has been further tooth surface loss. However, this would indicate fairly extensive surface loss.

General comparison with the study casts and the clinical photographs is also necessary. These records have a number of errors inherent in their methods, but can be useful in showing and educating patients about their erosion problems. There are more accurate methods such as replica techniques examined under the scanning electron microscope, but these have very limited use in general dental practice.

Prevention

- *Abrasion*: good oral hygiene instruction relating to toothbrushing procedures and use of toothpaste with minimal abrasivity
- *Attrition*: it is impossible to prevent parafunctional activity, but the consequent damage may be minimized by providing occlusal protection
- *Erosion*: the most important step in prevention is the determination of primary aetiological factors
  - Any reflux activity
  - Dietary assessment and counselling
  - Adequate follow-up to check whether the dentition is stable or deteriorating

Clinical implications

If there has been early diagnosis of tooth wear, and preventive measures are controlling the situation, then symptoms will be minimal and treatment, therefore, should be unnecessary. There may be cases, though, where patients are not compliant with preventive measures such as wearing occlusal guards or minimizing dietary acid intake. However, the aetiological factors need to be addressed first, before proceeding with complex restorative techniques, with all the implications for expensive maintenance that these incur. The exception to this may be with vomiting bulimia patients, in whom restorations are required in order to retain any remnants of the dentition.

The effects of tooth wear that may require treatment are aesthetics, tooth sensitivity, prevention of pulp exposure, fractured teeth and restorations and, occasionally, the improvement of masticatory function.

Treatment of tooth sensitivity can be a challenging problem if tooth wear is progressing. A variety of agents that are used to treat dentine hypersensitivity is given in Table 7.6. Some dental materials are themselves more susceptible to wear than others. For example, each composite material has its own wear resistance, which is improved by increasing the inorganic filler fraction and decreased by reducing the average filler particle size. However, it should be noted that *in vitro* testing of dental materials does not always show good correlation with clinical values. Additionally, although a composite might appear to have an optimal wear rate, its filler particles may increase the wear on opposing enamel and dentine surfaces, and lead to an increasing loss of vertical dimension. Adhesive materials based on (*bis*-glycidyl-methacrylate) *bis*-GMA-resins are also susceptible to chemical dissolution and may not have good long-term survival in situations of high acidic challenge. However, restoration with composite or compomer materials may be useful as an interim treatment with progression to adhesive metal castings and porcelain veneers if necessary.

Table 7.6 Treatment for sensitive dentine

Fluoride
• mouthrinses
• varnish
• toothpastes, with or without iontophoresis* (with low abrasivity)
Copal varnishes
Potassium oxalate
Strontium chloride
Dentine-bonding agents
Sealants
Restorative techniques
• Glass ionomers
• Compomers
• Composites

*Iontophoresis—use of a small electric current to introduce sodium fluoride and/or corticosteriods into the dentinal tubules.

An extensive discussion of restorative techniques is outside the scope of this chapter, but it needs to be emphasized that treatment of tooth wear will be ineffective in the long term, unless the aetiological factors are controlled or eliminated.

Treatment of tooth wear

- Address the aetiological factors first
- If diagnosis is made early and prevention is effective, then treatment will not be necessary
- If the tooth wear is not under control, attempts at restorative treatment will fail
- Restorative treatment may be necessary for
  - aesthetics
  - tooth sensitivity (dentine hypersensitivity)
  - prevention of pulp exposure
  - loss of structural integrity
  - fractured teeth
  - fractured/failing restorations

Conclusions

Tooth wear has been a long recognized phenomenon in adults and ascribed to the triumvirate of abrasion, attrition, and erosion. The aetiology of tooth wear is multifactorial, although one type of tooth wear and one specific aetiological factor may predominate.

Pathological tooth wear is now being seen more commonly in our ageing population, who are retaining their teeth longer. It is also becoming more prevalent in a younger population, probably largely related to erosion.

Although clinical measurement of tooth wear is difficult, with no universally accepted clinical diagnostic index, there is evidence that levels are rising and certainly patients' awareness of the problem is increasing. Dental professionals world-wide need to mirror that awareness and be more vigilant.

It is essential that early diagnosis and recognition of the problem is made so that the relevant preventive measures can be instituted. The aetiological factors need to be addressed first, so that the progression of tooth wear to pain and destruction can be avoided. Preventive programmes must remain the cornerstone in the management of dental erosion.

If there has been an early diagnosis of tooth wear and preventive measures have been successfully applied, then complex restorative treatment, with all its time-consuming implications, should be unnecessary.

Manufacturers have a responsibility to ensure that their products (dentifrices, soft drinks) are minimally dentally damaging.

References

Etiology, mechanisms and implications of dental erosion (1996). *Euro. J. Oral Sci.,* 104, Part II.

Hinds, K., and Gregory, J. (1994). *National Diet and Nutrition Survey: children aged 1 to 4 years. Volume 2: report of the dental survey.* Her Majesty's Stationery Office.

Kelleher, M., and Bishop, K. (1999). Tooth surface loss: an overview. *Br. Dent. J.,* 186, 61–66.

Milosevic, A., Young, P.J., and Lennon, M.A. (1994). The prevalence of tooth wear in 14-year-old school children in Liverpool. *Comm. Dent. Hlth.,* 11, 83–86.

Millward, A., Shaw, L., and Smith, A. (1994). Dental erosion in four year old children from differing socio-economic backgrounds. *J. Dent. Child.,* 61, 263–266.

O'Brien, M. (1994). *Children's Dental Health in the United Kingdom 1993,* London: Office of Population Censuses and Surveys, HMSO.

Pindborg, J.J. (1970). *Pathology of the dental hard tissues.* Copenhagen: Munksgaard. 312–321.

Shaw, L., and Smith, A.J. (1999). Dental erosion—the problem and some practical solutions. *Br. Dent. J.,* 186, 115–118.

Smith, B.G.N., and Knight, J.K. (1984). An index for measuring the wear of teeth. *Br. Dent. J.,* 156, 435–438.

Ten Cate J.M., and Imfeld, T. (Editors) (1996). Etiology, mechanisms and implications of dental erosion. *Euro. J. Oral Sci.,* 104: Part II, 151–244.

Walker, A., Gregory, J., Bradnock, G., Nunn, J.H., and White, D. (2000). *National Diet and Nutrition Survey: young people aged 4 to 18 years.* Volume 2: Report of the oral health survey. The Stationary Office 2000.

8

The prevention and control of periodontal disease

The prevention and control of periodontal disease

Bill Jenkins and Peter Heasman

Introduction

Periodontal disease, once established, is often time-consuming and costly to treat, while untreated or unsuccessfully treated periodontal disease is a significant cause of tooth loss. Approximately 10–15% of the populations of industrialized countries are affected by generalized severe chronic periodontitis, and evidence suggests that it may often have its onset during adolescence and early adulthood. Furthermore, gingivitis, which always precedes periodontitis, is widely prevalent in children. Preventive strategies which are targeted at children, adolescents, and young adults may, therefore, reduce the need for protracted and expensive treatment of established disease.

The aims of this chapter are to describe the nature, occurrence, and distribution of periodontal disease and then to review different aspects of management: health education; professional cleaning; plaque control; and supportive periodontal care. Preventive regimes that have been applied to adults and children will also be described.

How does periodontal disease progress?

The structure of normal healthy periodontium is illustrated in Figure 8.1a. The oral epithelium is keratinized but the crevicular (sulcular) epithelium and the junctional epithelium are not. The junctional epithelium is attached to the enamel surface and underlying connective tissue by a basal lamina and hemi-desmosomes, and its free surface (from which desquamation takes place) forms the bottom of the gingival crevice. The crevice is only about 0.5 mm deep—as seen in histological section. Clinically, however, the crevice depth is considered to be the distance to which a blunt probe will penetrate and, because it will readily disrupt the fragile junctional epithelium, the probing depth of the healthy gingival crevice reaches about 2 mm.

When plaque is allowed to accumulate freely, there is an acute exudative inflammatory response within 2–4 days in the connective tissue underlying the coronal portion of junctional epithelium. After 10–21 days of persistent plaque accumulation, marked collagen destruction and a dense infiltrate of chronic inflammatory cells can be observed in this zone. The clinical

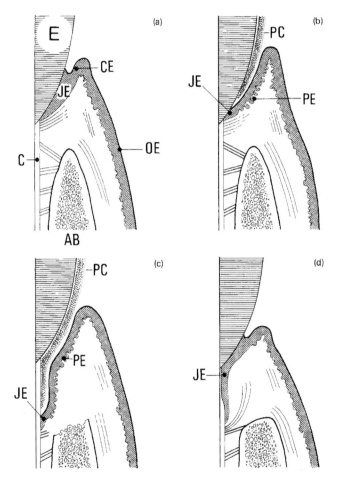

Key: AB, alveolar bone; C, cementum; CE, crevicular epithelium; E, enamel; JE, junctional epithelium; OE, oral epithelium; PC, plaque/calculus; PE, pocket epithelium

Figure 8-1 (a) Periodontal health, (b) chronic gingivitis (late phase), (c) chronic periodontitis, (d) repair following debridement.

changes of chronic gingivitis can now be detected: redness, swelling, reduced resistance to probing, and an increased tendency of the gingiva to bleed on probing or when the teeth are brushed.

Bacterial deposits do not extend below the gingival margin in the subclinical stages of developing gingivitis. The process of gingival enlargement, however, helps to create a subgingival flora and, gradually, apical advancement of subgingival plaque occurs (Fig. 8.1b) as the junctional epithelium separates from the tooth surface to become 'pocket epithelium', characterized by the formation and lateral extension of rete pegs, and by areas of micro-ulceration.

As chronic gingivitis develops, an equilibrium is usually established between the increased mass of bacteria and the host defences, maintaining a state of chronic gingivitis indefinitely. If and when periodontitis does supervene, it is thought to be precipitated either by a proportional increase in pathogenic microorganisms within the subgingival bacterial flora, by impaired host resistance, or by both factors in combination.

As soon as the destructive process extends apically to affect the alveolar bone and fibre attachment of the root surface, periodontitis is said to have developed (Fig. 8.1c). Thus, periodontitis is characterized by loss of (connective tissue) attachment. Junctional epithelium proliferates apically to maintain an epithelial barrier at the base of the deepening pocket, and the denuded cementum becomes contaminated by micro-organisms and their products. Periodontitis is detected most readily with a probe, a blood-stained or purulent exudate being elicited by probing to the base of the pocket beyond the amelo-cemental junction.

Chronic gingivitis is a condition that can be largely reversed by plaque control. On the other hand, the loss of fibre attachment, which is the principal feature of periodontitis, is virtually irreversible. Destruction may occur at a linear rate, proceeding very slowly, consistent with tooth survival, or progressing more quickly, leading eventually to tooth loss. Attachment loss may also occur at a continuous, but exponential rate. Alternatively, progression may be episodic, acute episodes being interspersed with periods of remission or repair. Different patterns of progression may affect the same site at different times, and prolonged remission may not be uncommon. Furthermore, the rate of periodontal destruction may vary at different stages of the disease, between single tooth surfaces and between individuals.

Periodontitis is treated by removal of plaque and calculus, together with pathologically altered cementum, and by establishing effective, daily plaque control. Following treatment of periodontitis, repair processes take place in which the junctional epithelium is re-established by involution of pocket epithelium, and supported by new gingival connective tissue, consisting of functionally orientated (but not tooth-attached) collagen fibres (Fig. 8.1d). More advanced lesions may not respond to treatment without surgical intervention.

Periodontal disease progression

- chronic gingivitis usually follows 10–21 days of plaque accumulation
- chronic periodontitis is always preceded by gingivitis
- chronic periodontitis is characterized by destruction of periodontal ligament and alveolar bone

Who is affected by periodontal disease?

Epidemiological studies are carried out to determine population trends in the occurrence and distribution of periodontal disease. However, the interpretation and comparison of data are fraught with difficulties. Fundamentally, there has been a lack of uniformly applied diagnostic criteria. Instead, epidemiological surveys have used a wide variety of disease markers. These include gingivitis levels, probing depths, clinical attachment level scores, and radiographically assessed alveolar bone loss, all expressed in a variety of different ways. Attachment loss with gingival recession may occur due to trauma from oral hygiene devices rather than inflammatory processes, making attachment loss on facial surfaces difficult to interpret. Partial recording systems which may not reflect full mouth conditions are commonly employed. Furthermore, there is great variation in choice of threshold values used to assign an individual subject as a 'case', that is, as suffering from periodontal disease. Finally, the periodontal disease experience of older populations with substantial tooth loss has been necessarily, but falsely, based on their surviving healthier teeth. The narrative which follows should be read with these methodological and analytical considerations in mind.

Periodontal disease in children and adolescents

This literature has been reviewed by Jenkins and Papapanou (2001) who reached the following conclusions:

- Gingivitis is common. Its prevalence, severity, and extent increase with age, beginning in the primary dentition and reaching a peak at puberty followed by a limited decline in adolescence. Lingual surfaces of molars and proximal surfaces, generally, are most frequently affected;

- The very limited data available on periodontitis in the primary dentition point to a subject prevalence of approximately 5% in children of European origin. Usually, few sites are affected and the amount of attachment loss is inconsequential;

- Very rarely, a generalized severe periodontitis may affect the primary dentition, possibly resulting in premature loss of teeth. These cases are usually associated with a major underlying systemic disorder;

- Periodontitis is common in the permanent dentition of most teenage populations, but usually only minor amounts of attachment loss or bone loss are found (see Table 8.1);

- A few teenage populations have been identified with periodontal destruction substantially beyond the 'norm'. These differences are attributed to race, ethnicity, and variation in the availability and uptake of preventive dental care;

- In both the primary and permanent dentitions, the proximal surfaces of the first molars are the sites most often affected by periodontitis and by progressive destruction;

Table 8.1 Prevalence, severity, and extent of loss of attachment on mesio-buccal surfaces of first molars, first premolars, and central incisors in 167 British teenagers examined over a 5-year period at ages 14, 16, and 19 years. (From Clerehugh et al. *Journal of Clinical Periodontology*, 17, 702–708. Published with kind permission of Blackwell Science Ltd.)

Age (years)	Loss of attachment			
	Prevalence (% subjects)		Extent (% teeth)	
	≥1 mm	=2 mm	≥1 mm	=2 mm
14	3	0	0.3	0
16	37	3	7	0.3
19	77	14	31	3.1

- A severe aggressive form of periodontitis (juvenile periodontitis) affects approximately 0.1% of white populations and up to 2.6% of black populations. Limited evidence suggests that the disease susceptibility of these subjects has its first manifestation in the primary dentition;

- At a population level, plaque and calculus deposition and levels of gingivitis and periodontitis are slightly greater in boys than in girls;

- Within the last 40 years, improvements in oral hygiene in childhood and adolescence, matched by reductions in gingivitis, have been observed in some developed countries. In others, oral hygiene has deteriorated and gingivitis levels have increased. There is no evidence of a change in the prevalence and severity of periodontitis.

Periodontal disease in adults

Gingivitis in adults is common and exists at the levels observed in older adolescents. Levels of periodontitis have been estimated from proximal radiographic bone levels and from probing attachment loss data, and, since prevalence estimates of periodontitis are a function of the criteria used for diagnosis, rates of almost 100 per cent are frequently obtained when assignment of a diagnosis of periodontitis depends on attachment loss or bone loss of only 1 mm. By selecting higher attachment loss thresholds, as shown in Table 8.2, the following is apparent:

- The prevalence and extent of clinically significant attachment loss are low in young adults and increase with age.

- Only a minority of teeth, affected by attachment loss, progress eventually to an advanced stage.

While the pattern of attachment loss demonstrated in Table 8.2 is confirmed by many other studies, the figures quoted should not be regarded as definitive, since probing was carried out only at mesio-buccal surfaces in the upper jaw and disto-lingual surfaces in the lower jaw. Such a partial recording system is likely to have underestimated both the proportion of subjects and the number of teeth affected by severe attachment loss.

Table 8.2 Prevalence, severity, and extent of loss of attachment in the United Kingdom in 1998. Adapted from the ONS survey, *Oral Health in the United Kingdom in 1998* (Walker and Cooper eds, 2000). (Reproduced with kind permission of the Controller of HMSO and the Queen's printer for Scotland.)

Loss of attachment

Age (years)	Prevalence (% subjects)		Extent (% teeth)	
	≥4 mm	≥6 mm	≥4 mm	≥6 mm
16–24	14	0	2	0
25–34	26	2	5	0
35–44	42	3	8	1
45–54	52	10	13	2
55–64	70	17	20	4
65 +	85	31	30	1

Table 8.3 Number of dentate individuals of each age and the percentage distribution according to severity of periodontal disease (From Hugoson et al. (1998) *Journal of Clinical Periodontology*, 25, 542–549.)

Age (years)	Number of dentates	Percentages Periodontal disease groups				
		1	2	3	4	5
20	100	37	63			
30	102	39	58	3		
40	93	23	44	28	3	2
50	97	10	28	40	14	7
60	83	15	17	44	18	6
70	77	4	8	5	26	7
	552	22	38	27	10	3

Although a high proportion of older people may have one or more teeth affected by advanced attachment loss, as shown in Table 8.2, a smaller proportion are affected by generalized advanced destruction as demonstrated in Table 8.3. The data for 552 dentate adult subjects, illustrated in Table 8.3, are from an epidemiological survey in 1993 of 584 randomly selected individuals, evenly distributed into age levels, from a medium-sized town in Sweden (Hugoson et al. 1998). Following a detailed clinical and radiographical examination, these individuals were assigned to one of five periodontal disease groups, according to their dominant disease characteristics:

Group 1—negligible gingivitis and no bone loss;

Group 2—gingivitis but no bone loss;

Group 3—early bone loss;

Group 4—moderately severe bone loss;

Group 5—advanced bone loss.

Table 8.3 shows that, out of the entire sample, 22% were essentially free of periodontal disease (Group 1), while a further 38% had gingivitis (Group 2). Early marginal bone loss (Group 3) affected 27%, while only 10% and 3% of the entire sample suffered from moderately severe (Group 4) and advanced bone loss (Group 5), respectively. The prevalence and severity of bone loss increased with increasing age. Early bone loss affected only 3% of 30-year-olds. Moderately severe bone loss was common only at older age levels affecting 14%, 18%, and 26% of 50-, 60-, and 70-year-olds, respectively. Advanced bone loss was not diagnosed before the age of 40 years and was uncommon at all ages thereafter.

In extrapolating the results of this Swedish study to other parts of the world, it must be remembered that these data were collected from a population with a high level of dental awareness. Nevertheless, there is good agreement with cross-sectional studies of various other adult populations that the risk of multiple tooth loss (due to generalized moderately severe or advanced bone loss) is confined to 10–15% of the whole adult population. Of course, although that statistic is widely acknowledged, it is relatively meaningless; periodontitis is a progressive disease so that, for individuals who survive into old age, there is a much higher risk of eventual tooth loss from periodontal disease.

It should also be appreciated that the assignment of each subject to one of five categories, based on the dominant disease characteristic is somewhat contrived (Table 8.3). While it is a useful means of illustrating how different amounts of periodontal disease are distributed in a population, this approach masks the considerable diversity of disease pattern in individual mouths; for example, severe gingivitis or severe periodontitis may be widespread in some mouths, but localized in others.

How common is periodontal disease?

- gingivitis is highly prevalent both in children and adults
- chronic periodontitis may be identified in teenagers
- the prevalence and severity of chronic periodontitis increase with age

Trends, outcomes, and influences

Periodontal disease trends

The changing patterns of periodontal disease prevalence over periods of time are difficult to evaluate accurately, because the methods and criteria of assessment may also vary from one study to the next. Nevertheless, data sets from successive national surveys allow some valuable observations with respect to basic disease trends to be made. For example in the UK, Children's Dental Health Surveys were undertaken in 1973, 1983, and 1993. These show that the number of children with plaque and debris on their teeth increased steadily between the ages of 5 and 8 years, reaching a plateau before decreasing slightly to the age of 15 years (Fig. 8.2a). This tendency with age is seen in all three surveys and

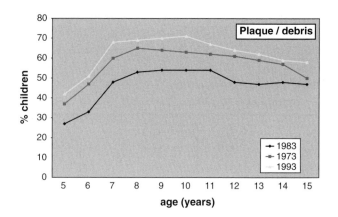

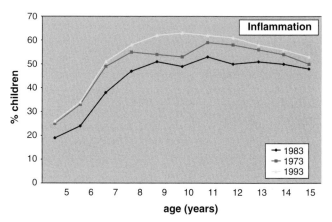

Figure 8.2 a and b Plaque debris and inflammation in children (National Surveys of Children's Dental Health, 1973, 83, and 93).

the well-recognized relationship between plaque and inflammation is also obvious (Fig. 8.2b). A very general overview of the three sets of data, however, suggests that there were more children with plaque and debris on their teeth in 1993 compared to previous years; furthermore, the age-related subject prevalence of gingivitis in children increased from 19% to peak at 53% in 1983 and from 26% to 63% in 1993. This suggests a deterioration in the gingival health of younger children over the 10 years, although the prevalence of gingival inflammation in 15-year-olds remained virtually unchanged over the same period (Fig. 8.2b).

The Adult Dental Health Surveys of 1988 and 1998 (Todd and Lader 1991, Walker and Cooper 2000) also demonstrate an interesting trend for periodontal disease in the UK. In 1988, pockets ≥ 4 mm were found in 51% of dentate adults between 16 and 24 years and in 76% of those in the 55–64 age range. In 1998, the respective figures were 34% and 62%. In 1988, pockets ≥ 6 mm were found in 2% of 16 to 24-year-olds and in 16% of 55 to 64-year-olds. In 1998, the prevalence rates had decreased to 1% and 9% respectively. It appears that at least in adults, there may have been an overall improvement in periodontal disease status between 1988 and 1998. Unfortunately, however, clinical attachment levels were measured only in the 1998 survey and so a direct comparison of the 'gold standard' for determining periodontal disease status over the 10 year period cannot be made.

Tooth mortality

There is great variation in tooth mortality statistics in different parts of the world, evidently reflecting preventive health behaviour and the availability and effectiveness of dental services. The dentist's and patient's attitude, together with technical difficulties associated with provision of treatment, may also be significant factors determining the timing of extractions. While caries and periodontal disease are the commonest reasons for adult tooth extraction, periodontal disease assumes less importance as a cause of tooth loss in populations with a high caries experience. This is illustrated by Fig. 8.3, which demonstrates that periodontal disease was a less frequent cause of extraction than caries, even in older age groups. In this Scottish study, caries and its sequelae accounted for 55% of extractions overall and periodontal disease was responsible for only 17% (McCaul *et al.* 2001).

Factors affecting the prevalence and severity of periodontal diseases

It is well established that, for gingivitis to occur and periodontitis to be initiated, plaque must be present. Indeed, there is a good correlation between standards of oral hygiene and the prevalence and severity of gingivitis. However, the absence of major differences in prevalence and extent of severe periodontitis between populations with different standards of plaque control suggests that only small amounts of plaque are required to initiate periodontitis in a susceptible patient and, once initiated, progressive destruction is largely independent of the patient's oral hygiene. It is believed, instead, that host response factors and the presence of specific pathogens within the subgingival microflora are responsible for progressive periodontitis.

Population studies have identified a variety of correlates (determinants) of periodontitis, a few of which may be risk factors, exposure to which increases the risk of disease. Thus, severe periodontitis has been positively associated with older age groups, male gender, black race, diabetes, osteoporosis, low educational status, smoking, infrequent dental attendance, and certain bacterial pathogens. Among this list of correlates, evidence for a causal role is greatest for smoking. Although some studies have shown that periodontitis is more severe in certain racial groups, it is not clear whether this association is attributable to some intrinsic effect of race, or is a function of confounding factors. Smoking, for example, could be a confounding factor in many cross-sectional studies, which have sought to link periodontitis with demographic variables. While old people have substantially more attachment loss than young people, this is thought to reflect the duration of exposure to aetiological agents, rather than the ageing process itself. Nevertheless, since biochemical and immunological processes of periodontal tissues are subject to age-associated changes, it is possible that the increased attachment loss of older people is a function of ageing as well as time.

Implications for prevention

Since gingivitis is caused by supragingival plaque accumulation, and since gingivitis is a prerequisite for the development of periodontitis, both diseases can be prevented by an adequate standard of plaque control. However, the standard of tooth cleanliness required to maintain periodontal health will be subject to great variation according to individual susceptibility. Ideally, individuals at high risk of developing the more aggressive forms of periodontitis should be singled out for priority preventive care. In the absence of reliable predictive tests, this may only be possible by repeated monitoring of regular dental attenders to identify inflammatory changes at an early and reversible stage.

Trends, outcomes, and influences

- The prevalence of gingivitis amongst 15-year-olds in the UK appears to have changed very little over the last 20 years, while tooth cleanliness has deteriorated
- The suggestion that periodontal disease rather than caries is responsible for the majority of dental extractions in older adults appears to be unfounded
- Exposure to certain factors such as diabetes and smoking increases significantly the risk of periodontal disease

What causes periodontal disease?

Dental plaque occupies the central role as the major aetiological factor in the pathogenesis of periodontal disease. It is, however, recognized that a number of factors which may predispose to

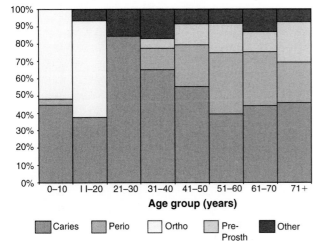

% of teeth extracted

Legend: Caries | Perio | Ortho | Pre-Prosth | Other

Age group (years)

Figure 8.3 Reasons for extraction of teeth.

plaque accumulation or which modify the host's response, also play a significant role in disease initiation and progression.

Dental plaque

Dental plaque is the non-mineralized, bacterial aggregation on the teeth and other solid structures in the mouth, which is so tenaciously adherent to the surfaces that it resists removal by salivary flow or a gentle spray of water across its surface.

Approximately 70% of the volume of plaque is composed of bacterial cells. The remainder comprises protein and extracellular polysaccharides, which act as a matrix for the cellular component. In addition, plaque contains small numbers of epithelial and white blood cells that are derived from the crevicular fluid. The exact structural, bacteriological, and biochemical composition of plaque is subject to great variation depending on: the concentration of bacteria in saliva; the site and duration of plaque formation; the nature of competitive resident flora; oxygen and nutrient availability; the composition of the diet; and the presence of periodontal disease.

The earliest deposit to form on a cleaned tooth surface is the 'acquired pellicle'. It is a structureless film of salivary glycoproteins selectively adsorbed to the surface of hydroxyapatite crystals, and is visible within minutes following a polish with pumice. The formation of pellicle is accompanied by bacterial colonization as micro-organisms in saliva adsorb to the pellicle. After 3 or 4 h a thin layer of plaque, composed mainly of Gram-positive cocci (principally streptococci) will be established. These remain the predominant micro-organisms for approximately 7 days although, during this time, there is a proportional increase in Gram-positive rods and in Gram-negative cocci and rods. After 7 days filaments, fusobacteria, and spirilla are found in greater numbers. As the plaque matures further, spirochaetes and vibrios appear, and filamentous bacteria, especially *Actinomyces,* may become predominant.

There appear to be many mechanisms for bacterial adherence: *Streptococcus sanguis* is adapted for adherence to hydroxyapatite and is among the pioneer bacteria to be found in the deepest layers of plaque; some organisms interact with salivary constituents which serve as the binding material; and the occurrence in plaque of *Streptococcus mutans* is dependent on sucrose from which it synthesizes the extracellular polysaccharides to mediate its attachment. The synthesis of surface polymers may also account for the ability of bacteria of one species to bind to one another or to bacteria of another species. Corn-cob structures, filamentous bacteria coated with cocci, represent an example of such interspecies binding. In addition to the extracellular polysaccharides, plaque contains intracellular polysaccharides in the form of storage granules synthesized from dietary sugars.

Bacteriological studies of dental plaque during the development of gingivitis suggest that there are more than 200 different species in mature plaque. Gingivitis is believed to result from quantitative changes in plaque rather than from the overgrowth of specific micro-organisms. Periodontitis is caused by the subgingival down growth of those bacteria that are best able to evade host defences

and survive in a low oxygen environment. Thus the composition of subgingival plaque differs from plaque on the adjacent visible tooth surface. For example, in subgingival plaque, Gram-positive bacteria are found in lower proportions; and Gram-negative bacteria in higher proportions than in supragingival plaque. The subgingival flora comprise a layer of tooth-attached plaque as well as a loosely adherent component in direct association with the pocket epithelium (Fig. 8.4). The tooth-attached plaque consists mainly of Gram-positive rods and cocci, while the unattached plaque consists predominantly of Gram-negative organisms including motile forms. Many different bacterial species are thought to be of significance in the aetiology of periodontal disease.

The mechanisms by which bacteria may provoke an inflammatory response and cause tissue damage are complex. Bacterial invasion of the tissues, if it occurs at all, is thought to be relatively unimportant. Instead, tissue damage is sustained mainly by penetration of the tissues by various soluble substances produced by the bacteria. These toxins have wide-ranging effects: in addition to toxic effects on host cells and enzymic degradation of tissue, chemotactic and antigenic effects occur as well as activation or suppression of inflammatory and immune mechanisms, and stimulation of bone resorption.

Dental calculus

Mineralization within plaque results in calculus formation. The inorganic content of calculus (70–90%) is mostly crystalline and amorphous calcium phosphate. The organic component includes

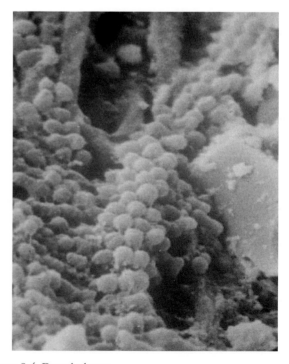

Figure 8.4 Dental plaque

protein, carbohydrates, lipid, and various non-vital micro-organisms, predominantly filamentous ones. The rate of calculus formation between individuals is very variable, and children form less calculus than adults. Calcification may commence in one-day-old plaque but the exact mechanism for calculus formation is not known. In supragingival locations, however, formation is thought to result from interactions between saliva, tooth surfaces, and plaque; whereas in subgingival locations, the inflammatory exudate within pockets is the fluid medium involved. Subgingival calculus forms more slowly and is usually more difficult to remove by virtue of the intimate relationship which it forms with the rougher root surface. Calculus itself is not causative of periodontal disease, but is always covered by plaque and retains toxic bacterial products.

Stains

Stains are caused by food substances such as tea, coffee, and red wine, by tobacco, by the products of chromogenic bacteria or by metallic particles. The pigments become absorbed by plaque or pellicle.

The cause of the problem

- In chronic periodonitis, the main challenge to the host comprises the Gram-negative, anaerobic micro-organisms
- calculus does not cause periodontal disease

Factors that increase the risk of periodontal disease

A number of factors can influence the risk of disease developing either on a site level by predisposing to local plaque accumulation, or by modifying the inflammatory response of the host.

Factors predisposing to plaque accumulation

Local accumulation and retention of plaque is enhanced by a number of well-recognized anatomical and iatrogenic (dental) factors which, therefore, may have a profound effect on periodontal health. Anatomical factors such as tooth malalignment, crowding, and tipped or rotated teeth may be very difficult to eliminate and the most appropriate treatment is to provide the patient with an effective method to improve plaque control. Iatrogenic factors, however, are often a result of poor quality dental treatment or treatment planning; and as such, are entirely preventable. Iatrogenic factors include:

- rough surfaces of restorations which accumulate plaque more readily than a well-finished or highly polished restoration (Fig. 8.5);
- overhanging or defective cervical margins of restorations which act as retention sites for dental plaque and, in particular, anaerobic periodontal pathogens;

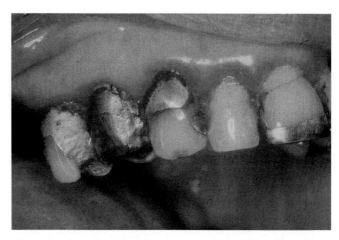

Figure 8.5 Rough surface of restoration and gingival inflammation.

- subgingival restoration margins which lead to greater plaque accumulation, and result in poorer gingival health than do restoration margins that are in level with, or remain above the gingival crest;
- removable partial dentures which often lead to an increase in the accumulation of plaque on the abutment teeth. Coverage of gingival margins may also lead to denture-induced gingival overgrowth;
- fixed orthodontic appliances, which are very difficult to keep clean and, in particular, when brackets, bands, wires, or elastics are very close to the gingival margin.

Clearly, all treatment should be carefully planned and undertaken to the highest standard in a manner which limits plaque accumulation. When partial dentures or orthodontic appliances are indicated, explicit instructions should be given with respect to their long-term care with a view to maintaining a level of plaque control that is compatible with periodontal health.

Factors modifying the inflammatory response

Host defence mechanisms appear to be both protective and destructive, but in most cases, the tissue damage sustained is minor relative to the protection provided. An intact and normal functioning host response would appear to be compatible with, at worst, slowly progressive periodontal disease. However, subtle changes in the capacity of various components of the host response to deal with the bacterial challenge may cause an increased susceptibility to periodontal disease. In addition, a number of identifiable risk factors are thought to affect the host response to local irritants, increasing the severity of periodontal disease. The most well-recognized and widely prevalent risk factors are smoking and diabetes.

Smoking

There is now unequivocal evidence to show that chronic periodontitis is two to five times more severe amongst smokers compared to non-smokers. Resolution of inflammation and long-term stability are also much less predictable following periodontal treatment in smokers, and there is a dose-dependent risk of disease recurrence during the maintenance phase. Increased in smokers, although, oral hygiene levels alone are no longer thought to be accountable for the increased severity of the disease.

Considerable research has established that nicotine may have wide ranging effects on the host's immune and inflammatory status by causing:

- vasoconstriction of the periodontal and gingival microvasculature;
- a reduction in neutrophil chemotaxis and phagocytosis;
- a reduction in the ability of neutrophils to adhere to capillary walls;
- in a dose-dependent manner, the production and release of cytokines such as interleukins, TNF_α and acute phase proteins;
- a reduction of the concentration of serum immunoglobulins, particularly in subjects with early onset periodontitis.

Diabetes

Both type 1 and type 2 diabetes increase the risk of severe periodontitis by 2–3 fold and this correlation seems to be linked to the status of diabetic control, the presence of complications and the duration of the syndrome. Poor or unstable glycaemic control leads to an increase in advanced glycated end products (AGEs), which are glucose-derived compounds that form when there is a chronic elevation in blood glucose. AGEs link with receptors on macrophages to upregulate the macrophages to release biological mediators of inflammation such as cytokines.

There is also, however, evidence to suggest that the association between diabetes and periodontal disease is a two-way process as periodontal infection increases the resistance to insulin, which induces further hyperglycaemia and thus further destabilizes glycaemic control. This implies that prevention or treatment of periodontal disease in diabetics may, in the long-term, help to stabilize glycaemic control and thus prevent further complications.

Risk factors

- Anatomical and iatrogenic factors may predispose to plaque accumulation
- In smokers and diabetics, the host's inflammatory response may be compromised significantly

Periodontal health education

Dental hygiene advice

The objective of oral hygiene education is to produce a change in behaviour, which will result in a reduction of plaque accumulation sufficient, if possible, to prevent the initiation and progression of dental caries and periodontal disease, and to make the patient as independent as possible of professional support. A successful outcome will depend not only on mastery of plaque control techniques but also on a change of behaviour and compliance with the suggested plaque control regime. Clearly, therefore, the clinician must use an educative approach aimed at changing the patient's attitude to periodontal disease and dental care, incorporating the following steps or principles:

- belief in susceptibility to the disease;
- belief that the disease is undesirable;
- belief that prevention is possible;
- belief that prevention is desirable.

Furthermore, plaque control skills must be taught using proper educational principles such as step-size advancement, self-pacing, repeated feedback, and reinforcement, as well as active participation by the patient.

Dental health education and instruction in oral hygiene are traditionally carried out by dental personnel at the chairside, but this process is labour-intensive and, with repetition, is likely to affect the mood of the instructor and, thereby, the effect of the instruction. In recent years, however, the need for oral hygiene instruction to be given at the chairside has been questioned. Self-educational programmes, comprising self-examination and instruction manuals, have been shown to be as effective as chairside instruction by dental personnel in changing oral hygiene habits.

The dental surgery has frightening overtones for many people, who then find it difficult to concentrate on advice being given. This fact alone might explain the success of self-education manuals—the freedom to assimilate information in a less hostile environment compensating for the lack of personal contact.

Regardless of the means employed, it is well known that oral hygiene instruction usually has no long-term effect unless periodically reinforced. Initial incentives for behavioural change appear to fade after the target behaviour has been achieved. According to the Committee on Oral Health Care for the Prevention and Control of Periodontal Disease (Committee Report 1966):

> Probably the most important and difficult problem that remains to be solved before much progress can be made in the prevention of periodontal disease is how to motivate the individual to follow a prescribed effective oral health-care programme throughout his life.

This remains true even today.

Improved oral hygiene alone has little effect on gingival condition, pocket depth, or subgingival flora of deep periodontal lesions. In patients with existing periodontal disease, therefore, dental health education must be supported by attention to the subgingival environment.

Dietary advice

Plaque formation is not dependent on the presence of food in the mouth. Furthermore, the effect of dietary sugars on plaque quantity in man is generally far less pronounced than could be anticipated from theoretical considerations. There is great individual variation in the amount of plaque formation, and its response to different dietary regimes. Although diet may influence the quantitative proportions of plaque micro-organisms, the clinical significance of such changes with respect to the initiation and progress of periodontal disease is not known.

The traditional concept of natural cleansing by abrasive foodstuffs is not valid. This is one example of a dental health message, popular in the past, which has little or no evidence to support it. Cervical tooth regions are not subject to much physical stress from food particles during mastication; and excessive chewing of raw vegetables and fruit has a limited effect on the quantity of plaque accumulating at these sites. Similarly, gum chewing does not have an effect at reducing plaque at the gingival margin or between the teeth.

The potential role of micro-nutrient supplements remains worthy of further consideration and research. Vitamins A, C, and E are recognized antioxidants, which have the capacity to scavenge the very powerful, host-damaging free radicals and oxygen reactive species, which are produced by the wave of neutrophils that infiltrate the tissues during periodontal disease.

Smoking cessation advice

In the UK, 70% of smokers have a desire to quit the habit. Every year 30% attempt to quit although only 2–3% are successful. There is clear evidence that advice from a general medical practitioner is a strong motivational force in getting patients to stop smoking and will achieve a quit rate of between 3 and 5%. In North America in particular, there is a growing acceptance of the responsibilities of dental health care professionals in providing advice in smoking cessation, a role which has been consolidated by the acceptance of the relationship between smoking and periodontitis. Indeed, the dental team is ideally placed to deliver smoking cessation advice to their patients; and in the UK, for example, the potential workforce to deliver such advice is considerable: 30 000 dentists; 40 000 dental nurses; 4000 dental hygienists.

The first step to adopting a successful team approach is straightforward:

- encourage all the dental team to undergo training in smoking cessation counselling;

- elect a team leader, who need not necessarily be a dentist, to co-ordinate working objectives and team strategies;

- enforce a smoke-free environment in the workplace;

- always take a full smoking history from patients;

- be prepared to assess the readiness of patients to quit.

It has been suggested that smokers fall into three categories:

Pre-contemplators—who are not interested in quitting;

Contemplators—who are interested in quitting but not ready to do so when asked;

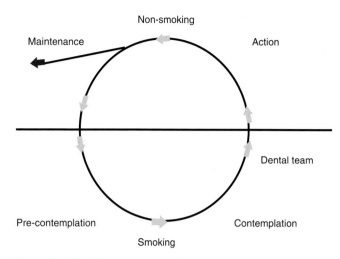

Figure 8.6 Smoking cessation cycle.

Active quitters—those who are ready to make an attempt.

Smokers are likely to move from one category to the next at any time (Fig. 8.6) and it should be the duty of any healthcare professional to be in a position to provide the necessary support when it might be needed. This support should follow the 4 'A's approach:

- ASK about smoking status and record details of the smoking history;

- ADVISE about the value of quitting, focusing on the link between smoking and periodontal disease, of which most patients are completely unaware;

- ASSIST those who wish to quit. Be willing to refer patients to their general medical practitioners, or to smoking cessation co-ordinators for further assistance if necessary. Be prepared to help patients set 'quit dates';

- ARRANGE follow-up appointments to reinforce advice and to monitor progress.

This approach, in many ways, is similar to that adopted by dentists, dental hygienists, dental therapists, and dental health educators when delivering oral hygiene advice to improve plaque control. The dental team may, therefore, be better placed than their medical counterparts to deliver a very cost-effective, healthcare message.

Advice to patients

- A change in dental hygiene behaviour must be sustained in the long-term

- Some of the established concepts linking diet and periodontal disease may be unfounded

- Smoking cessation advice must be offered to all smokers

Toothbrushing—types and techniques

Design characteristics

Design variations in toothbrushes include dimensions of the head, the length, diameter, and modulus of elasticity of the filaments and their number, distribution, and angulation. Operating efficiency may further depend on moisture content, temperature of the water used, and brushing technique. These variables confound comparison of the many investigations carried out to determine optimum toothbrush characteristics. Although current opinion favours a soft-textured, nylon, multi-tufted brush with a short head, there is no clear-cut evidence that one particular type of toothbrush is superior to others with respect to plaque removal and prevention of gingivitis. Frequent use of a hard-textured brush has been linked to gingival recession.

Toothbrushing methods

Toothbrushing methods are categorized according to the direction of the brushing stroke: (i) vertical; (ii) horizontal; (iii) roll technique; (iv) vibrating techniques (Charters, Stillman, Bass); (v) circular technique; (vi) physiological technique; (vii) scrub brush method. Comparative studies of these different methods have yielded conflicting results and each technique has its own protagonists. The Bass technique is one of the toothbrushing methods most widely recommended by dentists and hygienists. This involves placing the bristles of the brush at a 45° angle to the long axis of the teeth and vibrating the brush in an anterior–posterior direction to remove the plaque. In the general population, however, research shows that about one in three people use no definite brushing stroke, and of those who employ an identifiable stroke, almost half used the roll method.

Powered toothbrushes

There is evidence to suggest that powered toothbrushes will improve plaque control in specific patient groups: those with fixed orthodontic appliances; children and adolescents; those with a physical or learning disability; and institutionalized patients who depend upon care providers to brush their teeth. It is difficult to know whether the improvement in plaque control is due to increased efficiency in brushing, or whether it is likely to be more short-term, and due to the 'novelty effect' of brushing with a new, more exciting product.

Generally, the brush heads of powered toothbrushes tend to be more compact than those of conventional, manual brushes (Fig. 8.7). The bundles of bristles are arranged either in rows or in a circular pattern mounted in a round head. The bristles are also arranged as more compact single tufts, which facilitate interproximal cleaning and brushing in less accessible areas of the mouth. The traditional designs of brush head operate with a conventional side-to-side, arcuate or back and forth motions; whereas, the circular brush heads have oscillating, rotational, or counter-rotational movements.

A number of the newer generation powered toothbrushes also have novel design features which are aimed at further improving

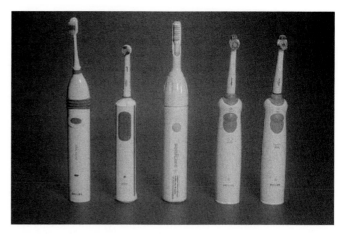

Figure 8.7 Powered toothbrushes.

the efficacy of cleaning while reducing the likelihood of gingival trauma. Such features include:

- an active brush tip to facilitate plaque control around posterior teeth;
- an orthodontic brush head for cleaning around the components of orthodontic appliances;
- rotating or spiraling filaments for improved interproximal cleaning;
- a clicking mechanism to warn when a pre-determined brushing force has been reached;
- timers, which usually indicate a brushing time of 2 min.

Toothpaste

It has long been established that brushing with a conventional fluoride toothpaste is a more effective means of plaque control than brushing with water alone. This effect may be attributed to detergents, abrasives, or the antimicrobial effect of fluoride. Nowadays, many toothpastes are formulated with more effective antimicrobial agents, which make significant contributions to plaque removal and reduction of gingivitis. Although the degree of abrasivity may not influence the amount of plaque removal achieved, the abrasive property of toothpaste keeps the pellicle layer thin and prevents the accumulation of surface stains. Toothpaste with a high dentine abrasion value may cause destructive lesions in the cervical tooth region, but the optimum degree of abrasivity, which will reduce surface pellicle without damaging tooth structure, has not been determined. Some toothpastes are now formulated with crystallization inhibitors such as soluble pyrophosphates, zinc citrate, or a polymer system (Gantrez), which have been shown to reduce supragingival calculus formation.

Cleaning between the teeth

It is well established that periodontal conditions are worst in interdental areas where standard toothbrushes are less effective at removing proximal surface plaque. Furthermore, bacterial deposits which remain after brushing will promote the regrowth of fresh plaque, and the establishment of a complex and presumably pathogenic flora on cleaned tooth surfaces may be accelerated when plaque remains on other tooth surfaces. The need for effective interdental cleaning has led to the manufacture of various devices. They should be recommended in accordance with individual dexterity and interdental anatomy.

Wood points (toothpicks)

The wood point is effective only where sufficient interdental space is available to accommodate it. Triangular wood points are superior to round or rectangular ones, which are ineffective on lingual aspects of proximal surfaces. Posterior teeth normally have wider lingual than buccal embrasures and although access is much more restricted, wood points can be fixed in a handle and inserted from the lingual side.

Dental floss

Although flossing requires more digital skill and is much more time-consuming than using wood points, there appears to be no alternative method of cleaning proximal surfaces when a normal, healthy papilla fills the interdental space. When toothbrushing is accompanied by flossing, more plaque tends to be removed from the proximal surfaces than by tooth-brushing alone (Kiger et al. 1991). Furthermore, a 2-week supervised clinical trial of patients with gingivitis, showed that interdental bleeding was reduced by about 67 per cent by flossing and brushing compared to a 35 per cent reduction achieved by toothbrushing alone (Graves et al. 1989).

There is little apparent difference in the cleaning ability of waxed and unwaxed floss, nor is there any difference between dental tape and waxed or unwaxed dental floss with regard to their effectiveness at reducing interdental gingival bleeding.

Interspace brush (single-tufted toothbrush)

This device was introduced to improve access to tipped, rotated, or displaced teeth and teeth affected by gingival recession. The combined use of the interspace brush and wood points compensates for the lack of effectiveness of wood points alone within lingual embrasures. The interspace brush is of limited value on its own at cleaning proximal surfaces except for surfaces adjacent to an extraction space.

The interdental brush (bottle brush)

Open interdental spaces are cleaned most thoroughly by the interdental brush which is manufactured in different shapes and sizes. The larger type is held by its wire handle while smaller versions are attachable to a metal or plastic handle. Studies comparing the interdental brush with dental floss have shown it to be superior in cleaning large interdental spaces and suggest that when the interdental brush is used habitually, supragingival proximal surfaces can be kept free of plaque, and subgingival plaque to a depth of 2–2.5 mm below the gingival margin may be removed.

In patients with gingivitis, swollen papillae may initially limit the choice of interdental aid to dental floss. If, however, any proximal attachment loss has occurred, the gingival recession, which will inevitably occur with treatment, should, in due course, allow interdental brushes to be used instead.

Irrigation devices

These provide a steady or pulsating stream of water escaping through a nozzle under pressure. Oral irrigators should not be used as a substitute for toothbrushing, and are time-consuming and messy to use. There is also a risk that patients using irrigation devices may believe them to be more effective than proved, and reduce their efforts in manual plaque control. Nevertheless, supragingival irrigation has a small adjunctive effect on plaque removal and gingivitis, particularly in areas of the dentition not readily accessed by conventional mechanical means. In special cases, irrigation devices may have a role in the delivery of chemical agents to the oral cavity.

Which oral hygiene aids?

- A manual toothbrush is appropriate for most people
- Powered toothbrushes may improve tooth cleaning efficiency but also have a 'novelty effect', which may diminish with time
- The selection of one or more adjunctive aids for tooth cleaning should be based upon local anatomy and the manual dexterity and compliance of the patient

Tooth-cleaning—How often should we and how often do we?

Frequency of tooth-cleaning

Plaque forms continuously and tooth surfaces cannot be maintained in a plaque-free state by conventional mechanical means. The object of plaque control in prevention of periodontal disease is, therefore, the periodic removal of accumulated plaque at intervals which are sufficiently frequent to prevent pathological effects arising from recurrent plaque formation. While the optimum frequency of tooth-cleaning is unknown, it would appear that individuals with healthy gingivae and no history of periodontal disease can prevent gingivitis by very thorough mechanical plaque removal every 48 h. On the other hand, if the prevailing standard of plaque control is less than ideal or if inflammation is already present, colonization of the cleaned tooth surface occurs much sooner, and plaque grows more rapidly and matures faster. This may be attributable to the presence of bacterial growth factors in gingival fluid, which is secreted in larger amounts by inflamed gingival tissues. Dental plaque accumulation may also increase adjacent to swollen gingival tissues due to impaired natural cleansing by the tongue, cheeks, and lips. Therefore, more frequent plaque removal may be necessary to control gingivitis, rather than prevent its onset.

Individual susceptibility to gingivitis and periodontitis may be another important factor to consider in selecting a suitable frequency of tooth cleaning. In their original experimental gingivitis model, Löe and co-workers (1965) showed that, following the first clinical signs of inflammation, the introduction of thorough oral hygiene measures, twice daily, achieved resolution of gingivitis within a few days. This was true even of the more susceptible individuals, who had developed gingivitis at an early stage of plaque accumulation. Accordingly, to achieve gingival health, the recommended interval between tooth-cleaning sessions should, in theory, depend on the expected thoroughness of cleaning, on prevailing gingival conditions and on individual susceptibility to periodontal disease. In practice, most patients are conditioned to believe in a cleaning frequency of twice daily and there would appear to be no good reason to alter that perception. In the UK, three out of every four dentate adults questioned claimed to clean their teeth at least twice a day with only 4% cleaning less than once a day. The prevalence of visible plaque, dental calculus, and primary carious lesions is greater in those subjects who brush on one or fewer occasions a day compared to twice daily brushers (Adult Dental Health Survey—Oral Health in the United Kingdom 1998).

Dental hygiene behaviour—techniques of tooth-cleaning

Fifty-two per cent of dentate adults report using dental hygiene products additional to a toothbrush and toothpaste, with dental floss being the most frequently used method. Twenty-eight per cent claim to use dental floss and 24% to use a mouthwash. All other methods of, or aids to tooth cleaning are used by between only 1 and 5% of subjects: wood points; smokers' toothpaste; disclosing tablets; interspace brush; and chewing gum. There are no data regarding interdental brushes.

Remarkably, over a third of the population do not recall having been given any advice regarding care of the 'gums' or having been shown how to brush their teeth, either by a dentist or a dental hygienist.

Facts about tooth cleaning

- 75% of adults in the UK brush 'twice a day'
- Over 50% of adults use an adjunctive method for plaque removal

Chemicals that can help to reduce plaque formation

Plaque control by mechanical debridement is highly labour-intensive, whether professionally administered or practiced personally. Satisfactory home-care further demands a measure of manual dexterity and a high degree of motivation, which many individuals do not possess. Not surprisingly, therefore, a large number of chemical agents have been tested for their ability to reduce plaque accumulation. Some chemicals act by preventing colonization of the enamel or by removing attached organisms but, on the whole, these have shown less promise than antimicrobial agents. This section will be limited to a consideration of those chemicals which have been tested as preventive agents for their effects on supragingival plaque accumulation.

Chemical antiplaque agents are assessed in several different ways: *in vitro* studies may be employed to evaluate antimicrobial action; short-term studies of a few days can assess the ability of the chemical agent to inhibit plaque formation *in vivo*; however, studies of 2–3 weeks are necessary to establish an inhibitory or therapeutic effect on gingivitis; and long-term studies of unsupervised use for several months are required to assess fully the adjunctive value of the agent when used in conjunction with toothbrushing.

In spite of the wide range of antimicrobial substances of proven effectiveness in the treatment of many different infections, the nature of dental plaque infection limits the usefulness of chemical agents. Of major significance are the apparent non-specific nature of chronic gingivitis and the proliferative capacity of oral bacteria. Therefore, while various antiseptic mouthwashes can achieve a temporary reduction in the number of bacteria in plaque, only those agents that remain active in the mouth, to exert a prolonged effect after administration, are capable of significant plaque inhibition. Thus, the cationic bisbiguanide, chlorhexidine, appears to be a much more effective plaque-inhibitor *in vivo* than other antiseptics with equal or better *in vitro* activity. Indeed, it is well established that the antiplaque effect of chlorhexidine is unsurpassed by all other chemical agents. Phenolic agents (Listerine) and triclosan are moderately effective, whereas quaternary ammonium compounds, metal salts, fluorides, sanguinarine, oxygenating agents, hexetidine, and enzymes are of little value.

Chlorhexidine

How does chlorhexidine work?

Chlorhexidine has a broad spectrum of bactericidal activity against Gram-positive and Gram-negative organisms. It was first marketed by ICI (Macclesfield, England) in 1953 as a general disinfectant for skin and mucous membranes. It is used principally in the form of chlorhexidine digluconate.

The positively charged chlorhexidine binds to bacterial cell walls and to various oral surfaces including the hydroxyapatite of tooth enamel, the organic pellicle covering the tooth surface, mucous membrane, and salivary protein. Besides acting immediately on oral bacteria, it is retained on the tooth surface to exert a prolonged bactericidal effect, and subsequently, as its concentration falls, a bacteriostatic effect for several hours. It interacts with bacteria, damaging permeability barriers and precipitating cytoplasm. The pharmacodynamics of chlorhexidine in the mouth indicate that the frequency of application should not be less than twice daily. A 0.2 per cent aqueous mouth rinse in 10 ml doses for 1 min, twice daily, has been shown to reduce the salivary bacterial count by 85–95 per cent and, essentially, to prevent plaque accumulation and gingivitis development in subjects whose habitual mechanical cleaning is suspended. Suppression of the salivary flora, however, does not appear to play a major part in dental plaque inhibition, which is primarily a result of the local antibacterial activity of chlorhexidine that is bound to tooth surface components.

How is chlorhexidine administered?

Chlorhexidine may be administered as a mouth rinse, as a toothpaste or gel, in an oral irrigator, or as a spray (Fig. 8.8). Inconvenient local side effects make it unsuitable for long-term use.

The antiplaque effects of chlorhexidine are dose-, not concentration-related. Thus, optimum plaque control is achieved by using a mouthwash with a divided daily dose of 18–20 mg; for example, 10 ml of 0.2 per cent chlorhexidine twice daily, or 15 ml of 0.12 per cent chlorhexidine twice daily. Significant, although suboptimal, effects may be obtained with reduced dosage and frequency of use, namely 15 ml of 0.2 per cent chlorhexidine once daily; 10 ml of 0.1 per cent chlorhexidine twice daily; and 15 ml of 0.1 per cent chlorhexidine once daily. In theory, those side effects, such as taste disturbance, which are concentration-dependent, should be less when using reduced concentrations of the drug, thereby leading to better compliance for long-term usage. It should be stressed that antimicrobial agents, chlorhexidine included, have little or no effect on established plaque in doses intended for inhibition of new plaque formation. Furthermore, chlorhexidine mouthwashes,

although producing a large reduction in supragingival plaque development, have a less dramatic effect on established gingivitis where subgingival plaque has already formed.

Taste disturbance can be reduced by reducing the concentration of chlorhexidine, and to achieve an effective dose; an oral irrigator can be used to deliver a larger volume, for example, 400 ml of 0.02% chlorhexidine. Indeed, by improving the distribution of chlorhexidine to the more inaccessible areas of the dentition, this use of an oral irrigator may achieve better plaque control than a 0.2 per cent mouthwash.

Many toothpaste ingredients, notably anionic detergents, will interact with, and inactivate chlorhexidine. As a result, attempts to formulate an active chlorhexidine-containing toothpaste have, on the whole, met with little success. When anionic detergents are omitted from toothpaste formulations of 1% chlorhexidine, modest reductions in plaque and gingivitis can be achieved. Staining and calculus, however, remain problematic side effects.

Aqueous gels containing 1 per cent chlorhexidine have been commercially available for many years. Clinical trials have demonstrated modest reductions in plaque and gingivitis among participants who brushed with the gel. However, the necessary absence of detergents and abrasives from gel formulations of chlorhexidine reduces patient acceptance, since there is then nothing in the product to counteract stain formation.

Although chlorhexidine gel is of little adjunctive value in individuals with moderate or good oral hygiene, it may have a greater therapeutic effect among those with high plaque levels and frank gingivitis. Chlorhexidine gel may also be applied in trays to the teeth of severely handicapped individuals, for whom conventional cleaning methods are difficult or unacceptable. The application technique can be awkward, and this is likely to reduce compliance in the long term.

Another option for those with a severe disability is a spray application of chlorhexidine solution. This has been proven to be more popular than the mouthwash or gel, although studies have shown that when a low dose (1.5–2.0 ml of 0.2 per cent solution) of chlorhexidine is applied in a spray to the teeth of handicapped children by their parents or care workers, it is less effective than gel application in trays. However, when applied under optimal conditions by dental professionals, there is a marked inhibitory effect comparable to the standard mouthwash regimen. Therefore, if sufficient professional support is provided, a spray application of chlorhexidine would appear to have some advantage over more traditional methods of chemical plaque control. Studies also show that, when teeth are targeted to receive chlorhexidine, much lower doses are required for plaque control, the proportion of drug, which becomes bound to the oral mucosa, being minimized.

Is chlorhexidine safe?

Bacteriological studies conducted after long-term use of chlorhexidine mouthwash have shown that, although the number of salivary and plaque organisms is reduced, there is

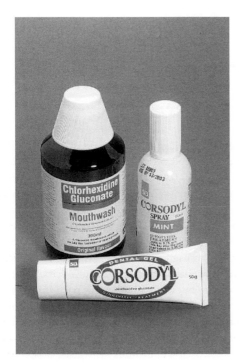

Figure 8.8

no detectable shift in microbial populations, no residual effects on salivary or plaque bacteria after cessation of rinsing and little evidence of bacterial mutation or selection of resistant strains. The total salivary bacterial counts tend to rebound to control levels within 48 h and plaque forms again at normal rates after 24 h.

Chlorhexidine is known to have low irritancy and is most unlikely to produce sensitization. Absorption after oral ingestion is very low and long-term use has produced no changes in haematological or biochemical parameters. Prolonged application has failed to show carcinogenic or teratogenic effects.

What are the side effects?

The majority of side effects are of a local nature. It has an unpleasant taste and produces disturbances in taste sensation, which may last for several hours. Desquamative lesions of the oral mucosa occur in a small number of individuals, perhaps due to precipitation of acidic mucins and proteins that cover and protect mucous membranes. This makes the epithelium vulnerable to mechanical trauma or to the cytotoxic effect of chemicals, including chlorhexidine itself. A few cases of unilateral or bilateral parotid gland swelling have been reported after use of chlorhexidine mouth rinses. The clinical features are suggestive of mechanical obstruction of the parotid duct. The unpleasant taste and mucosal effects can be diminished by reducing the concentration (and using a larger volume to maintain clinical efficacy).

Brown discolouration of teeth and fillings is common, both with mouthwash and gel preparations of chlorhexidine, a side effect which is shared with other cationic antiseptics. Brown staining of the dorsum of the tongue occurs with the mouthwash, but not with the toothpaste/gel. There is an interaction between locally adsorbed chlorhexidine and factors derived from diet such as the tannin-like substances in red wine, tea, and coffee. This interaction is responsible for the characteristic stain. There is also a tendency for more supragingival calculus to be formed, which counteracts the benefits of chlorhexidine. The mechanism for this effect may involve the suppression of acidogenic plaque bacteria and the pH at the tooth surface being raised, leading to precipitation of calcium and phosphate.

Stain and calculus formation are dose-dependent and cannot be reduced significantly without loss of antiplaque effects.

When should chlorhexidine be used?

Although the side effects are minor, their existence has placed limitations on the application of chlorhexidine to clinical practice. Nevertheless, chlorhexidine has been shown to serve a useful function in the following circumstances:

- post-operative management of periodontal wounds;
- management of desquamative forms of gingivitis—individuals with painful gingival lesions may be placed on a chlorhexidine mouthwash regimen instead of toothbrushing;
- plaque control during intermaxillary fixation;
- long-term plaque control in handicapped individuals or medically compromised patients.

Unfortunately, the success of chlorhexidine in these specific situations is not equalled by its effect on established periodontal disease. As previously noted, the standard mouthwash regimen will not remove existing supragingival plaque, or penetrate below the gingival margin to remove subgingival plaque. Indeed, it is also apparent that chlorhexidine does not penetrate the interdental space sufficiently well to have any significant effect on interdental gingivitis. Furthermore, if chlorhexidine mouthwash is used during the initial phase of hygiene therapy, it will mask the effects of personal mechanical plaque control upon which successful long-term treatment of periodontal disease is dependent, and make proper evaluation of the patient's efforts impossible. Chlorhexidine, therefore, should be reserved for prevention of plaque accumulation only where mechanical plaque removal is impracticable.

Chlorhexidine

- Chlorhexidine is the most effective method of chemical plaque control
- Chlorhexidine may be applied in different ways, most commonly as a mouthwash, a gel, or a spray

Phenolic compounds

Listerine®, a combination of the phenol-related essential oils, thymol and eucalyptol, mixed with menthol and methyl salicylate in a hydroalcoholic vehicle, is a well-established commercial mouthwash. Early studies, both short- and long-term, confirm moderate antiplaque and antigingivitis effects, with a bitter taste and occasional staining as the principal side effects. Short-term comparative studies, with chlorhexidine as a positive control, have shown listerine to be somewhat less effective. There are no data on the substantivity of Listerine.

Triclosan, another non-ionic phenol, has been a common constituent of soaps and deodorants for the last 25 years. It is a broad-spectrum antimicrobial agent of moderate activity and substantivity. It has been formulated with a copolymer (Gantrez) to improve its substantivity and 0.03 per cent triclosan/Gantrez mouthwash achieves moderate reductions in plaque and gingivitis of limited magnitude without side effects when used as a pre-brushing rinse. Being non-ionic, triclosan is compatible with toothpaste ingredients, and is now a common constituent of toothpaste in combination with other chemical substances such as Gantrez, pyrophosphate, or zinc citrate. Pyrophosphate is a weak antimicrobial agent. It has low substantivity but acts synergistically with triclosan to give an enhanced antimicrobial effect *in vitro*. Zinc, in common with other metal ions, is a highly substantive antimicrobial agent. It is formulated with citrate to reduce the metallic taste and, when combined with triclosan, exhibits synergistic action comparable *in vitro* to the triclosan/pyrophosphate combination. Gantrez, zinc salts, and pyrophosphates are also crystallization inhibitors and, by interfering with the mineralization of plaque, they reduce supragingival calculus formation. Data are available which demonstrate that the efficacy of toothpastes containing Gantrez/triclosan or zinc citrate/triclosan have modest effects as inhibitors of plaque and gingivitis, and limited evidence would suggest that the former toothpaste may also inhibit the progression of periodontitis.

It appears from numerous studies that triclosan in toothpaste does not reduce the bioavailability of fluoride or disrupt the natural microbial ecology of the mouth.

Professional cleaning

Scaling and root planing

Scaling alone is sufficient to completely remove plaque and calculus from enamel leaving a smooth clean surface. Root surfaces, however, whether supra- or subgingival, may have deposits of calculus embedded in cemental irregularities (Fig. 8.9a). A portion of cementum must, therefore, be removed to eliminate these deposits (Fig. 8.9b). Furthermore, plaque accumulation results in contamination of cementum by toxic substances, notably endotoxins. Some evidence suggests that this cementum may be biologically unacceptable to adjacent gingival tissue and should be removed by root planing, a procedure which may result in exposure of dentine. While this is not the aim of treatment, it may be unavoidable. There is little evidence that the degree of root smoothing per se is of biological importance although it

gives the best clinical indication that calculus and altered cementum have been completely removed.

Subgingival debridement should result in a sufficiently plaque-free environment to allow renewal of junctional epithelium and the epithelial attachment. The degree of subgingival root surface cleansing necessary to achieve this is likely to vary from patient-to-patient and from site-to-site. Although it is well established that non-surgical instrumentation often fails to achieve complete removal of plaque and calculus, incomplete debridement may still be compatible with clinical periodontal health in many cases. In other cases, failure to achieve complete plaque removal will allow recolonization of the root surface to take place, and inflammation to persist or recur.

Following subgingival instrumentation, good supragingival plaque control is a prerequisite for pocket healing. At sites of persistent supragingival plaque accumulation, pocket debridement has no effect on gingivitis; an initial, small reduction in probing depth is reversed within 8 weeks and the main periodontal pathogens are re-established within 4–8 weeks in the proportions observed prior to debridement.

Polishing

Polishing enamel may result in reorientation of surface crystals to create a smoother surface. However, although early experimental studies have shown that polishing to a high gloss inhibits formation of pellicle, plaque, and calculus, there is no documented evidence of periodontal health benefits from this practice. Removal of extrinsic tooth stains for cosmetic reasons, and the psychological

(a) 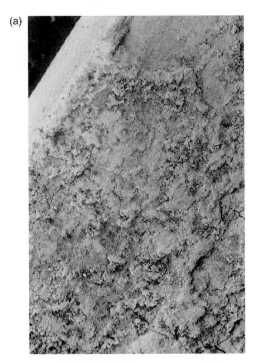 (b)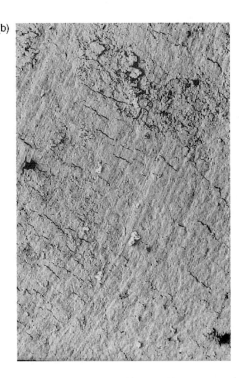

Figure 8.9 Root surfaces and calculus deposits.

effect of having clean teeth after a dental appointment may be the principal benefits of polishing, while removal of fluoride from superficial layers of the enamel could be a significant drawback. Clearly, tooth polishing cannot be supported on scientific grounds as a routine procedure, but may be indicated in special instances where plaque removal is obviously inhibited by surface roughness.

Tooth surface instrumentation

- Scaling and, if necessary, polishing should produce a smooth surface which will facilitate plaque removal for the patient
- Mechanical instrumentation of the root aims to produce a surface that is biologically acceptable to the periodontal tissues

Supportive periodontal care

When periodontal treatment is complete, the long-term stability of the periodontal tissues is achieved with a programme of supportive periodontal or maintenance care. The overall aims of supportive care are to:

- prevent the recurrence and progression of periodontal diseases;
- prevent or reduce tooth loss;
- increase the probability of diagnosing and treating, in a timely manner, other oral diseases.

In order to achieve these aims, the attainment of a high level of plaque control is essential and selective re-treatment is also often necessary to remove recurring deposits of plaque and calculus. It is customary to commence supportive care by adopting a standard approach until a degree of stability has been assessed. Then, each supportive care programme should be tailored to meet the individual's precise needs. The intervention may include reinforcement of oral hygiene instruction with either supragingival scaling, subgingival debridement or perhaps, a combination of the two regimes.

There appears to be no clear evidence to indicate what frequency of recall interval is likely to give the best long-term results, although a 3 month recall interval for patients seems to be favoured in most clinical trials and dental practice. This interval, however, appears to have evolved as a matter of convenience to both clinicians and patients rather than being based upon specific clinical and, or microbiological data. Clearly, this is an area where further research is needed to inform clinical practice.

It must be emphasized that existing periodontal disease must first be treated and optimal periodontal health established by a sustained course of treatment before scheduling a recall programme of professional cleaning. This is because a maintenance schedule comprising single-visit sessions of scaling and oral hygiene instruction at widely spaced intervals is unlikely to restore periodontal health or prevent progressive attachment loss when a significant amount of disease is present at the outset.

Supportive care

- After it has been successfully treated, periodontal disease will likely recur unless adequate plaque control is maintained
- Professional support is essential both to maintain good plaque control and intercept recurrent disease while still at an early stage

Preventive programmes—the classic studies

The components of an effective preventive programme based on plaque control are dental health education, oral hygiene instruction, and professional tooth cleaning. The relative importance of each component has been assessed in a number of classic studies predominantly in the 1960s and 1970s. These have measured various parameters of oral cleanliness and periodontal health, namely, plaque and calculus accumulation, gingival inflammation, gingival bleeding, pocket depths, attachment levels, and bone resorption. This work has been carried out both in children and adults. The discussion which follows concerns non-surgical methods of periodontal care, which have been standardized for testing on large groups of individuals. The participants were 'ordinary' members of the public rather than periodontal patients per se, and the various procedures were tested both for their effects on pre-existing periodontal disease and for their ability to prevent new or recurrent disease. Because of the 'treatment' element, these programmes cannot be solely regarded as primary prevention.

Preventive programmes in children

It is generally assumed that good oral hygiene practices are best acquired in childhood when they may be integrated with other developing health habits. Preventive programmes in schools provide continual opportunities for peer influence and the stimulating effect of daily personal interaction.

Evidence for the effectiveness of dental health education programmes in schools is equivocal, although there may be significant improvements in knowledge and attitudes, changes in behaviour, as measured by reduction in plaque and gingivitis, are usually short-lived. The 'Natural Nashers' health education programme in the UK was a large trial involving 6700 13–14-year-olds who received a teacher-mediated dental health education programme comprising three 70–80 minute sessions, at weekly intervals (Craft 1984). The programme employed active learning principles and included a slide presentation, experimental work, and use of work sheets. Improvement in plaque and gingivitis levels, while statistically significant, was small and faded considerably between the 5- and 28-week observation periods. Nevertheless, the exposure to such a dental health programme might conceivably improve the uptake of subsequent practice-based preventive care.

Supervised toothbrushing in schools is an alternative approach, which has been evaluated in several studies. For example, in a study of 12–13-year-old schoolchildren, a 3-year supervised daily brushing regimen reduced gingivitis in 56 per cent of all tooth areas examined (in the last year), whereas a control group showed a 75 per cent increase in gingivitis, typical of this stage of childhood (Lindhe *et al.* 1966).

Although supervised toothbrushing may produce an overall improvement in gingival health, a number of additional observations have been made in several studies:

- the reduction of gingivitis is often unevenly distributed within the dentition with, for example, the upper anterior part of the mouth showing greater resolution of inflammation than the posterior, less accessible areas;
- gingivitis scores tend to remain somewhat higher for proximal surfaces than for buccal and lingual surfaces;
- this type of preventive programme lacks any prolonged effect after it is withdrawn.

These limitations of supervised toothbrushing have, to some extent, been overcome in clinical trials in which dental personnel have introduced various other preventive strategies to children on an individual basis.

In 1974, Axelsson and Lindhe reported the effect of a rigorous preventive programme in school children aged initially 7–14 years. The test groups received professional tooth cleaning, oral hygiene instruction, and topical fluoride applications every 2 weeks. Parental involvement was obtained at the beginning of the study and after 1 year. The experimental group demonstrated low plaque scores and negligible signs of gingivitis after 2 years and there were no significant differences between gingivitis scores of proximal and buccal/lingual areas. Children in the control group, on the other hand, had much higher plaque and gingivitis scores. Thus, it appears that careful fortnightly interproximal cleaning with floss or polishing tips prevents gingivitis in those areas in children. Furthermore, the plaque control programme was equally effective for molars and incisors.

This study was continued for two further years. During the third year, the interval between prophylactic sessions was prolonged to 4 weeks in the younger age groups and to 8 weeks in the oldest age group and during the fourth year, all children were recalled every 8 weeks (Lindhe *et al.* 1975, Axelsson and Lindhe 1977). The excellent standard of oral hygiene was maintained during the third and fourth years and there was no significant change in gingival condition. Significant differences, however, were once again observed between test and control groups. This introductory 2-year programme of fortnightly professional tooth-cleaning and oral hygiene sessions, followed by recall at intervals of one or two months during the third and fourth years, practically eliminated all signs of gingivitis in school children.

A trial with a similar design assessed primarily the effect of preventive measures in a large group (1100) of schoolchildren between the ages of 7 and 17 years. Specially trained dental nurses administered oral hygiene instructions and professional tooth cleaning, and applied topical fluoride every third week. Over the 3-year trial period, the frequency of plaque-infected surfaces in the experimental group fell from 64.1 per cent to 29.2 per cent, and the frequency of inflamed gingival units from 41.1 per cent to 18.8 per cent. Differences between test and control groups were highly significant at re-examination (Hamp *et al.* 1978).

Further studies were designed to ascertain the separate effect of each component of the prophylactic regimen.

Poulsen *et al.* (1976) attempted to determine the benefits that might be obtained by professional tooth-cleaning alone in 78, 7-year-old children. Thus the experimental group received thorough mechanical cleaning every 2 weeks while a control group were given no professional tooth-cleaning. Both groups received fortnightly supervised fluoride rinsing. Throughout the study, home-care standards were not intentionally influenced. After 1 year, there was a statistically significant difference in plaque accumulation between the groups and an improvement in gingivitis in the test group. This study was continued for one further year during which the interval between professional tooth-cleaning sessions was increased to 3 weeks. Plaque and gingivitis scores increased in the experimental group but remained significantly lower than in the control group, where there was no appreciable change in oral cleanliness or gingival health (Agerbaek *et al.* 1978).

These studies demonstrate that the frequency of professional tooth-cleaning is of major importance when it is the only plaque control measure used, although it is difficult to assess the value of tooth-cleaning per se because the involvement of the children itself may have motivated them to practice better home care.

That the benefits of fortnightly professional tooth-cleaning cannot be attributed entirely to the repeated removal of 2-week old plaque has also been demonstrated in a later study involving 13–14-year-old children who received fortnightly professional tooth-cleaning in a split-mouth design (Axelsson and Lindhe 1981). The children were divided into two groups only one of which received oral hygiene instruction at 2-week intervals. There was an equal reduction in plaque and gingivitis in the untreated quadrants of both groups of children suggesting that the subjective impression of tooth cleanliness, as identified in the cleaned jaw quadrants of the group not receiving oral hygiene instruction, was sufficient to motivate the children towards a standard of home care that was equal to that achieved by the group which did receive oral hygiene instruction.

The fortnightly preventive programme of Axelsson and Lindhe (1974) which produced the most impressive reductions not only of gingivitis but also of caries, required about 160 min/child per year. Traditional dental treatment, for children not participating in the trial, required about 140 min/child per year and cost over twice as much as the preventive programme. Furthermore, the trial participants achieved a much better standard of dental health—gingivitis was negligible and practically no caries developed. Attempts by others to match these results have, however, been unsuccessful. Although other studies have achieved similar reductions in plaque and gingivitis, their effect on caries has not been sufficiently large to make such programmes cost-effective.

Preventive programmes in adults

From a practical standpoint, it is more important to prevent the progression of periodontitis, which is widespread in adults, than to abolish gingivitis. However, as gingivitis either precedes or accompanies destructive periodontal disease and plaque is the common aetiological agent, those measures which effect a reduction of gingivitis in children are pertinent also for adults. On the other hand, in adults, subgingival as well as supragingival deposits of plaque and calculus are common so that professional tooth-cleaning may include an element of subgingival instrumentation to treat early destructive lesions.

The success of a preventive regimen depends largely on the extent to which it will preserve attachment levels. In children, attachment loss occurs infrequently and the consequences of plaque accumulation must be measured predominantly by its effect on the gingivae. Preventive regimens in adults, however, may be assessed by comparing changes in attachment level with untreated control values.

The fundamental importance of oral hygiene instruction in preventing periodontitis was demonstrated in the 1970s when it was shown that, when scaling and polishing is unsupported by oral hygiene instruction, then gingivitis and progressive attachment loss occurs, regardless of whether the procedure is repeated annually, 6-monthly, or 3-monthly (Suomi *et al.* 1973*a*).

The need for scaling will clearly depend to a large extent on the rate of calculus formation and the presence of pathological pockets, which harbour subgingival deposits of plaque and calculus. When pockets are less than 3 mm deep, therefore, gingivitis may be substantially reduced by oral hygiene instruction alone even when abundant supragingival calculus is present. Pockets of 4–5 mm, on the other hand, will not respond to oral hygiene instruction until subgingival debridement has been performed and, once pocket depths exceed 5 mm, adequate non-surgical treatment becomes much less predictable.

The effect of a prophylactic regimen, not only on gingival health but also on attachment levels, was reported in a 3-year, classic study (Suomi *et al.* 1971*a,b*, Suomi *et al.* 1973*b*) in which a test group was given dental health education, oral hygiene instruction, and professional tooth-cleaning at 2–4 month intervals. Control subjects, who were not recruited to the preventive programme, had substantially greater plaque scores, more gingivitis, and their rate of attachment loss, at 0.1 mm/year, was more than 3½ times greater than their experimental counterparts. Furthermore, during the 3-year trial period, the experimental group showed almost no radiographic evidence of bone loss in the region studied—the lower right posterior segment—whereas the controls exhibited 0.19 mm of marginal bone destruction. Two and a half years after the experiment had been discontinued and the preventive regimen disbanded, the former experimental group continued to demonstrate cleaner teeth and better periodontal health than the former control group. Nevertheless, the difference between groups with respect to oral hygiene and gingivitis had diminished.

Another, similar 3-year study included an investigation on caries increment (Axelsson and Lindhe 1978). An experimental group of 375 adults received oral hygiene instructions and thorough scaling and root planing at the beginning of the study. These measures were repeated as necessary at 2-month intervals for the first 2 years, and at 3-month intervals during the third year. A total of 180 matched controls received only traditional dental care at yearly intervals and, during this period, demonstrated persistent gingivitis and progressive loss of periodontal attachment. The experimental group showed negligible signs of gingivitis and no loss of periodontal support.

This maintenance schedule was discontinued after 6 years. Then, during the following 9 years, the recall programme was designed to be needs-related. Thus, 65 per cent of the subjects were recalled once per year, 30 per cent twice per year, and 5 per cent (those with a recent history of progressive attachment loss) were recalled 3–6 times per year, and the low incidence of periodontal disease and caries was maintained (Axelsson *et al.* 1991). This showed that by tailoring supportive measures to individual requirements, it is possible to reduce greatly the overall professional input to a standardized preventive programme without detriment to dental or periodontal health. Furthermore, this type of study serves as a model for periodontal care; initial treatment to achieve optimum periodontal conditions, followed by a standard programme of maintenance care during which stability is assessed, ending with needs-related preventive maintenance.

In a 10-year longitudinal study, 454 Swedish shipyard workers received traditional dental care and then, for an additional 4 years they were enrolled instead on a treatment programme with a strong preventive emphasis, which included scaling and oral hygiene instruction at 3-monthly intervals (Söderholm 1979). The preventive programme reduced the proportion of tooth surfaces coated in plaque from 60 per cent to approximately 20 per cent, and the rate of periodontal bone loss from about 0.1 mm per year to zero; the rate of tooth loss was halved, at 0.1 teeth per individual per year. A cost-benefit analysis showed that traditional dental care required 2 h of 'dentist time' and 16 min of 'dental auxiliary time' per year, while the preventive programme needed 54 min of 'dentist time' and 1 h 54 min of 'dental auxiliary time' per year. Although the participants spent 32 min more per year in the dental chair during the preventive programme, their dental care cost 10–20 per cent less, because the greater proportion of dental care was performed by a dental auxiliary. Furthermore,

Prevention is better than cure

- Controlled clinical trials have shown that gingivitis in children can be reduced by oral hygiene instruction and professional tooth-cleaning

- In adults, individually-tailored, needs-related preventive care is consistent with long-term periodontal stability

- The rate of attachment loss is reduced significantly when subjects are enrolled into programmes of regular oral hygiene instruction and professional tooth-cleaning during the 4 years of prevention, the participants enjoyed a much better standard of periodontal health and an improved periodontal prognosis (Björn 1982).

Conclusions

Susceptibility to periodontal break down varies considerably both between and within individuals and potential risk factors must be assessed professionally before selecting a suitable preventive strategy. Periodontal health education must be reinforced periodically with the establishment of thorough daily interdental cleaning as a principal goal for the susceptible patient. Existing periodontal disease should be treated and periodontal health re-established before embarking on a programme of supportive periodontal care. At this stage, the interval between recall visits must also be determined by individual needs and susceptibilities. Preventive strategies, treatment of periodontal disease, and supportive care regimes may all be supplemented in certain circumstances by chemical methods of plaque control although chemical antiplaque agents should not be regarded as a convenient replacement for the more traditional, mechanical means of eliminating dental plaque.

References

Agerbaek, N., Poulsen, S., Melsen, B., and Glavind, L. (1978). Effect of professional tooth cleansing every third week on gingivitis and dental caries in children. *Commun. Dent. Oral. Epidemiol.*, 6, 40–41.

Axelsson, P., and Lindhe, J. (1974). The effect of a preventive programme on dental plaque, gingivitis, and caries in schoolchildren. *J. Clin. Periodontol.*, 1, 126–138.

Axelsson, P., and Lindhe, J. (1977). The effect of a plaque control programme on gingivitis and dental caries in schoolchildren. *J. Dent. Res.*, 56, 142–148.

Axelsson, P., and Lindhe, J. (1981). Effect of oral hygiene instruction and professional tooth cleaning on caries and gingivitis in schoolchildren. *Commun. Dent. Oral. Epidemiol.*, 9, 251–255.

Axelsson, P., Lindhe, J., and Nyström, B. (1991). On the prevention of caries and periodontal disease. Results of a 15 year longitudinal study in adults. *J. Clin. Periodontol.*, 18, 182–189.

Björn, A.-L. (1982). Economy aspects of preventive dentistry. In: *Dental Health Care in Scandinavia* (ed. A. Frandsen). pp. 217–224. Quintessence, Chicago.

Clerehugh, V., Lennon, M.A., and Worthington, H.V. (1990). 5-year results of a longitudinal study of early periodontitis in 14 to 19-year-old adolescents. *J. Clin. Periodontol.*, 17, 702–708.

Committee Report (1966). Oral Health Care for the Prevention and Control of Periodontal Disease. In: *World Workshop in Periodontics* (ed. S.P. Ramfjord, D.A. Kerr, M.M. Ash). pp. 444–453. University of Michigan Press, Ann Arbor.

Craft, M.H. (1984). Dental health education and periodontal disease: health policies, disease trends, target groups and strategies. In: *Public Health Aspects of Periodontal Disease* (ed. A. Frandsen). pp. 149–160. Quintessence, Chicago.

Graves, R.C., Disney, J.A., and Stamm, J.W. (1989). Comparative effectiveness of flossing and brushing in reducing interproximal bleeding. *J. Periodontol.*, 60, 243–247.

Hamp, S.-E., Lindhe, J., Fornell, J., Johansson, L.Å., and Karlsson, E. (1978). Effect of a field programme based on systematic plaque control on caries and gingivitis in schoolchildren after 3 years. *Commun. Dent. Oral. Epidemiol.*, 6, 17–23.

Hugoson, A., Norderyd, O., Slotte, C., and Thorstenssen, H. (1998). Distribution of periodontal disease in a Swedish adult population 1973, 1983 and 1993. *J. Clin. Periodontol.*, 25, 542–548.

Jenkins, W.M.M., Papapanou, P.N. (2001). Epidemiology of periodontal disease in children and adolescents. *Periodontology 2000*, 26, 16–32.

Kiger, R.D., Nylund, K., and Feller, R.P. (1991). A comparison of proximal plaque removal using floss and interdental brushes. *J. Clin. Periodontol.*, 18, 681–684.

Lindhe, J., Koch, G., and Månsson, J. (1966). The effect of supervised oral hygiene on the gingiva of children. *J. Periodontal. Res.*, 1, 268–275.

Lindhe, J., Axelsson, P., and Tollskog, G. (1975). Effect of proper oral hygiene on gingivitis and dental caries in Swedish schoolchildren. *Commun. Dent. Oral. Epidemiol.*, 3, 150–155.

Löe, H., Theilade, E., and Jensen, S.B. (1965). Experimental gingivitis in man. *J. Periodontol.*, 36, 177–187.

McCaul, L.K., Jenkins, W.M.M., and Kay, E.J. (2001). The reasons for extraction of permanent teeth in Scotland: a 15-year follow-up study. *Br. Dent. J.*, 190, 658–662.

O'Brien, M. (1994). Children's dental health in the United Kingdom 1993. London: The Stationery Office.

Poulsen, S., Agerbaek, N., Melsen, B., Korts, D.C., Glavind, L., and Rolla, G. (1976). The effect of professional tooth cleansing on gingivitis and dental caries in children after 1 year. *Commun. Dent. Oral. Epidemiol.*, 4, 195–199.

Söderholm, G. (1979). Effect of a dental care programme on dental health conditions. A study of employees of a Swedish shipyard. Thesis, University of Lund, Sweden.

Suomi, J.D., Greene, J.C., Vermillion, J.R., Doyle, J., Chang, J.J., and Leatherwood, E.C. (1971a). The effect of controlled oral hygiene procedures on the progression of periodontal disease in adults: results after third and final year. *J. Periodontol.*, 42, 152–160.

Suomi, J.D., West, T.D., Chang, J.J., and McClendon, B.J. (1971b). The effect of controlled oral hygiene procedures on the progression of periodontal disease in adults: radiographic findings. *J. Periodontol.*, 42, 562–564.

Suomi, J.D., Smith, L.W., Chang, J.J., and Barbano, J.P. (1973a). Study of the effect of different prophylaxis frequencies on the periodontium of young adult males. *J. Periodontol.*, 44, 406–410.

Suomi, J.D., Leatherwood, E.C., Chang, J.J. (1973b). A follow-up study of former participants in a controlled oral hygiene study. *J. Periodontol.*, 44, 662–666.

Todd, J.E. (1975). *Children's dental health in the United Kingdom 1973*. London: The Stationery Office.

Todd, J.E., and Lader, D. (1991). *Adult Dental Health 1988. United Kingdom*. London: The Stationery Office.

Todd, J.E., and Dodd, D. (1985). *Children's Dental Health in the United Kingdom 1983*. London: The Stationery Office.

Walker, A., Cooper, I. (2000). *Oral Health in the United Kingdom 1998*, London: The Stationery Office.

Additional reading

Fairbrother, K.J., and Heasman, P.A. (2000). Anti-calculus agents. *J. Clin. Periodontol.*, 27, 285–301.

Jenkins, W.M.M., and Papapanou, P.N. (2001). Epidemiology of periodontal disease in children and adolescents. *Periodontology 2000*, 26, 16–32.

Kinane, D.F., and Chestnutt, I.G. (2000). Smoking and periodontal disease. *Crit. Rev. Oral. Biol. Med.*, 11, 356–365.

Heasman, P.A., and Seymour, R.A. (1994). Pharmacological control of periodontal disease. *J. Dent.*, 22, 323–335.

Heasman, P.A. (1998). Powered toothbrushes. *Brit. Dent. J.* 184, 168–169.

Soskolne, W.A. (1998). Epidemiological and clinical aspects of periodontal diseases in diabetics. *Ann. Periodontol.* 3, 3–12.

Prevention of dental trauma

9

Prevention of dental trauma

Richard Welbury

Introduction

Dramatic improvements have been made over the last 25–30 years in our understanding of wound healing and the techniques available to treat traumatized teeth. Dr Jens Andreasen summarized some of these developments in the following way.

> The acid etch technique and composite resin restorations demanded rethinking on the part of the profession and this led to the concept of very conservative preventive restorations, tunnel preparations and the like to preserve tooth structure. Recent and on-going research into dentin bonding agents and pulpal responses to a bacteria-tight seal under dental restorations once again force us to rethink treatment strategy in order to save tooth structure and maintain pulp vitality. Recent advances in the understanding of wound healing related to dental trauma, tooth and bone transplantation and implantation have opened up new treatment avenues which for the first time make it possible to fully restore even the most severely traumatized dentition. (Andreasen 1994)

Developments have also occurred in our approach to the prevention of dental trauma. This chapter considers the epidemiology of dental trauma and ways in which it can be prevented.

Epidemiology

Trauma to children's teeth occurs quite frequently. Previous studies in the UK (Todd and Dodd 1985) suggested that the incidence of trauma to teeth was increasing, but more recent studies have indicated a fall (O'Brien 1994). It is suggested that this may be due to a more sedentary lifestyle for children with less active participation in organized sport and more recreational reliability on computer games. However, it is evident from the world literature that dental trauma is a global entity. At the age of 5 years some 31–40 per cent of boys and 16–30 per cent of girls will have suffered dental trauma. By the age of 12 years the corresponding figures are 12–33 per cent of boys and 4–19 per cent of girls. Traumatic injuries are twice as common in boys in both the permanent and the primary dentitions. The major causes of these injuries vary considerably and include accidents in and around the home, falls during normal play, injuries sustained during sport, and injuries as a direct result of violence (Table 9.1). The main 'peak periods' for dental injury are described as being between the ages of 1 and 3, and again between the ages of 7 and 10. For children under 3 years of age, who are usually both unsteady on their legs and lacking in a proper sense of caution, falls are the most common cause of injury. In school-age children, bicycle, skateboard, micro-scooters, and road accidents are the most significant factors, while in adolescence there is another, although less marked, peak largely due to sports injuries. Most of these sports injuries result from participation in contact sports such as American football, rugby, soccer, boxing, wrestling, diving or stick sports. However, other sports like skiing, skating, cycling, and horse riding, which do not necessarily involve player contact, may also place the participant at risk.

The Fédération Dentaire International (FDI) have recently classified organized sport into two categories: (1) high-risk sports that include American football, hockey, ice-hockey, lacrosse, martial sports, rugby, football, and skating; and (2) medium-risk sports that include basketball, diving, squash, gymnastics, parachuting, and waterpolo (FDI 1990). In childhood a small percentage of injuries can be attributed to violence, but once adulthood is reached, violence is a commoner cause of dental trauma than sports (Table 9.2). An iatrogenic cause of trauma, particularly in younger patients where the anterior teeth are only partially erupted and root length is not complete, is avulsion reportedly caused by excessive pressure from a laryngoscope during intubation anaesthesia.

Broadly speaking, approaches to unintentional injury prevention can be divided into education (provision of information and training), environmental change (modification of products/environment, or use of additional safety devices), and enforcement (usually through regulation or legislation).

Table 9.1 The causes of dental trauma in children in the UK (*British Dental Journal* 1989)

Causes	Percent
Falls	43
Bicycle/road accidents	35
Sports	14
Fights	3

Table 9.2 The causes of dental trauma in adults in the UK (*British Dental Journal* 1989)

Causes	Per cent
Rugby	24
Soccer	20
Cricket	20
Fights	36

As the aetiology of dental injuries is multifactorial it is difficult to institute effective empirical preventive measures. Although there is not much that can be done about asphalted primary school playgrounds, wooden gymnasia floors, or steel bicycle handlebars, it is possible to make sure that equipment in pre-school play areas and public parks is constructed to established safety guidelines. In addition, it has been shown that individuals who take part in contact sports, and those who have an increased overjet and inadequate lip coverage have an increased prevalence of dental trauma and injuries also tend to be more severe. Interestingly, a recent study showed an increased incidence of trauma in obese children compared to normal counterparts. This was said to be due to less well-developed protective reflexes while falling. It has also been suggested that sportswomen may be more susceptible than men to injury as it has not been traditional for them to wear any form of mouth protection in sports.

As with other areas of medical disease prevention, the prevention of dental injuries may be primary, secondary, or tertiary. Primary prevention is the prevention of circumstances that lead to injury. Secondary prevention is the prevention or reduction of injury severity in incidents which do happen. Tertiary prevention is the optimal treatment and rehabilitation of the injured person to minimize the impact of the injury.

Trauma to the primary dentition

- occurs commonly between the ages of 1 and 3
- is commonly caused by falls during normal play
- is twice as common in boys than girls

Primary prevention

Playground surfaces

The most common cause of tooth injury in children is falling on a hard surface. The British Standard for new play equipment for permanent installation outdoors, BS 5696 (1990), strongly recommends that any organization responsible for the purchase of play equipment should ensure that an impact-absorbing surface is provided around the items from which children are most likely to fall. Studies of accidents to children in playgrounds have shown that the majority of the more serious cases were head injuries caused through striking hard ground. Playgrounds should be all

about fun and be as safe as practically possible; however, no matter how safe the equipment or the playground's layout, there is always a risk that children will trip or stumble, run into each other or a piece of equipment, miss their footing or loose their grip, or more seriously, fall from a height. If a child falls from an item of play equipment, then he or she falls subject to the forces of gravity. This acceleration throughout a 2.5 m fall will result in a fall speed of 7 m/s or 15.7 mph at the point of ground contact. The purpose of safer surfacing in a play area is to absorb the impact of such a fall and to prevent a child suffering a head impact, which could be life threatening. The ability of a surface to absorb an impact is measured by its Critical Fall Height (CFH). British Standard 7188 (1991) gives details for CFH testing criteria as well as tests for a surface's resistance and ease of ignition. BS 7188 uses the Severity Index (SI) as a means of calculating CFH, but a new European standard for playground surfacing is currently being drafted, which will use Head Injury Criteria (HIC) as its means of calculating CFH. The test, which determines a human's tolerance to an impact SI, is based on research into road vehicle design and the NASA manned space programme. They estimated the severity of a blow to the head by mathematical integration of the area under a plot of deceleration versus time for the entire duration of the impact event (Wayne State University Curve). This curve produces a theory of 'short duration, high acceleration' tolerance. The deceleration suffered by a child's head as it is brought to a stop, and the period of time over which the deceleration acts must be considered. For brain damage not to occur, it is summated that the child's head should not be subject to a prolonged deceleration of more than 50 g.

Impact-absorbing surfaces are tested by dropping a headform representation of a child's head from a series of heights on to the surface. Accurate electronic deceleration measurements are taken during the period of impact in order to obtain the SIs for these falls, which are then plotted. A surface's CFH represents the greatest height of a head-first fall from which a child, landing on a surface, could be expected to avoid sustaining a critical head injury. The height of the curve at which the SI or HIC is 1000 represents the surface's CFH. In addition to the measurement of a surface CFH, BS 7188 also describes the measurement of four other parameters:

1. the ability of the surface to resist abrasive wear;
2. the slip resistance of the material;
3. the resistance to indentation by part landing and recovery from sustained landing; and
4. the response of the material to one particular source of ignition.

The resilient or compliant elastomeric composition of impact-absorbing surfaces is expensive. A cheaper alternative is tree bark chippings, but these have the disadvantage of needing daily raking to remove, for example, broken glass and dog faeces. In addition to consideration of the playground surface, all playground equipment should meet British Standard Safety Criteria (Fig. 9.1). Slides

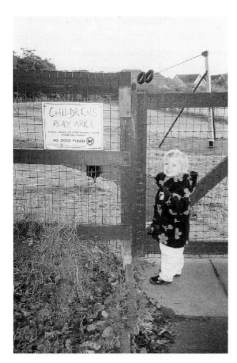

Figure 9.1 Children's playgrounds should be specially designed areas that conform to accepted safety standards.

should not be free standing, but should be built into earth mounds. Climbing frames should be no higher than 2.5 m high and built over an acceptable surface (Fig. 9.2). Supervision of small children at play (parental or professional) is very important, and probably the most effective way of preventing serious injury.

In playgrounds children should

- have equipment that conforms to British Standards
- have surfaces that conform to British Standards
- be supervised by adults

Early (mixed dentition) treatment of large overjets

In the UK, the incidence of accidental damage to permanent incisors significantly increases with overjets greater than 9 mm (Table 9.3, Fig. 9.3). Even though the proportion of children with an overjet of 7 mm or more, never exceeds 9 per cent (Table 9.4), this is still a significant number of children at high risk from traumatic injury. However, the relationship between overjet size and the concomitant risk of trauma remains unclear. A recent systematic review has shown that overjets of >3 mm may pose a significant risk for dental trauma, and there is support for including such a measurement in an orthodontic treatment index (Nyugen *et al.* 1999). However, the roles of some confounders (lip posture, sports participation, tendency for accidents) remains to be elucidated. The same authors concluded that overjet may actually play

Table 9.3 The percentage of children in the UK with accidental damage to permanent incisors by size of overjet and age (Todd and Dodd 1985)

Age (years)	Children with overjet <5 mm	Children with overjet ≥5 mm	Children with overjet ≥9 mm
8–9	10	17	7
10–11	14	31	34
12–13	22	32	45
14–15	22	39	44

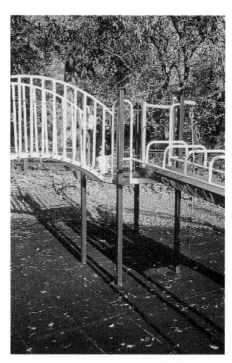

Figure 9.2 Impact-absorbing surfaces in playgrounds is essential.

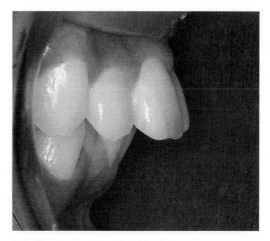

Figure 9.3 Overjet increases the risk of trauma.

Table 9.4 The percentage of children by age with an overjet of 7 mm or more in the UK in 1983 (Todd and Dodd 1985)

Age (years)	Percentage with overjet ≥ 7 mm
8–9	9
10–11	9
12–13	8
14–15	5

less of a role as a risk factor in boys, probably because the nature of their activities overrides any effect of overjet!

It should be the aim of any caring society to prevent disfigurement from loss of or damage to a permanent incisor and for this reason alone early treatment of large overjets is justified.

Orthodontic treatment in the early mixed dentition is classically carried out in uncrowded arches using functional appliances or extra oral traction. Both treatments work best during active growth and may have a favourable influence on growth in some cases. An early start to treatment does not always mean an early finish, and treatments can be prolonged. However, if treatment is done in crowded arches then it is inevitably longer and involves two stages:

1. Primary canine extraction and overjet reduction.
2. Relief of crowding in the permanent dentition by extraction followed by arch realignment with fixed orthodontic appliances.

Therefore, while it may be feasible to correct incisor oral relationship in the early mixed dentition, a number of problems may arise, and treatment should not be attempted unless there are strong indications for doing so, and certainly not without a precise orthodontic diagnosis and treatment plan (Richardson 1989).

Overjets

- predispose to dental trauma
- can be reduced in the early mixed dentition
- reduction in uncrowded arches is with functional appliances or extra oral traction
- reduction in crowded arches involves extractions in both dentitions

Provision of mouth protection in sports

Dental injuries associated with sports in British children under 15 years of age account for only 14 per cent of all injuries. The incidence in Sweden in the same age group is 25 per cent due to the popularity of ice hockey. In the majority of cases it is the front teeth of the upper jaw that are affected, and usually more than one tooth is damaged. It is rare that a dental injury heals spontaneously without treatment and such injuries in children should be considered as serious, since injuries to the teeth and jaws that are not fully developed can lead to their being adversely affected for life. The use of mouth protectors has been made mandatory by the controlling bodies of some sports in different countries. In 1962, it was made compulsory for American football players, high schools, and junior colleges, to wear mouthguards, and in 1973 mandatory for university teams by the National Collegiate Athletics Association (NCAA). In addition, in 1990 the NCAA made it mandatory for all players to wear yellow mouthguards so that they were easily visible to all players, officials, and coaching staff. In 1986, it was estimated that 2.26 per cent of all American football wounds involved injuries to the dental or facial tissues. Studies in other sports have shown a dramatic reduction in the number of dental injuries when a mouthguard was worn and their advocation by the dental profession for all persons, especially children and adolescents involved in contact sports, is justified (Fig. 9.4).

Impact to the maxilla and/or mandible during sport is usually by a direct blow from a fist, elbow, or knee. The injury patterns sustained have led to the development of mouthguards, protective helmets, and faceguards. The different functions of mouthguards are:

1. They hold the soft tissues of the lips and cheeks away from the teeth, preventing laceration or bruising of the lips and cheeks against the hard and irregular teeth during impact.
2. They cushion the teeth from direct frontal blows and redistribute the forces that would otherwise cause fracture or dislocation of anterior teeth.
3. They prevent opposing teeth from coming into violent contact, reducing the risk of tooth fracture, or damage to supporting structures.
4. They provide the mandible with resilient support, which absorbs impacts that might fracture the unsupported angle or condyle of the mandible.
5. They help prevent neurological injury by holding the jaws apart, and act as shock absorbers to prevent upward and backward displacement of the mandibular condyles against the base of the skull. Under experimental conditions they may reduce intracranial pressure and bone deformation due to impact.
6. They provide protection against neck injuries. It has been demonstrated on cephaloametric radiographs that repositioning of the mandibular condyle, cervical vertebrae, and other cervical anatomic structures takes place when a mouthguard is in place.
7. They are psychological assets to contact sport athletes.
8. They fill the space and support adjacent teeth, so that removeable prostheses can be taken out during contact sports. This prevents possible fracture of the prostheses and accidental swallowing or inhaling of the fragments.

Criteria for mouthguard construction

The FDI has listed the following criteria for constructing an effective mouthguard (FDI 1990):

- The mouthguard should be made of a resilient material which can be easily washed, cleaned, and readily disinfected.

- It should have adequate retention to remain in position during sporting activity, and allow for a normal occlusal relationship to give maximum protection.

- It should absorb and dispense the energy of a shock by: covering the maxillary dental arch; excluding interferences; reproducing the occlusal relationship; allow mouth breathing; protecting the soft tissues.

The FDI also recommends that mouthguards should, preferably, be made by dentists from an impression of the athlete's teeth.

Mouthguard design

The accepted design is based on that suggested by Turner (1977). The mouthguard is normally fitted to the maxillary arch except in Class III malocclusion. It should be close-fitting and should cover the occlusal surfaces of the teeth, except where it is anticipated that the exfoliation of primary teeth or further eruption of teeth will occur. It should extend at least as far back as the distal surface of the first permanent molar. The flanges of the mouthguard should extend beyond the gingival attachment, but short of the muco-buccal fold. The flange should be no greater than 2 mm thick over the labial mucosa to avoid stretching the lips, which could lead to them splitting on impact. The buccal edge of the flange should be smooth and rounded, and carefully relieved around the frena and muscle attachments (Fig. 9.5). The palatal aspect of the mouthguard should extend approximately 5 mm on to the palate and should be tapered to a smooth, thin, rounded edge to avoid interference with speech and breathing, or stimulation of the 'gagging' reflex. The occlusal thickness of the guard should not exceed the width of the freeway space, and should occlude evenly and comfortably with the opposing arch.

An alternative design advocated by Chapman (1985) describes a bimaxillary mouthguard that covers both arches and holds the mandible in a position that allows maximum oral air flow (Fig. 9.6). It is claimed that this design offers several advantages by allowing complete protection of the teeth, as well as the intra- and extra-oral tissues, from injury. It is also suggested that this mouthguard offers increased mandibular protection by giving it rigid support, reducing the likelihood of concussion by preventing the transmission of forces through the tempromandibular joint to the base of the skull. However, this type of mouthguard is bulky and may not be well tolerated in sports that require a lot of running and communication. Further studies are necessary to fully evaluate the design of mouthguards.

Mouthguard materials

The most commonly used material is polyvinyl acetate–poly ethylene copolymer (PVAc-PE). Polyurethane (PU) was popular, but is now less frequently used. The physical and mechanical properties of the materials vary with their chemical composition. The properties can be different with different brands of the same material, and this may be due to a variation in the degree of cross-linking between polymer chains, the proportion of plasticizer present, and the volume of the filler particle.

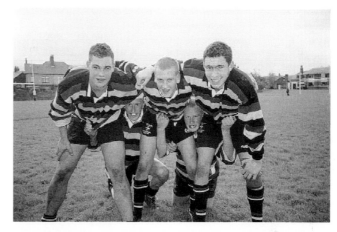

Figure 9.4 Mouthguards are essential in contact sports!

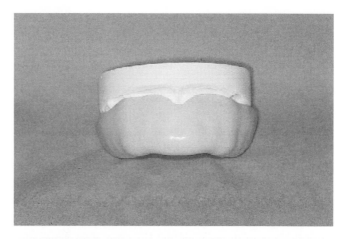

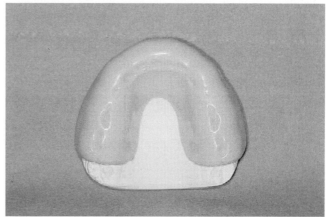

Figure 9.5 a and b Correctly extended upper mouthguard with registration of lower teeth on the occlusal surface.

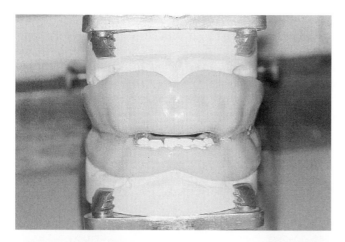
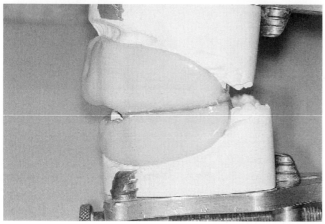

Figure 9.6 a and b Buxillary mouthguard relieved anteriorly.

Types of mouthguards

Mouthguards can be classified into three types: (1) stock, (2) mouth-formed, and (3) custom-made.

Stock

Stock mouthguards made of latex rubber or polyvinyl chloride, and available in small, medium, and large sizes were commonly used in the boxing profession. They can only be kept in place by biting the teeth together, have no inherent retentive properties, impede speech and breathing, and are a danger to the airway, especially when consciousness is impaired. There is no evidence that they are effective in redistributing forces of impact, and soft tissue injury may result from rough or sharp edges. A stock mouthguard is currently available from an orthodontic manufacturer for use while wearing a fixed appliance. It is bulky and there is no evidence that it is of any practical benefit.

Mouth-formed

Mouth-formed guards are available in two types. The first is made with a firm white outer shell of a plasticized vinyl chloride plastic in the form of a dental arch, which is filled with a soft chemo- or thermosetting acrylic resin that is adapted to the teeth. The outer shell is fitted and trimmed, if necessary, around the frenal

attachments prior to filling with soft lining and seating in the mouth. The resin sets in the mouth after 3–5 minutes and remains resilient at mouth temperature. Unfortunately, this appliance is extremely bulky and it makes normal speech virtually impossible. The margins of the outer shell may also be sharp unless protected by an adequate thickness of the lining material. The second most commonly used type of mouth-formed guard ('boil and bite' type) is constructed from a preformed thermoplastic shell of PVAc-PE copolymer or PVC that is softened in warm water, and then moulded in the mouth by the athlete using tongue and fingers. Even under professional supervision it is difficult to mould this type effectively. The temperature necessary to allow adequate adaptation for the teeth is fairly high and there is a risk of burning the mouth. In addition, if it is not centred correctly during moulding, it will be thinner in some areas, thus reducing its effectiveness.

Custom-made

Custom-made mouthguards are made by a heating-vacuum unit on dental casts poured from impressions of the player's mouth. This is the most satisfactory mouthguard in terms of acceptability and comfort to the athlete. Alginate impressions are taken of both arches together with a wax jaw registration, with the mandible in the physiological rest position. The mouthguard is constructed with an even occlusal imprint, which enables the athlete to brace the muscles of the head and neck as the teeth come into uniform contact with the mouthguard. This increases the separation between the cranial base and the condyle, and reduces the risk of brain concussion. An optimal thickness of 4.5 mm for the occlusal surface has been recommended. Proper extension of the mouthguard is very important, but all fraenum attachments must be sufficiently relieved. It should be extended just short of the mucobuccal fold and distally to cover the second molars (Fig. 9.5). The edges should be smoothed with a polishing stone, and flamed with an alcohol torch on the cast prior to placement in the mouth.

Hoffman et al. (1999) describe a 'heavy pro' custom-made mouthguard that has a 0.8 mm hard plastic layer (covering the facial gingiva, facial aspect of crowns and incisal edges of the anterior six teeth), which is sandwiched between two layers of PVAc-PE copolymer. This type of custom-made guard performed best after *in vitro* studies comparing it with two 'boil and bite' guards, and light, medium, and heavy custom-made guards. The guards were placed on a specially constructed dentoform that recorded: projectile impact at the incisal edge; projectile impact at the marginal gingiva; transmission of force from the central incisor to the lateral incisor; force transmission to the canines; force transmission to the second molars. Forces of 250, 350, and 500 N were tested five times for each guard. The 'boil and bite' guards offered the least protection compared to the custom-made guards.

Care of mouthguards

Bacteriological studies have led to the recommendation that mouthguards should: (a) be washed with soap and water immediately after use, (b) be dried thoroughly and stored in a perforated box, and (c) be rinsed in mouthwash or mild antiseptic (e.g. 0.2 per cent chlorhexidine) immediately before use again. Practically, most dentists would advise that the mouthguard be thoroughly rinsed after use and stored in a sturdy identifiable container.

Life of mouthguards

A mouthguard constructed for a child in the mixed dentition, and up until about 15 years old, may need to be renewed once a year. Once the occlusion is established, there is no reason why a polyvinyl acetate–polyethylene mouthguard, if well looked after, should not last for between two and three years.

Mouthguards

- give essential protection in all contact sports
- should be custom-made for retention, comfort, and safety
- may involve a bimaxillary design

Special considerations in mouthguard design

Partially dentate athletes should not wear removable prostheses while participating in sports, in order to prevent injury or aspiration of fragments if the appliance were to fracture. Occlusal rims may be constructed on a thermoplastic base to replace the missing teeth.

Athletes undergoing fixed orthodontic treatment can have a mouthguard constructed provided that the brackets and arch wires are covered with wax prior to taking an impression. Care should be taken not to place the lips or other soft tissues under tension by making the mouthguard too thick. While the design of mouthguards and the materials from which they are made need further investigation to produce more effective and inexpensive guards, there can be little doubt that evidence to date suggests that a correctly made mouthguard reduces considerably the severity of oral injuries.

Provision of mouth protection for special groups

Self-inflicted injuries have been reported in individuals who are intellectually compromised as a result of neurological damage. This may be due to brain anoxia at birth or congenital syndromes. There are a number of methods for the treatment of self-induced oral injuries, and these include processed hard acrylic splints, wire and acrylic splints, and double thickness soft vinyl mouthguards. Mouthguards have also been recommended for patients with Parkinson's disease whose involuntary movements may traumatize oral soft tissues. Comatose patients can be protected from intra-oral injury by wiring a tongue stent to the mandible. These treatments will be discussed more fully in Chapter 13.

The use of laryngoscopes during intubation anaesthesia have been associated with dental injuries. Teeth may be fractured or displaced by using the incisal edges of the anterior teeth as a fulcrum when inserting a laryngoscope, retractors or endoscopes. Mouth-formed and custom-made guards and adhesive oral bandage have been used to prevent these oral injuries.

Pre-term infants who need prolonged oral intubation may suffer long-term damage to their palates. Damage may range from inducement of cleft palates to dilaceration of primary incisor teeth. Appliances have been described which aim to protect the palatal tissue in this group of vulnerable neonates. Furthermore, now very flexible nasal tubes are used, so this problem should not occur.

Secondary prevention

Dentoalveolar trauma

Prompt intervention following accidental damage to teeth can have a secondary preventive effect by reducing the complications of trauma. The development of both the acid-etch technique, dentine bonding agents, and more recently compomer technology, where a bonded restoration can be achieved without washing and drying, means that there is no excuse for leaving exposed dentine for any length of time in coronal fractures. The recognition that non-setting calcium hydroxide is capable of allowing continued root growth and apexification in non-vital immature incisors has made both treatment and long-term prognosis more predictable for these teeth. Recently, however, a new product, Mineral Trioxide Aggregate (MTA), promises to replace the time spent achieving an apical barrier with non-setting calcium hydroxide by creating a barrier in one appointment. This would save considerable patient and operator time. The avulsed tooth is now a viable proposition, and if stored correctly and replanted soon after injury may be retained as a functioning member of the dentition with a healthy periodontal ligament for life. Even the avulsed tooth with an extra-alveolar dry time of greater than 60 min, which has had its necrotic periodontal ligament removed, may grow a new periodontal ligament with the help of Emdogain Gel. Such advances in the field of dental traumatology are exciting, and enable the clinician to retain teeth which would previously have been extracted. These advances in the diagnosis, treatment, and prognosis of dental traumatic injuries have been most significant over the last 25 years and current knowledge is essential to treat appropriately (Welbury 2001).

Traumatized teeth should be

- accurately diagnosed
- treated quickly
- treated appropriately

The role of the dental practitioner in child protection

The incidence of orofacial injuries in children who have been physically abused is in excess of 65%. In all types of abuse, the incidence of orofacial injuries which are visible to the dental practitioner is of the order of 35%. The dental practitioner may be the first professional to see or suspect abuse. Injuries may take the form of contusions and ecchymoses, abrasions and lacerations, burns, bites or dental trauma.

The following eleven points should be considered by the dentist whenever doubts or suspicions are aroused:

- Could the injury have been caused accidentally and if so how?
- Does the explanation for the injury fit the age and the clinical findings?
- If the explanation of cause is consistent with the injury, is this itself within normally acceptable limits of behaviour?
- If there has been any delay seeking advice, are there good reasons for this?
- Does the story of the accident vary?
- The nature of the relationship between parents and child.
- The child's reaction to other people.
- The child's reaction to any medical or dental examination.
- The general demeanour of the child.
- Any comments made by the child and/or parents that cause concern about the child's upbringing or life-style.
- History of previous injury.

Dental practitioners should be aware of local procedural guidelines set up by Area Child Protection Committees (ACPC's). In the UK, each area must have an ACPC by law as a result of the Children Act (1989), which came into force in 1991. Ideally each ACPC should have a dental member who will provide the local dental expertise, and the best pathways of referral for dentists will be agreed. There is published data in the United States and the UK that shows clearly that dental practitioners would prefer to speak to a dental colleague with expertise in the topic before making a referral to either social services or the medical profession. There is an apprehension to refer because of lack of training. The dental profession needs to be involved in inter-agency training in child protection issues. Without such training and an appreciation of the work of other agencies, we are likely to continue to miss opportunities to help children in need.

Tertiary prevention

Advances in dental materials science, especially in the fields of implantology and porcelain technology, has meant that injuries sustained in childhood and adolescence can be expect to be treated in early adulthood with advanced techniques that often make the original injury imperceptable to the layman's eye. In this way the impact of the original injury is significantly minimized.

Conclusions

The prevention of oral trauma and the maintenance of a healthy complete dentition for life should be the aim of any caring parent and dental practitioner. Playgrounds and play areas should be carefully designed and constructed. Young children's play should be supervised. Large overjets should be treated in the mixed dentition. Correctly fitting 'custom-made' mouthguards should be worn for contact sports. Traumatized teeth should be treated to the highest clinical standards. Local procedural guidelines for child protection should be known.

References

British Dental Journal (1989). Patient and practice newsletter, 15 April.

BS 5696. *Play equipment intended for permanent installation outdoors*. Part 1: methods of test, 1986. Amended 1990; Part 2: specification for construction and performance, 1986. Amended 1990; Part 3: code of practice for installation and maintenance, 1979. Amended 1990. British Standards Institution, London.

BS 7188. British Standard methods of test for impact absorbing playground surfaces, 1989. Amended 1991. British Standards Institution, London.

Chapman, P.J. (1985). The bimaxillary mouthguard: increase protection against orofacial and head injuries in sport. *Australian J. Sci. Med. Sport* 17: 25–29.

FDI (Fédération Dentaire Internationale) (1990). *Commission on Dental Products*. Working Party No. 7. I.D.I. World Dental Press: London.

Hoffmann, J., Alfter, G., Rudolph, N.K., and Goz, G. (1999). Experimental comparative study of various mouthguards. *Endod. Dent. Traumatol,* 15: 157–163.

Nyugen, Q.V., Bezemer, P.D., Habets, L., and Prahl-Andersen, B. (1999). A systematic review of the relationship between overjet size and traumatic dental injuries. *Eur. J. Orthod.* 21: 503–515.

O'Brien, M. (1994). *Children's Dental Health in the United Kingdom 1993*. HMSO: London.

Richardson, A. (1989). *Interceptive Orthodontics* (2nd edn) BDJ Publications: London.

Todd, J.E. and Dodd, T. (1985). *Children's Dental Health in the United Kingdom, 1983*. HMSO: London.

Turner, C.H. (1977). Mouth protectors. *Br. Dent. J.* 143: 82–86.

Welbury, R.R. (2001) Traumatic injuries to the teeth In: *Paediatric Dentistry* (2nd edn) (ed. R.R.Welbury) Oxford University Press: Oxford, UK.

Prevention of malocclusion

10

Prevention of malocclusion

Peter Gordon

Introduction

Malocclusion of the teeth is not really a disease in the way that dental caries and periodontitis are, it is more a reflection of the natural variation that occurs in any biological system. True prevention of malocclusion is difficult to envisage, as there is a strong genetic component in the make-up of most malocclusions (Mills 1978). Preventive measures may be effective in dealing with environmental factors, but are unlikely to influence the outcome in cases where the genetic background is one of the more important determining factors.

The interception and early treatment of developing malocclusions has come to be regarded as being almost synonymous with the prevention of malocclusion, but interception is, of course, early treatment of malocclusion rather than prevention. True prevention is virtually impossible, but early treatment may prevent the full expression of a malocclusion or may result in easier treatment, or less treatment. On the other hand, it sometimes results in two courses of orthodontic treatment rather than one. The decision as to whether to treat a malocclusion early rather than late has to be taken bearing in mind the likely benefit to the subject, balanced against the costs. In this review of the role of interceptive orthodontics the various situations will be considered in which interceptive or early treatment of a developing malocclusion is likely to prove helpful.

Normal development

The primary incisor teeth erupt at approximately 6 months of age (Foster and Hamilton 1969), followed by the primary first molars at approximately 12 months of age. These are followed by the primary canine teeth at around 16 months and the primary second molars at around 24 months. There are particular occlusal features that occur commonly in the primary dentition, as outlined by Friel (1954) and by Foster and Hamilton (1969). These are the presence of anthropoid spacing, mesial to the upper primary canine and distal to the lower primary canine, the presence of generalized spacing in the incisor region, and the molar teeth occluding so that the distal surfaces of the upper and lower primary second molars are in the same vertical plane. Variation in the eruption sequence of the primary teeth is relatively uncommon, though there is considerable variation in the age at which the teeth erupt into the mouth. Variation in the occlusion of the primary teeth is relatively common. Crowding of primary teeth is not usually a problem, though absence of spacing between the primary incisor teeth is a reliable indication that the permanent teeth in that area will be crowded in due course (Baume 1950, Leighton 1971). Variation in the occlusion of the molar teeth, either in the antero-posterior or the transverse plane is commonplace, but is seldom treated in the primary dentition, as it does not seem to give rise to any functional problem.

The permanent teeth start to erupt at about the age of six years (Houston et al. 1992). The first tooth to erupt is generally the lower first permanent molar, followed by the upper first molar and the lower central incisor. The upper central incisor, lower lateral incisor, and upper lateral incisor usually erupt between the ages of 7 and 9 years. The lower canine and the four first premolar teeth erupt at about the age of 10 or 11, followed by the second premolars, the upper canine, and the second permanent molars.

The distal surfaces of the second primary molar teeth guide the erupting first permanent molars into a cusp-to-cusp occlusion with their opposing teeth (i.e. 1/2 unit Class II). The permanent upper incisors are more proclined than their primary predecessors and this allows some forward repositioning of the mandible, which encourages the formation of a Class I molar occlusion (Friel 1954). The lower second primary molar is larger than the corresponding tooth in the upper arch, and when these teeth are shed, the lower first permanent molar moves mesially rather more than the upper first molar. This also encourages the establishment of a Class I molar occlusion.

The above account is very much simplified and idealized; in real life the occlusion is seldom so well organized and there are several factors, inherited and environmental, which can influence the development of the occlusion.

Aetiology of malocclusion

Skeletal factors

The skeletal pattern (i.e. the relationship of the mandible to the maxilla in the antero-posterior, transverse, and vertical dimensions) is one of the most important factors governing the presence or absence of a malocclusion of the teeth, being intimately related to both incisor overjet and overbite and to the occlusion of the teeth in the buccal segments. There are two aspects of the skeletal pattern which have to be taken into account: one is the size of the mandible, relative to the size of the maxilla; the other is the position of the mandible, relative to the maxilla. Since the latter part of the nineteenth century, clinicians and research workers have made determined efforts to influence the developing skeletal pattern. A variety of myo-functional appliances have been developed and exercises proposed, with the intention of modifying the muscular environment of the developing bones, in the hope thereby of influencing their final size and position. These determined efforts have met with some limited success. It does seem possible to modify the position of the mandible relative to the maxilla, mainly by restraining the downwards and forwards translation of the maxilla during growth, but this change in skeletal pattern occurs only to a minor extent. Even less are the alterations produced in the size of the maxilla or the mandible—these changes are barely measurable.

Myo-functional orthodontic appliances can undoubtedly influence the developing dentition, but they seem to produce their effects mainly by inducing dento-alveolar changes, rather than by modifying the underlying skeletal pattern.

Similarly, the use of extra-oral appliances to apply relatively high forces to the maxilla, during growth, can influence the position of the maxilla to a certain extent, but these forces are generally applied to the maxilla via the teeth. The teeth tend to move, under the influence of these forces, producing dento-alveolar changes, rather than any substantial modification of the underlying skeletal pattern.

The changes in occlusion produced by the use of myo-functional appliances and head-gear are achieved only with a major expenditure of time and effort. It is probably more appropriate to regard the use of these appliances as active treatment of a developing malocclusion rather than as any kind of preventive or interceptive measure.

Soft tissue form and function

Skeletal pattern is one factor that can influence the position of the teeth, but it is by no means the only factor. The dental arches and, indeed, the skeletal pattern itself, develop within a soft-tissue environment. Muscular activity in the lips, cheeks, and tongue, and in the muscles of mastication, has a profound effect on the occlusion of the teeth, influencing, as it does, the labio-lingual inclination of the anterior teeth and the development of buccal segment cross-bites (Wilmott 1984).

Sucking habits

Digit-sucking habits can cause malocclusion, though they are probably a less important cause than is perceived by the general public. The majority of young children have a sucking habit, either digit-sucking, or sucking on a dummy (Johnson and Larson 1993). The effect of this activity on the position of the teeth is very variable; in some cases a very determined habit will have no noticeable effect, in other cases the sucking habit will produce a change in the position of the teeth. The effect will vary according to what it is that is being sucked. Thumb-sucking, if only one thumb is being sucked, will tend to produce a Class II division 1 type of incisor relationship, with an asymmetric increase in the incisor overjet, produced by proclination of the upper incisors and retroclination of the lowers (Melsen et al. 1979). The incisor overbite will tend to be incomplete, and there will be a tendency towards a crossbite of the buccal segment teeth. While the child is indulging in the habit, there is a lowering of the intra-oral air pressure accompanied by a lowered tongue position (Day and Foster 1971). These are the two factors, associated with digit-sucking, that tend to produce a buccal segment crossbite. Sucking both thumbs (at the same time) will tend to produce a more symmetrical increase in incisor overjet. Finger-sucking may have less effect on the incisor overjet.

The changes produced by the sucking habit are dento-alveolar changes, the angulation of the teeth is changed with little or no impact on the underlying skeletal pattern (Larsson 1972). When the sucking habit is continued into the mixed dentition it may start to give rise to concern. If the upper incisor teeth are proclined and the lower teeth retroclined, then the lower lip may start to function behind the upper incisors, maintaining the position of the teeth after cessation of the habit. This arrangement is not self-correcting and will require a course of orthodontic treatment to re-establish a Class I incisor occlusion. If the habit is producing an obvious proclination of the upper incisors, it would be sensible to discourage the habit before the establishing of a lip-trap. Interceptive treatment of a sucking habit will only be useful in Class I cases—thumb-sucking is very often blamed for an increased incisor overjet that is really the result of an underlying Class II skeletal pattern.

Interceptive measures usually involve the provision of some sort of intra-oral appliance, together with the application of a bit of psychological pressure. The appliance may be an acrylic baseplate, retained by Adam's clasps, possibly with a bulge of acrylic in the middle of the palate. This serves as a reminder to the child that they should stop sucking their thumb and may reduce the satisfaction obtained by continuation of the habit. Psychological pressure, or encouragement, may be brought to bear by pointing out to the parent, in the presence of the child, that thumb-sucking is something that all young children do, and something that they tend to stop doing as they grow older and more mature.

Aetiology of malocclussion

- Skeletal pattern is one of the most important factors in the aetiology of malocclusion. It is very difficult to alter the skeletal pattern
- Thumb-sucking is often accused of producing an increased incisor overjet that is really the result of an underlying Class II skeletal pattern

Interceptive measures

Dento-alveolar factors, the *local* causes of malocclusion, are the causes that are most amenable to an interceptive approach. Early detection of an anomaly, followed by early treatment, can sometimes avoid the need for more complex treatment at a later date. The various factors that can adversely affect the development of an otherwise normal occlusion can be categorized according to the developmental age at which a problem becomes evident.

Primary dentition

Relatively little interceptive orthodontic treatment is carried out in the primary dentition, before the eruption of any permanent teeth. The dental arches are generally well aligned. There may be an increased incisor overjet, or a Class III incisor relationship, but these occlusal features are seldom so pronounced that they give rise to comment. Crowding of the primary dentition is usually expressed as an absence of spacing—the primary teeth are well aligned and unspaced—crowding will become evident when the permanent teeth erupt.

Early loss of a primary first molar may allow mesial drift of the second molar. This is difficult to prevent when the child is so young. The techniques employed are the same as those suggested for use in the mixed dentition, but the space maintainers have to be worn for an extended period of time. If the primary second molar is lost prior to the eruption of the permanent first molar, then it is very difficult, though not absolutely impossible, to prevent mesial movement of the unerupted permanent tooth (Fields 1999).

Early loss of a primary incisor should have little effect on the arrangement of the permanent teeth. If the primary incisors are spaced, then one would not expect much mesial movement of the teeth distal to the lost incisor. Some space closure may well take place if the primary incisors are not spaced, but it can be argued that, in this situation, the permanent incisors are already short of space and the early loss of the primary tooth has merely served to localize the pre-existing crowding of the permanent teeth.

Mixed dentition

It is in the mixed dentition that most attempts have been made to intercept the development of malocclusion, with the aim of simplifying later orthodontic treatment, or even of avoiding the need for orthodontic treatment at a later date.

Early loss of primary molar teeth

The effect, in the mixed dentition, of early loss of primary molar teeth depends on the amount of crowding in the dental arches, and on which tooth it is that has been lost (Richardson 1965). If the dentition is crowded, then the crowding tends to become apparent either in the incisor region, or else in the region of the permanent molar teeth. The cumulative size of the primary canine and molar teeth exceeds the cumulative size of the permanent canine and premolar teeth (Houston et al. 1992), so that if the primary teeth are retained until they are shed in the ordinary way

as the permanent teeth erupt, then there will be sufficient space for the permanent canine and premolar teeth. If a primary molar tooth is lost prematurely, through caries and if the teeth are crowded, the teeth adjacent to the tooth that is extracted will tend to drift into the space that has become available, reducing the amount of space available for the developing permanent canine and premolar teeth.

If a primary second molar is lost and the teeth are crowded, the first permanent molar will move forward into the space, reducing the space available for the second premolar. There may be some shift of the centre-line, with the crowded incisor teeth moving around to the side of the missing primary molar, but most of the space loss occurs by mesial movement of the first permanent molar. If a primary first molar or canine is lost and the teeth are crowded, then the permanent incisor teeth will move round to that side, resulting in a more pronounced shift of the centre-line (van der Linden 1990). There may be some forward movement of the first permanent molar, but more loss of space occurs as a result of drifting of the incisor teeth.

Balancing and compensating extractions

The shift in centre-line, which occurs when a tooth is lost on one side, in a crowded dentition, is difficult to correct once established. A balancing extraction (extracting a second tooth, on the opposite side of the same dental arch) is sometimes recommended, in crowded arches, to prevent the centre-line shift (Ball 1993). The tooth extracted to balance the first extraction is not necessarily the same tooth on the opposite side—the operator is guided in the first instance by the condition of the teeth.

If the occlusion of the buccal segment teeth is Class I, with good interdigitation of the cusps, then the loss of a tooth in one arch will allow mesial drift of the posterior teeth in that arch, on that side, leading to disruption of the buccal segment occlusion. A compensating extraction, that is the extraction of a tooth from the opposing arch, will allow both upper and lower buccal segment teeth to drift forwards together, maintaining the Class I occlusion. A compensating extraction may also be carried out in the case of the early loss of a lower first permanent molar from a dentition with a Class I occlusion, in which case the upper first molar may have no opposing tooth with which to occlude and will over-erupt.

Balancing extractions, to prevent centre-line shifts in occlusions with crowded teeth, are commonly carried out. No matter what the inter-arch relationship, centre-line discrepancies are difficult to correct once established; the prevention of a centre-line shift may prevent the need for quite comprehensive orthodontic treatment at a later stage. Compensating extractions are less frequently indicated; they are potentially useful mainly in Class I occlusions.

Serial extractions

Kjellgren (1948), proposed a treatment for crowded Class I occlusions that illustrates well the concept of balancing and compensating extractions. In the case of a crowded Class I occlusion, the occlusal problem generally becomes apparent following the eruption of the permanent lateral incisors, when it can be seen that there is insufficient space to accommodate the anterior teeth. Kjellgren suggested that the four primary canine teeth should be extracted in these cases, at around the age of eight or nine years. This would allow the four incisor teeth in each arch to move distally into the space made available by the extractions, thereby improving the alignment of these teeth. It would be anticipated that the buccal segment teeth would move mesially, to some extent, helping to close any residual space. This mesial movement would occur in both upper and lower arches, maintaining the Class I buccal segment occlusion.

The intention is to obtain good alignment of the teeth and relief of crowding by the eventual extraction of all four first premolars. Early loss of these teeth will afford the maximum opportunity for spontaneous alignment of the permanent canine teeth, and Kjellgren suggested that the four primary first molars should be extracted when their roots were approximately half resorbed, in order to encourage early eruption of the first premolars, so that they, in turn, could be extracted at the earliest possible moment.

The problem here is that there is no guarantee that the extraction of the first primary molars will lead to early eruption of the first premolars (Kerr 1980). In addition, it is unlikely that the roots of the primary molars will all be resorbing at the same rate, so the recommendation that these teeth be extracted at just the right moment, when their roots are half resorbed, is difficult to implement. Another difficulty lies in the fact that the eruption of the lower premolar occurs, on average, at approximately the same time as the eruption of the permanent canine in that arch. These teeth are competing for the same space and the canine tooth is often displaced labially, to the extent that it unlikely to align spontaneously following the extraction of the first premolar.

Serial extraction, as the technique came to be known, is not practiced nowadays in the way originally described by Kjellgren. In particular, the primary first molars are not extracted, since it has been found that these extractions confer no additional benefit. Occasionally, if these teeth are in poor condition, the primary first molars may be extracted instead of the primary canine teeth. The alignment of the permanent incisors proceeds more slowly than if the primary canines had been removed, but the final alignment will be much the same. Extraction of primary canine teeth to allow alignment of the incisors is sometimes practiced, especially if the maxillary lateral incisors are instanding, and if extractions are required in one arch, in a Class I case, then they are generally carried out in both arches. Spontaneous alignment will result in an improvement in the position of the incisors, but sometimes only to a limited extent. If perfect alignment is required, a fixed appliance will generally be necessary, once the permanent teeth have erupted.

The treatment of anterior crossbites

An anterior crossbite (one or more maxillary incisors occluding lingually to the opposing teeth) may become apparent when the incisor teeth erupt. There may be dento-alveolar factors involved in the development of this anomaly, or the crossbites may be an indication of an underlying skeletal discrepancy. Crowding, resulting in the lingual displacement of the upper lateral incisors may possibly be treated with a modified serial extraction technique. An anterior crossbite may result from the prolonged retention of a primary incisor (possibly a non-vital tooth that has failed to undergo root resorption) and the subsequent lingual deflection of the permanent tooth. In this case the prompt removal of the offending primary tooth may allow spontaneous alignment of the erupting permanent incisor, provided that the incisor overbite has not produced an occlusal lock.

Early treatment of instanding upper incisor teeth may be indicated for a variety of reasons. The inevitable occlusal interferences can lead to mandibular displacement; the opposing lower tooth or teeth are liable to move labially, producing a marked gingival recession on the labial aspect of these teeth. In addition, the labial surface of the instanding upper incisor can undergo marked attrition, with the production of a noticeable facet or 'chisel edge' incisally. Treatment usually involves proclination of the instanding tooth, probably with a removable orthodontic appliance. If it is necessary to create space in the dental arch in order to accomplish this tooth movement, then a form of serial extraction treatment will probably be needed to provide sufficient space.

There are a number of pitfalls that may prevent the successful execution of these apparently simple tooth movements. If the teeth are crowded, then the unerupted permanent canine tooth may impede labial movement of the upper lateral incisor. More often, lack of incisor overbite may prevent the establishment of a stable Class I incisor relationship. This is particularly likely if there is an underlying Class III skeletal relationship, in which case interceptive measures are unlikely to prove successful and the malocclusion is best left for definitive treatment at a later date.

The treatment of posterior crossbites

Crossbites involving posterior teeth are generally associated with a discrepancy in width of the upper and lower dental arches. In the case of a buccal crossbite, the buccal cusps of the lower teeth occlude outside the buccal cusps of the upper teeth, with the lower arch being disproportionately wide, or the upper narrow. In the case of a lingual crossbite, the buccal cusp of the lower tooth occludes lingual to the palatal cusp of the opposing upper tooth, with the upper arch wide or the lower narrow. The discrepancy in width may be dento-alveolar in origin, or it may be a sign of a skeletal discrepancy. Buccal segment crossbites may be bilateral or unilateral and the two tend to be treated differently.

Interceptive measures

- The early treatment of crowding involves the extraction of at least four primary teeth, and does not prevent the need for further treatment at a later age
- Unilateral posterior crossbites are sometimes treated in order to provide sufficient space for the anterior teeth

A unilateral buccal crossbite may be associated with a mandibular displacement. The discrepancy in arch widths produces a cusp-to-cusp transverse relationship between the dental arches when the teeth occlude in the retruded contact position. In order to achieve a better occlusion, the mandible is postured to one side when moving to the intercuspal position. This produces a normal buccal segment occlusion on one side and a buccal crossbite on the other. In such a case, if the maxillary arch were expanded in the transverse dimension until it was wide enough to accommodate the lower in the retruded contact position, then both the buccal segment crossbite and the mandibular displacement would be corrected. A narrowness of the upper arch may also be associated with lack of space for the incisor teeth, and the expansion of the upper arch may also provide sufficient space to correct this problem. Early treatment of unilateral buccal segment crossbite may be indicated in the early mixed dentition, after the eruption of the first permanent molar, when it becomes apparent that there is insufficient space for the upper incisor teeth.

This line of treatment is attractive only if the skeletal pattern is Class I, so that there is no need to correct the incisor relationship and only if the expansion will provide sufficient space for the upper incisor teeth. This can be assessed by using the space available for the lower incisor teeth as a guide to the space available for the upper incisors. If the incisor relationship requires correction, or the teeth are crowded, then an interceptive approach to correct the buccal crossbite will involve two courses of treatment rather than one. For the same reason the interceptive approach is more often indicated when the crossbite has a dento-alveolar basis rather than having its origin in the skeletal pattern. In the latter case there is likely to be some other orthodontic treatment needed at a later date, and this reduces the benefit of an interceptive approach.

Bilateral crossbites are seldom amenable to treatment at an early age. There is usually a skeletal component in the aetiology of the condition; there is often no associated mandibular displacement and, therefore, less indication for treatment. In addition, the amount of correction required is considerably greater than is the case with a unilateral crossbite and any correction is more likely to relapse. If a bilateral crossbite is treated at all, the correction is usually done as part of a comprehensive course of orthodontic treatment, rather than as an interceptive measure. In the same way, a lingual crossbite, if not due to the deflection of a single tooth by a retained primary predecessor, is generally associated with a marked Class II skeletal pattern, and is not amenable to treatment using an interceptive approach.

Permanent dentition

Planned loss of first permanent molar teeth

Haphazard loss of first permanent molar teeth can have a detrimental effect on the developing occlusion. The worst effects are usually seen in the lower arch, when mesial tipping and mesio-lingual rotation of the second molar is usually evident, with a poor contact or no contact between the second molar and the second premolar (Crabb and Rock 1971). In addition, the upper first molar can over-erupt into the space left by the extraction of the lower tooth. In the case of early loss of an upper first molar, the upper second molar will usually move mesially, rotating about its palatal root, but with relatively little tipping. If it is evident at an early age that the first permanent molars have a poor long-term prognosis, then careful planning of the timing of the extraction of these teeth can help minimize the deleterious effects.

If the first molar is lost early, before the formation of the root of the unerupted second molar, then the second molar will generally move forwards before it erupts, coming through to replace the first molar (Thilander et al. 1963). If the extraction of the first molar is delayed until the second molar is erupted or is on the point of eruption, there will be little forward movement of the second molar, which will then proceed to tip and rotate in the manner described above.

It follows, then, that the timing of the extractions should be varied according to the space requirements of the case in question. If there is no malocclusion and the first permanent molars are being extracted simply because of caries or hypoplasia, then early extraction of all four teeth, when the bifurcation of the roots of the lower second molar is just visible on a radiograph (at about the age of ten years) will allow forward movement of the unerupted second molars, which in this case is just what is wanted. If the incisor overjet is increased, or the anterior teeth are crowded, so that the space created by the extraction of the first molars is needed for the alignment of the teeth, then the extractions should be delayed. In the case of the upper arch, in such a situation, it would be prudent to delay the extraction of the first molars until after the eruption of the second molars. It would then be possible to use an orthodontic appliance, incorporating the second molars, to make best use of the space created by the extractions.

Loss of first permanent molar teeth

- Early loss of first permanent molar teeth will allow mesial movement of the second molar

- Late loss of the first molar will provide space for the correction of a malocclusion, but in the absence of crowding, the space resulting from the late loss of a lower first molar may be difficult to close

Tooth anomalies

Supernumerary teeth

Supernumerary teeth can occur anywhere in the mouth, but are particularly common in the maxillary labial segment. They are usually classified by their shape, as supplemental, conical, or tuberculate (Taylor 1972). Supplemental teeth resemble those of the normal series found in that area of the mouth—it is often difficult to determine which is the supernumerary tooth. Conical supernumerary teeth have conical crowns and are usually found in the maxillary labial segment; they are sometimes inverted and may remain unerupted, more or less indefinitely. Supplemental and conical teeth seldom interfere with the eruption of the permanent teeth of the normal series. If the supernumerary teeth erupt, the teeth are usually crowded and extractions, with or without appliance therapy, will be needed to allow alignment of the remaining teeth.

Tuberculate supernumerary teeth, which occur palatal to the developing maxillary incisors, usually the central incisors, seem to prevent the eruption of the developing permanent teeth. It is very important that the presence of these teeth is recognized at an early age. The unerupted tuberculate supernumerary teeth should be extracted, surgically, as soon as possible. It is not necessary to uncover the unerupted permanent incisors; the mucoperiosteal flap should be replaced and the incisors left to erupt spontaneously. This is what is gained by early diagnosis—if detected early, the prompt removal of the tuberculate supernumerary teeth will allow spontaneous eruption of the permanent incisors. If detected late, then removal of the supernumerary teeth is less likely to result in spontaneous eruption of the central incisors. Their subsequent surgical exposure, followed by orthodontic alignment, produces a less satisfactory result. Orthodontic extrusion of unerupted teeth tends to leave a long clinical crown, with an unsatisfactory gingival margin and reduced periodontal support.

Hypodontia

Hypodontia, when one or more of the teeth fails to develop, is a relatively common condition which is almost certainly hereditary in origin; as such, there is little scope for prevention. If we disregard missing third molars, the prevalence of which is difficult to assess, then approximately 6 per cent of people have one or more missing teeth (Grahnen 1956). Early treatment is seldom indicated, but if the teeth are crowded, then the absence of a permanent tooth will influence the decision as to which teeth are selected for extraction.

Ectopic and anomalous teeth

Malpositioned maxillary canine teeth

Malpositioned canines are a considerable nuisance, from the point of view of both the patient and the practitioner. They are difficult to treat, the treatment is lengthy and demanding in terms of co-operation on the part of the patient and in terms of technical expertise on the part of the operator. The malpositioned tooth can be left alone, or it can be extracted; it can be aligned by means of orthodontic treatment, or it can be aligned surgically. Each of these remedies has its own disadvantages. Is it possible to intercept the developing problem and, by early intervention, persuade the malpositioned canine to erupt into the correct position?

The commonest line of interceptive treatment that has been recommended is extraction of the primary canine tooth. This approach is usually justified on empirical grounds rather than scientific—clinical experience is cited as the authority rather than the results of any prospective randomized clinical trial. There

have, however, been retrospective studies that have lent support to this line of treatment (Ericson and Kurol 1988). Cases in which the primary tooth has been extracted are compared to cases in which it has not, and it is claimed that the extraction of the primary tooth has been beneficial. The treatment in these retrospective studies has never been randomized and the groups in which the primary tooth has been left *in situ* always contain cases in which the reason the primary tooth was left in place was that the permanent tooth was in a truly hopeless position and there was no prospect whatsoever of aligning it. The milder the displacement, the more likely it is that the primary tooth will have been extracted, on the grounds that the displacement of the permanent canine may be due in part to some failure of resorption of the root of the primary tooth.

The presence of a palatally displaced maxillary canine may be associated with the presence of a diminutive upper lateral incisor, or a missing lateral incisor. It would appear that the root of the lateral incisor may play some part in guiding the eruption of the developing canine. The maxillary canine teeth should be palpable in the labial sulcus from the age of ten years onwards. If these teeth are not palpable at this age, then radiographs should be taken, to determine the position of the unerupted teeth. If a permanent canine is palatally displaced to a relatively mild degree and there appears to be a lack of root resorption of the primary canine, then extraction of the primary canine would be an acceptable line of treatment, provided that it is intended eventually to align the permanent tooth. This will probably involve the use of a fixed orthodontic appliance, possibly preceded by the surgical exposure of the tooth, should it fail to erupt spontaneously. The extraction of the primary tooth will seldom result in spontaneous alignment of the unerupted, displaced canine, but may allow some improvement in its position. The extraction of the primary tooth commits the operator to a particular line of treatment at a later date. If the root of the primary tooth has not started to resorb, then the primary canine may have a better long-term prognosis than a permanent canine that has been repositioned surgically, since transplanted canine teeth tend to undergo root resorption.

Helpful interventions

- Prompt diagnosis and treatment of tuberculate supernumerary teeth is very important. They will prevent the eruption of the permanent upper central incisors

- Extraction of an upper primary canine tooth, when the permanent canine is palatally displaced, may allow some spontaneous improvement in the position of the permanent tooth

Transposition of teeth

Transposition of teeth occurs when two adjacent teeth attempt to erupt with their positions interchanged. For some reason the teeth that are usually affected are the permanent canine and first premolar in the upper arch and the permanent canine and lateral incisor in the lower arch. Once again there is little that can be done to prevent the problem; early treatment is sometimes carried out in the lower arch where the lateral incisor is usually extracted, following its ectopic eruption.

Dilaceration of incisors

Supernumerary teeth can prevent the eruption of upper central incisor teeth. Another reason these teeth may fail to erupt is that the developing tooth is dilacerated. This developmental anomaly produces an angle between the crown of the tooth and its root. This could be caused by trauma to the primary upper incisors causing their impaction; the primary teeth are driven up into the gum and displace the calcified crown of the developing permanent incisor, producing an angle between the crown of the tooth and its root, which continues to develop in its original position. The permanent tooth then fails to erupt. While this is a plausible explanation for the production of this anomaly, it has to be said that dilacerated incisors frequently develop in situations where there is absolutely no history of trauma to the primary teeth and the aetiology of the condition is quite obscure (Stewart 1978).

There is not much that can be done to prevent the dilaceration of incisors, but early diagnosis of the reason for failure of eruption of the permanent incisor will allow proper planning of any subsequent treatment. The dilacerated tooth is usually extracted, though in some cases it may be possible to align the tooth orthodontically, following its surgical exposure. This may, however, produce a disappointing result. If there is a marked bend in the root of the central incisor it may be difficult to align the tooth without interfering with the position of its neighbours.

Risk assessment

Screening

It has sometimes been suggested that children should be screened for the presence of occlusal anomalies, at about the age of ten years (Chung and Kerr 1987). The argument has been that this would expedite the early detection of these anomalies, allowing any preventive action or early treatment to be taken at the appropriate moment. The type of screening process that has usually been advocated would involve a clinical orthodontic assessment and the taking of a pan-oral radiograph. Studies of the efficacy of such a screening process have indicated that routine screening of children for occlusal anomalies would not be a cost-effective exercise (Hiles 1985). There are two reasons for this: the occlusal anomalies tend to be detected in any case, whether or not the children are screened and if an anomaly is detected as a result of the screening process, there are relatively few cases in which the child would benefit from early interceptive treatment (Popovich and Thompson, 1975, Ackermann and Proffit, 1980). In other words, the screening process does not affect the outcome in the majority of cases.

Whether or not a screening programme would result in the early detection of occlusal problems that would otherwise go un-noticed depends on the level of provision and uptake of dental

Early treatment

- Early treatment of a developing malocclusion will sometimes entail the provision of two courses of orthodontic treatment instead of one

services (Al Nimri and Richardson, 2000). If a population of children is exposed to a high level of provision of dental services, then they are likely to receive a dental examination in any case. The 'screening' for malocclusion then becomes part of that process, and is the responsibility of the examining dentist. If the level of provision of dental services, or the uptake of services is low, then the resources that could be spent on the provision of a screening programme for occlusal anomalies would probably be better directed at improving the general dental condition of the children, rather than on screening for malocclusion.

Conclusions

- It is difficult to prevent malocclusion—most of the effort that is expended on interceptive orthodontics is directed towards early treatment rather than prevention.

- Careful timing of the extraction of poor quality first permanent molars can prevent the development of local malocclusions, as can prompt extraction of retained primary teeth that are deflecting the eruption of their permanent successors.

- Early treatment of tuberculate supernumerary teeth will certainly encourage spontaneous eruption of the permanent incisors, and greatly simplify their subsequent alignment.

- There are some situations in which early orthodontic treatment may be beneficial, resulting in a simpler treatment plan or in a more rapid course of treatment, but all too often, early treatment means more treatment, extending over a longer period of time, or in the provision of two consecutive courses of treatment.

- The use of myo-functional appliances to correct developing Class II malocclusions is probably better regarded as a full-blown course of orthodontic treatment than as an interceptive measure.

- The distinction between interceptive treatment and prevention may not be helpful. The aim of both interceptive treatment and of preventive treatment should be to minimize the total amount of treatment that needs to be provided.

References

Ackerman, J.L., and Proffit, W.R. (1980). Preventive and interceptive orthodontics: a strong theory proves weak in practice. *Angle Orthod.*, **50**, 75–87.

Al Nimri, K., and Richardson, A. (2000). Interceptive orthodontics in the real world of community dentistry. *J. Paed. Dent.*, **10**, 99–108.

Ball, I.A. (1993). Balancing the extraction of primary teeth: a review. *Int. J. Paed. Dent.*, **3**, 179–185.

Baume, L.J. (1950). Physiologic tooth migration and its significance for the development of occlusion. *J. Dent. Res.*, **29**, 123.

Chung, C.K., and Kerr, W.J.S. (1987). Interceptive orthodontics: application and outcome in a demand population. *Brit. Dent. J.*, **162**, 73–76.

Crabb, J.J., and Rock, W.P. (1971). Treatment planning in relation to the first permanent molar. *Brit. Dent. J.*, **131**, 396–401.

Day, A.J.W., and Foster, T.D. (1971). An investigation into the prevalence of molar crossbite and some associated aetiological conditions. *Dent. Practit.*, **21**, 402–410.

Ericson, S., and Kurol, J. (1988). Early treatment of palatally erupting maxillary canines treated by extraction of the primary canines. *Eur. J. Orthod.*, **10**, 283–295.

Fields, H.W. (1999). Moderate nonskeletal problems. In: *Contemporary Orthodontics*, 3rd Ed., Chapter 13 (W.R. Proffit ed.). Mosby: St. Louis.

Foster, T.D., and Hamilton, M.C. (1969). Occlusion in the primary dentition. *Brit. Dent. J.*, **126**, 76–79.

Friel, S. (1954). The development of ideal occlusions of the gum pads and the teeth. *Amer. J. Orthod.*, **40**, 196.

Grahnen, H. (1956). Hypodontia in the permanent dentition. *Odont. Revy*, **7** (Suppl. 3).

Hiles, A.M. (1985). Is orthodontic screening of 9-yr-old school children cost effective? *Brit. Dent. J.*, **159**, 41–44.

Houston, W.J.B., Stephens, C.D., and Tulley, W.J. (1992). *A Textbook of Orthodontics*, 2nd Edn., (Table 3.1, p. 31 and Table 3.2, p. 37), Wright: Oxford.

Johnson, E.D., and Larson, B.E. (1993). Thumb-sucking: literature review. *J. Dent. Child.*, **60**, 385–391.

Kerr, W.J.S. (1980). The effect of the premature loss of deciduous canines and molars on the eruption of their successors. *Eur. J. Orthod.*, **2**, 123–128.

Kjellgren, B. (1948). Serial extraction as a corrective procedure in dental orthopaedic therapy. *Acta Odont. Scand.*, **8**, 17–43.

Larsson, E. (1972). Dummy- and finger-sucking habits with special attention to their significance for facial growth and occlusion. 4. Effect on facial growth and occlusion. *Sven. Tandlak. Tidskr.*, **65**, 605–634.

Leighton, B.C. (1969). The early signs of malocclusion. *Trans. Eur. Orthod. Soc.*, **45**, 353–368.

van der Linden, F.P.G.M. (1990). *Problems and Procedures in Dentofacial Orthopedics*, pp. 27–38. Quintessence: Chicago.

Melsen, S., Stensgaard, K.. and Pedersen, J. (1979). Sucking habits and their influence on swallowing pattern and prevalence of malocclusion. *Eur. J. Orthod.*, **1**, 271–280.

Mills, J.R.E. (1978). The effect of orthodontic treatment on the skeletal pattern. *Brit. J. Orthod.*, **5**, 133–143.

Popovich, F., and Thompson, G.W. (1975). Evaluation of preventive and interceptive orthodontic treatment between three and eighteen years of age. Chapt 26, J.T. Cook (ed), Transactions of the Third International Orthodontic Congress, St. Louis, C.V. Mosby.

Richardson, M.E. (1965). The relationship between the relative amount of space present in the deciduous dental arch and the rate and degree of space closure subsequent to the extraction of a decidous molar. *Dent. Practit.*, **16**, 111–118.

Stewart, D.J. (1978). Dilacerate unerupted maxillary central incisors. *Brit. Dent. J.*, **145**, 229–233.

Taylor, G.S. (1972). Characteristics of supernumerary teeth in the primary and permanent dentition. *Dent. Practit.*, **22**, 203–208.

Thilander, B., Jakobsson, S.O., and Skagius, S. (1963). Orthodontic sequelae of extraction of permanent first molars. *Scand. Dent. J.*, **71**, 380–412.

Wilmott, D.R. (1984). Thumb sucking habit and associated dental differences in one of monozygous twins. *Brit. J. Orthod.*, **11**, 195–199.

11

Prevention of oral mucosal disease

Prevention of oral mucosal disease

Crispian Scully and Anne Hegarty

Introduction

Most conditions that affect oral mucosal health are acquired, through environmental or lifestyle factors, albeit the genetic constitution may well influence the result of an onslaught by some agent such as a micro-organism. Various biological, physical, and chemical factors may act singly or in concert to cause disease, some of which is preventable. A range of infections can affect the oral mucosa, but few are more devastating than HIV, which can result in oral and other fungal, viral, or other mucosal infections, or neoplasms.

Mucosal integrity is central to protecting the mouth against infections, or insults from the environment and lifestyle. Adequate nutrition and intact immune and other defences are, in turn, central to mucosal integrity. This chapter deals with the major preventable threats to the oral mucosa in four sections. The first relates to preventing oral infections, particularly in vulnerable patients. The second deals with preventable threats from lifestyle. There then follow sections on iatrogenic disease, particularly preventing and managing mucositis (an area in which there is new evidence emerging), and on nutrition. The latter is a large and complex subject, but the role of good nutrition in preventing mucosal disease occurs at many levels.

Causes of oral mucosal diseases

- Genetic
- Environment/lifestyle
- Biological, physical, chemical factors
- Infections

Infections

The prevention of oral mucosal infections in an immunocompetent person is a relatively minor problem mostly effectively achieved by avoiding contact. Only candidiasis is really open to preventive intervention, and in some cases this may be indicated. For immunocompromised patients though, the impact of both endogenous and exogenous infections can be considerable, and the range of organisms that can cause problematic infection is large. In such cases steps to prevent infections, or to limit them, may be indicated. The most common mucosal infections are candidiasis and herpesvirus.

Oral infections in the immunocompetent person

Candidiasis

Endogenous mucosal infections are not common, except for candidiasis—especially chronic atrophic candidiasis (denture-related stomatitis). Candidiasis is predisposed to by xerostomia, the use of antibiotics, and the use of corticosteroids. Denture-related stomatitis presents as chronic mucosal erythema beneath an upper denture, mainly full dentures. It is most common in the elderly, especially females, and particularly if dentures are worn at night. The earliest lesions are pinpoint areas of hyperaemia, which progress to diffuse uniform erythema of the hard palate, not extending beyond the limits of the denture-bearing area. Few patients have soreness unless there is also angular cheilitis. *Candida albicans* may be implicated and *Candida* species colonize the fitting surface of the denture. Removal of the denture plaque usually leads to resolution of the stomatitis.

It is unclear why only some denture wearers get chronic atrophic candidiasis since *C. albicans* is a common oral commensal. Factors that may be important include the local environment beneath a denture, diet, the spectrum or type of other organisms in denture plaque, and the host immune and other defences. Trauma may sometimes contribute to a small extent, but hypotheses such as allergy to denture materials have been discounted.

Denture-related stomatitis usually resolves, or can be prevented, if the dentures are left out of the mouth at night, plaque is removed by brushing, and the dentures disinfected. Yeast lytic enzymes and proteolytic enzymes are the most effective agents against candida. Denture-soaking solution containing benzoic acid completely eradicates *C. albicans* from the denture surface as it is taken up into the acrylic resin and eliminates the organism from the internal surface of the prosthesis. Chlorhexidine gluconate is an effective disinfectant. A solution of at least 0.12% chlorhexidine gluconate can eliminate *C. albicans* on the acrylic resin surface of the denture, and reduce palatal inflammation. A protease-containing denture soak (Alcalase protease) is also an effective way of removing denture plaque, especially when combined with brushing.

Chronic atrophic candidiasis which does not resolve (especially if there is an angular cheilitis) may require treatment with topical antifungals such as nystatin, amphotericin, or miconazole. Fluconazole is also effective, particularly when administered concurrently with an oral antiseptic such as chlorhexidine, but should not be used in patients on Warfarin therapy.

Other infections

Apart from high standards of personal hygiene, the use of barriers, and the avoidance of contact with those with communicable diseases and their bodily fluids such as saliva, little can be done to prevent exogenous infections with pathogenic agents that cause mucosal lesions, most of which are herpesviruses or enteroviruses.

Oral infections in the immunocompromised person

There are dramatic increases in the number of immunocompromised persons both as a consequence of the effects of infection by HIV and of treatment of organ transplant patients with immunosuppressive agents. Both are characterized by a predominantly T lymphocyte immune defect. T cells are essential to protection against infection with fungi, viruses, and some bacteria—mainly mycobacteria: immunocompromised patients are thus liable to infection both with fungal, mycobacterial, and viral pathogens (if they come into contact with them) and with opportunistic organisms, particularly, candida and herpesviruses.

Infections in immunocompromised persons tend to be recurrent or protracted, severe, and sometimes resistant to treatment. Occasionally they disseminate. In general, the spectrum of infections is wider, and their severity greater, the more profound the immune defect.

Oral fungal infections

Superficial oral fungal infections (mycoses), especially candidiasis, are extremely common in immunocompromised persons. Candidiasis accounts for nearly 80 per cent of hospital-acquired serious fungal infections. Most candidiasis is caused by *C. albicans* but other species are increasingly found. Candidiasis presents with or without soreness, as typical white or cream-coloured lesions of thrush on an erythematous background (pseudomembraneous candidiasis), or as erythematous candidiasis. Some patients may develop angular cheilitis.

Oral candidiasis is usually preventable with, or responsive to, standard topical antifungals but relapses are increasingly seen and there is consequently a trend towards the use of systemic imidazoles (ketoconazole) and bis-triazoles (fluconazole and itraconazole). If antibiotics or corticosteroids (oral or inhaled) are contributing causes, reducing the dose or changing the treatment may help. Intermittent or prolonged use of topical antifungals may be necessary where the underlying cause is unavoidable or incurable. Antifungal prophylaxis may well be indicated in immunocompromised persons.

Polyene antifungal agents

The polyene agents, derived from streptomyces species, include mainly nystatin and amphotericin. They are relatively cheap, effective topically, but have an unpleasant taste. Flucytosine may be useful as oral prophylaxis or therapy in a dose of 50–150 mg/kg/day, in divided doses, four times daily. Toxicity, due to metabolic effects on bone marrow cells, nausea, vomiting, and hepatic dysfunction have discouraged its use as a first-line agent.

Azole agents

Azoles are synthetic antifungals which are expensive. The currently available azoles are clotrimazole, miconazole, econazole, ketoconazole, fluconazole, itraconazole, and voticonazole. All the azoles are fungistatic, not fungicidal. This is especially important to consider when used in the chronically immunosuppressed, such as those with AIDS. None of the azoles are entirely benign. Hepatotoxicity may be common to all of them, and the potential for endocrine toxicities exists, particularly at high doses. Furthermore, as with any new agent, novel toxicities may yet be discovered.

Oral herpesvirus infections

Herpes simplex virus (HSV) infections are the most commonly recognized oral viral infections: 50–75 per cent of immunocompromised patients or those on chemotherapy develop oral HSV lesions. Chronic, extensive, and painful mouth ulcers affecting especially the keratinized mucosa are the most common intraoral lesions, and severe herpes labialis may be seen. Most infections result from reactivation of latent viruses (for example, in the trigeminal ganglion) and the viruses are often shed in saliva.

Though patients with HSV-induced oral lesions are managed mainly with supportive treatment, particularly maintenance of fluid intake, antipyretics and analgesics, and topical antiseptics to prevent bacterial superinfection, antivirals are indicated in immunocompromised patients or in others where there are frequent severe recurrences or complications. Antiviral prophylaxis, therefore, may well be indicated in immunocompromised patients.

Aciclovir is a potent acyclic guanosine derivative of very low toxicity. Adverse effects are rare and extremely minor though rashes, nausea, and other gastrointestinal effects have been reported in some patients receiving the drug orally, and rises in blood urea and creatinine levels may be seen after intravenous administration. Aciclovir has significant clinical benefit against HSV and is far more effective than previous nucleoside analogues such as idoxuridine or vidarabine.

Aciclovir has been advocated for prophylaxis in immunocompromised adults using an oral dose of 200mg three to four times daily or aciclovir topically. In established lesions viral shedding, pain, and duration of lesions are substantially reduced using aciclovir, either intravenously at a dose of 250mg every 8 hours, or orally 400mg 5 times a day. Aciclovir resistance is now becoming a clinical problem, particularly in patients with leukaemia, after tissue and organ transplants, and with HIV disease. Most aciclovir-resistant HSV isolates are fortunately, sensitive to foscarnet (trisodium phophonoformate hexahydrate). Valaciclovir, the pro-drug is sometimes used.

Penciclovir, a relatively new synthetic acyclic guanine derivative which

- possesses the same antiviral spectrum as aciclovir
- has similar mechanism of action to that of aciclovir, in that it undergoes phosphorylation in response to HSV viral thymidine kinase, is then further phosphorylated by host cell enzymes into a triphosphate, which selectively inhibits HSV viral DNA replication
- has considerably more bioavailability—up to 77% against the 10–20% for aciclovir.
- has a longer intracellular effect than aciclovir
- is more effective clinically than aciclovir
- is cheaper than aciclovir
- as a 1 per cent cream applied every 2 hours for 4 days is effective in herpes labialis
- Famciclovir, the pro-drug, is sometimes used.

New anti-herpes agents for herpes labialis include 10 per cent docosanol cream.

Other viral infections

Varicella-zoster virus (VZV) oral infections are less common than HSV infections. VZV is latent in sensory root ganglia and reactivation may cause zoster (shingles). The lesions are ulcerative and extremely painful, may lead to scarring and post-herpetic neuralgia, and occasionally result in dissemination of VZV. Aciclovir is the most reliable therapy, and may reduce the incidence of post-herpetic neuralgia, but aciclovir-resistant VZV are now being identified. Vaccines against HSV and VZV are now available.

Human cytomegalovirus (HCMV) is one of the leading causes of morbidity and mortality in immunocompromised patients. It is latent in salivary glands, but only recently has been recognized as causing oral lesions: these are usually chronic painful oral ulcers. No absolutely reliable, effective vaccine is available against HCMV but the Towne vaccine—a live, passaged HCMV—may confer useful protection in at-risk patients such as transplant recipients. Passive immunization using specific immunoglobulin with high-titre, anti-HCMV antibody after accidental exposure to the virus may provide a degree of protection against primary infection in seronegative subjects at risk. Interferon has not been found to be protective.

Low doses of aciclovir (250 mg 3 times a day or 5 mg/kg 2 times a day have not been effective in treatment of HCMV reactivation in bone marrow transplant patients but oral aciclovir (200 mg, 4 times a day) significantly reduces HCMV shedding and, high-dose aciclovir (450 mg; 4 times a day) can prevent reactivation of latent HCMV. *Ganciclovir*, a guanosine analogue, is active against cytomegalovirus, but is more toxic than aciclovir, can produce neutropenia, may have carcinogenic activity and, if given with zidovudine, can produce profound myelosuppression.

It is used for serious HCMV infections such as retinitis and pneumonitis.

Oral bacterial infections

A wide range of bacteria can, in immunocompromised patients, occasionally colonize the mouth and may sometimes cause oral infections, or be the portal for septicaemia. Broad-spectrum antimicrobials can also cause shifts but such drugs are primarily responsible for this. Bacteria that are typically found elsewhere, such as lower in the gastrointestinal tract (*Escherichia coli*, *Pseudomonas aeruginosa*, *Enterobacter cloacae*, *Klebsiella pneumoniae*, *Salmonella enteritidis*) may colonize the mouth, and septicaemias involving viridans streptococci, coagulase-negative staphylococci, capnocytophaga and other micro-organisms originating in the mouth are increasingly recognized in leukaemic, neutropenic, or other immunocompromised patients.

In addition to bacterial infections of the oral mucosa, neutropenic patients may develop periodontal infections and organisms commonly viewed as pathogenic such as *Staphylococcus epidermidis*, *C. albicans*, *S. aureus*, and *P. aeruginosa* may be detected in high concentrations in subgingival plaque.

Dental plaque control may therefore be critical in the immunocompromised cancer patient. Conventional toothbrushing is typically contraindicated during periods of myelosuppression due to the risk of bleeding and infection; but, since foam brush substitutes are not as effective in controlling plaque and gingivitis, chemical decontaminating regimens (such as aqueous chlorhexidine) are also required. Odontogenic infections are potentially life-threatening in the immunosuppressed patient, and broad-spectrum cover is needed (such as penicillin plus gentamicin).

Infective agents of importance in immunocompromised patients are:

- *Candida albicans*
- Herpes simplex
- Herpes varicella zoster
- Human cytomegalovirus
- *Escherichia coli*
- *Pseudomonas aeruginosa*
- *Enterobacter cloacae*
- *Klebsiella pneumoniae*
- *Salmonella enteritidis*
- Streptococci
- Staphylococci
- Capnocytophaga

Lifestyle issues in preventing oral mucosal disease

Lifestyle, or changes in lifestyle, can have a major impact in preventing disease in many systems, including the oral mucosa, but it is in the area of oral epithelial dysplasia and cancer that lifestyle factors are most significant in preventing oral disease.

Trauma, Chemicals, or Burns

Trauma from appliances or prostheses may cause oral ulceration and, very rarely, neoplastic change. Oral mutilation may be seen in some psychiatrically disturbed patients or those with learning disability. In some Chinese and Hindu cultures the lips, cheeks, or tongue are ceremonially pierced by spears or other objects while the person is in a state of trance. In some East-African groups, the uvula is removed in children in the belief that health will be improved.

Adverse oral effects of dental amalgam may include allergy, lichenoid reactions, electro-galvanism, and amalgam tattoos. Amalgam 'tattoos' are the most common oral tattoos, but are not discussed here. In the developing world, a range of different types of tattoos can be seen, some deliberately induced, others accidental. Accidental tattooing can originate from use of the bark of a plant *Juglans regia* (Derum or Dendava) used as an oral hygiene aid. One particularly obvious tattoo is that of the labial and buccal maxillary gingiva created using soot. In Eritrea, females are tattooed on the anterior maxillary gingiva in childhood: males are tattooed only in the canine regions. In parts of North Africa, the lip may be tattooed and in some parts of West Africa, the skin at the commissure is tattooed. In the developed world, deliberate tattoos not uncommonly use tribal or personal names especially in the lower labial mucosa.

Chemically induced lesions often present as mucosal burns or white lesions. They can be caused by:

- Drugs
  - analgesic tablets
  - cocaine, snuff or smokeless tobacco deliberately rubbed into the gingivae or vestibule
  - pancreatin can cause ulceration
- Mouthwashes
  - Chlorhexidine
  - Others, especially alcohol-containing washes
- Dental procedures
  - acids (chromic, trichloracetic, phosphoric)
  - self-curing resins, especially epoxy resins
- Natural products
  - Tobacco products
  - Areca nut
  - the houseplant Dieffenbachia
  - the enzyme bromelin in pineapple
  - others

Diagnosis is from the history and clinical features.

Thermally induced lesions often present as mucosal burns or white lesions, and can be caused by hot foods or drinks, hot instruments (dental handpiece or extraction forceps, for example), electrical burns, cryosurgery, or radiation. Those seen especially on the palate or tongue, for example, 'pizza-palate', present as white lesions, blisters, or ulcers. Diagnosis is from history and clinical features.

In some groups in developing countries such as in some Amazonian tribes and in the Surma tribe of Ethiopia, large plates are worn in the lower lip. Others wear lip plugs. Some African tribes such as the Toposa of Sudan wear a piece of wire, others such as the Dogon of Mali wear rings, in their lower lip. In the western countries, jewellery is usually applied to the lips (labret) but the practice of lingual piercing is a cause of some concern since oedema can be pronounced and may be hazardous to the airway.

Mucosal damage can be caused by

- Trauma
- Chemicals
- Burns

Epithelial dysplasia and cancer

Oral epithelial dysplasia

Studies in Western populations confirm the associations of oral epithelial dysplasia (OED) with tobacco and alcohol use. Analysis of the effects of chewing or smoking tobacco, alcohol consumption, body mass index, and vegetable, fruit, and vitamin/iron intake on the risk of erythroplakia in Indian populations also showed that tobacco chewing and alcohol drinking are strong risk factors for erythroplakia.

The role of diet in preventing oral epithelial dysplasia is less clear. Fruit and vegetable intake are considered important variables in lowering the risk of oral cancer, but this may not necessarily always be the case with oral epithelial dysplasia. A study of female tobacco/betel chewers in South India suggested that a diet deficient in foods of animal origin was a more significant risk factor for oral premalignancy than is a diet deficient in fruits and vegetables.

Oral squamous cell carcinoma: risk factors

Sun exposure
Working outdoors increases the risk of lip cancer: fair complexion may be a cofactor.

Tobacco use
Tobacco contains nicotine and other alkaloids. *N*-nitrosamines are the compounds thought to be the major carcinogenic agents in tobacco. Volatile and other nitrosamines may also be contributors.

The excessive use of tobacco products has been associated with various lesions in the oral cavity. Tobacco smoking can have a range of adverse effects on oral health including predisposing to candida carriage, candidiasis, and leukoplakia. Other tobacco-associated lesions include tooth stains, abrasions, smoker's melanosis, acute necrotizing ulcerative gingivitis, and other periodontal conditions, burns and keratotic patches, black hairy tongue, nicotinic stomatitis, palatal erosions, epithelial dysplasia, and squamous-cell carcinoma.

Tobacco is smoked as cigarettes, cigars, or in a pipe and, in some instances may be treated in a variety of ways, or contain additives. Alcohol synergizes with tobacco as a risk factor for all upper aerodigestive tract squamous cell carcinomas. The effect of smoking falls off soon after smoking ceases.

Analytical studies strongly suggest that tobacco smoking of any type, but especially pipe smoking significantly increases the risk of lip cancer. Details of tar yield of cigarettes, and type of cigarette used for the longest period can be used as the basis of a classification to examine the effects of different types of cigarette. Cigarettes can be classified as low or medium if the tar yield is below 22 mg, and as high if tar yield is above 22 mg. Compared with non-smokers, the risk of oral cancer for smokers using low to medium cigarettes is 8.5 and for high tar cigarettes is 16.4.

As regards intra-oral carcinoma, the sites of tongue, mouth, oropharynx, and hypopharynx are so often grouped together in analytical studies, or grouped in a variety of different combinations, that it is difficult to discuss these tumours individually.

Smokeless tobacco

Smokeless tobacco contains a number of carcinogens and its use is to be deprecated. There is clear concern about the possible carcinogenicity and other adverse effects of the snuff sold in small 'teabag' pouches. There is some limited evidence for an association between the use of such smokeless tobacco and oral cancer: there is no doubt, however, that smokeless tobacco can induce oral keratosis and gingival recession. The fact that this form of smokeless tobacco is held in the mouth for very long periods, and is popular with children and adolescents is a cause for concern.

Alcohol

A study of alcohol misusers from south London showed a high incidence of tooth wear and trauma to the dentition, and a small minority had oral mucosal lesions, including two previously treated carcinomas (Harris *et al.* 1997). Alcoholics have demonstrable cytological abnormalities on oral smears, though whether these are due to a direct effect of alcohol or an effect secondary to associated malnutrition is unclear (Table 11.1).

Oral cancer risk factors

- Sun exposure
- Tobacco
- Alcohol
- Betel use
- Socioeconomic status
- Occupation

Tobacco plus alcohol

The epidemiology of oral cancer and the worrying increases in some populations have been discussed elsewhere. The reasons for an increasing incidence of oral cancer, particularly among younger persons is unclear. A survey of young persons with oral cancer suggest that most are exposed to traditional risk factors of tobacco smoking, drinking alcohol, and a low consumption of fruit and vegetables. By 1988, both tobacco smoking and alcohol consumption had been accepted as independent risk factors for oral cancer (oral squamous cell carcinoma). Convincing evidence also now exists that the combined effect of alcohol and tobacco is greater than the sum of the two effects independently. Given the large attributable risk for the two habits of smoking and alcohol

Table 11.1 Dietary components that may either cause or protect against the development of cancer in humans*

	Causative	Protective
Classes of food	Alcoholic drinks, meat, (?) coffee (?)	Vegetables, fruit (?), milk (?)
Nutrients Major nutrients	Total energy, fat (?), complex carbohydrates (?), alcohol (?)	Fibre (?)
Minor nutrients	Cadmium (?)	Vitamin A, vitamin C (?) riboflavin (?), iodine (?), iron (?), selenium (?)
Non-nutrients		
Natural components	Cycasin (?)	Certain indoles (?)
Additives	Nitrates and nitrites (?), saccharin (?), cyclamate (?)	(?)
Contaminants	Aflatoxins, N-nitroso compounds (?), polycyclic aromatic hydrocarbons (?)	—

Adapted from Armstrong, B.K., McMichael, A.J., and MacLennan, R. (1982). The causes of cancer—diet. In: *Cancer Epidemiology and Prevention*. (D. Schottenfeld, and J.F. Fraumeni, eds.) W. B. Saunders, Philadelphia, p 429.

*Not necessarily oral cancer. Disputed, speculative, and less well-established effects are indicated by a question mark (?).

drinking, the dramatic reduction in risk (within 5–10 years of quitting) provides great hope for the prevention and control of the growing menace of oral cancer.

Betel use and other habits

There is some confusion over the use of the term betel. Betel leaf is derived from the betel vine, while nuts from the betel palm are termed areca nuts. These two products may be used orally alone, together, or together with other material such as tobacco, slaked lime, and other additives. In Papua New Guinea slaked lime (but not tobacco) is a prominent component of 'betel'; in other areas tobacco may be a main component.

While there is clear evidence of carcinogenicity from tobacco, the risk of oral cancer is also increased in persons who chew betel with or without tobacco. Areca nut use clearly predisposes to oral submucous fibrosis, a recognized premalignant condition, can cause cytogenetic changes whether tobacco is or is not used, and can result in the appearance of N-nitroso compounds in the saliva including N-nitrosoguvacine and nitrosamines such as 3-(methyl nitrosamino) propionitrite—a powerful carcinogen in rats. Areca nut-specific N-nitroso compounds can also cause epithelial changes *in vitro* and can promote experimental carcinogenesis.

Results of use of betel

- Tooth and mucosa staining
- Epithelial atrophy and ulceration
- Submucous fibrosis
- Leukoplakia and/or carcinoma where tobacco is included
- Oral cancer where slaked lime is used

Mouthwash use

In a study based on cases of oral cancer in women and a control group, both cigarette smoking and alcohol consumption were confirmed as independent risk factors, but no association was found for mouthwash use. Patients with oral cancer reported more frequently than did controls that they used mouthwash to 'disguise the smell of tobacco … (and) … alcohol' and mouthwash use was found to be strongly associated with smoking and drinking. Thus, using a mouthwash appeared in these instances to be a proxy for exposure to tobacco or alcohol, themselves risk determinants of oral cancer. However, a study from the USA reported that, after adjustment for tobacco and alochol use, the risk of oral cancer among users of mouthwash was found to be increased by 40 per cent in men and 60 per cent in women. The increased risk was apparent only when using mouthwashes of a high alcohol content (25 per cent or higher). Thus, it appears that the risk from alcohol in mouthwashes is similar, at least qualitatively, to that of alcohol used for drinking, although in terms of

attributable risk the contribution of mouthwash use to oral cancer remains small.

Other liquids

Particular types of tea (maté) consumed in Latin America may be associated with oral cancer. Studies from Brazil and Uruguay have demonstrated this association.

Marijuana use

There have been some case reports of oral cancers in marijuana smokers, but these have yet to be supported by data from an epidemiological study.

Socioeconomic status

The relationship between socioeconomic status and oral cancer risk has been explored. Three indicators of socioeconomic status were considered (education, occupational status, and percentage of potential working life in employment). After adjustment for established risk factors, the third index (percentage of potential working life in employment) only was found to have an independent association with oral cancer risk consistent with the hypothesis that behaviours leading to social instability, or social instability itself, are linked to an increased risk of oral and pharyngeal cancer.

Occupation

Limited epidemiological evidence suggests increased risk for oral and pharyngeal cancer for workers exposed to formaldehyde, workers with access to alcohol (such as bartenders and restaurant workers), electrical and electronics workers, textile and apparel workers, and manmade mineral fibre workers. Most of this evidence comes from occupational disease surveillance studies and from retrospective cohort studies in which the number of cases of oral cancer is small.

Oral squamous cell carcinoma: protective factors

Diet

The most favourable diet for reducing oral cancer risk is given by infrequent consumption of red and processed meat and eggs and, most of all, by frequent vegetable and fruit intake. The role of specific food groups and diet variety on the risk of oral and pharyngeal cancer has been considered in a case–control study in the Swiss Canton of Vaud. After allowance for education, alcohol, tobacco, and total energy intake, significant trends of increasing risk with more frequent intake emerged for eggs, red meat and pork, and processed meat. Inverse trends in risk were observed for milk, fish, raw vegetables, cooked vegetables, citrus fruit, and other fruits. There was a reduction of approximately 50 per cent in oral cancer risk with the addition of a serving per day of fruit or vegetables.

The relation between selected micronutrients and oral and pharyngeal cancer risk was investigated using data from a case–control study in Italy and Switzerland (Negri *et al.* 2000). In general, the more a micronutrient was correlated to total vegetable and fruit intake, the stronger was its protective effect against oral cancer.

Retinoids

The risk of oral cancer has been inversely associated with consumption of fruit and vegetables in several studies and with consumption of vitamins. Retinoids such as 13-cis-retinoic acid (isotretinoin) and fenretinide and carotenoids such as α-carotene can suppress oral leukoplakias. Isotretinoin may also prevent the development of carcinoma and can also prevent second primary tumours in patients with oral squamous carcinomas but does not prevent recurrences of the primary neoplasm. Retinoids suppress oral premalignant lesions and decrease the incidence of second primary tumors in head and neck cancer patients. There is some evidence that 13-cis-retinoic acid (isotretinoin) enhances cell mediated immunity and Langerhans cells and that beta carotene induces a mononuclear infiltrate in the tumour suggesting that immunomodulation may be a protective mechanism against the tumour. Retinoids, however, also regulate gene expression, which may be a further, or alternative, mechanism. It is thought that retinoids restore normal cell growth and differentiation by means of nuclear retinoic acid (RA) receptors (RAR alpha, beta, and gamma) and retinoid X receptors (RXR alpha, beta, and gamma).

Tea

Oral administration of 1.5 per cent green tea, 0.1 per cent tea pigments, and 0.5 per cent mixed tea (a composite of whole water extract of green tea, tea polyphenols, and tea pigments) as the sole source of drinking water for two weeks before initiation of 7,12-dimethyl-benz[a]anthracene (DMBA) treatment and until the end of the experiment in golden Syrian hamsters, significantly reduced the incidence of dysplasia and oral carcinoma (Li *et al.* 1999). Protection from DNA damage and suppression of cell proliferation could be important mechanisms to account for the anticarcinogenic effects of the tea preparations. EGCG [(−)-epigallocatechin-3-gallate], the major constituent of green tea, affects cell populations, inhibiting growth, with a decrease in efficacy as cells progressed from normal to cancer.

Cancer chemoprevention: Bowman–Birk inhibitor

Bowman-Birk inhibitor is soybean-derived protease inhibitor that has demonstrable chemopreventive activity in a number of *in vitro* and animal systems. When the factor was administered to 32 subjects with oral leukoplakia for 1 month there was a positive clinical response in 31 per cent (Armstrong *et al.* 2000) possibly via an effect on *neu* oncogene expression (Wan *et al.* 1999).

Oral cancer: possible protective factors

- Vegetables and fruit
- Tea
- Bowman-Birk inhibitor

Preventing Iatrogenic Oral Disease

The range of oral lesions now recognized as iatrogenic complications is increasing, and undoubtedly will increase in the future, but mucositis is symptomatically the most profound. Drug-induced lesions are also important.

Mucositis

Oral mucositis is a major dose-limited toxic effect of intensive cancer therapy, and various aspects have been reviewed over the past few years (Scully *et al.* 2003). Mucositis, sometimes termed mucosal barrier injury or MBI, is the term given to the widespread oral erythema, ulceration, and soreness, which is a common complication of a number of therapeutic procedures involving chemo-, radio-, or chemoradiotherapy, used largely for cancer therapy but also in the conditioning prior to bone marrow transplantation—haemopoietic stem cell transplantation (HSCT). Mucositis invariably follows external beam radiotherapy involving the orofacial tissues, and may follow chemotherapy. At least 40 per cent of chemotherapy patients can be affected by mucositis, and there is often underestimation of severity or underreporting. In patients on fluorouracil and cisplatin, 90 per cent develop mucositis, and etoposide and melphalan cause particularly severe mucositis. Oral mucositis is seen in over 75% of patients and is particularly severe after HSCT because of radiation damage and myeloablation. The course follows the polymorphonuclear leukocyte count, where conditioning with total body irradiation (TBI), and methotrexate for prophylaxis of graft versus host disease as in allograft patients, causes profound myelosuppression, and severe mucositis. The latter is a common sequelae of high-dose chemotherapy and upper mantle head and neck irradiation, particularly with TBI.

Mucositis may have a significant effect on the quality of life, in terms of pain; ability to eat, swallow and talk, and there is often, therefore, the need to interupt or curtail the therapy, reduce the dose or delay therapy. In one study some 30–50% of patients with HSCT felt that mucositis was their most significant toxicity, and was particularly a problem after TBI.

Mucositis can be caused directly by cytotoxic effects and indirectly by sustained neutropenia after cytostatic therapy with changes in mucosal immune regulation, colonizing microflora, and wound-healing. Mucositis can arise as a consequence of the

- Direct effect of the interventive regimen on cell division
- Release of cytokines (such as interleukin-1 and tumour necrosis factor alpha)
- Oral infections that may ensue
- Aggravation by trauma

Not only does MBI open the way to adherence and invasion by oral commensals, but the flora changes seen in such patients leads to the appearance or increase in potential pathogens such as alpha haemolytic streptococci which can lead to bacteraemia.

Streptococcus mitis can cause bacteraemia and, especially in those on high dose cytarabine, adult respiratory distress syndrome. Any fall in neutrophil count clearly aggravates the situation, while recovery of the count is mirrored in resolution and healing of the mucositis, so that healing is complete by 2–3 weeks.

Mucositis appears from 3 to 15 days after cancer treatment, earlier after chemotherapy than after radiotherapy. The pain from mucositis can be so intense as to interfere with eating, and significantly affect the quality of life frequently leading to the need for opioid analgesics and sometimes to interruption of the planned cancer therapy. In addition to causing pain, ulcerative mucositis can provide a portal for microbial entry, and can thus lead to local and sometimes systemic infections, which may even be life-threatening.

Mucositis—characteristics

- Erythema, ulceration, soreness
- Up to 40% of chemo and radiotherapy patients affected
- Up to 75% of haemopoietic stem cell transplant patients affected
- Directly caused by cytotoxic effects of therapy
- Indirectly caused by neutropoenia consequent upon therapy

Prophylaxis

The basic strategies in management of mucositis aim at pain relief, efforts to hasten healing, and prevention of infectious complications. Prophylaxis is however, the goal. Clinical trials of agents aimed at preventing or ameliorating mucositis have not, however, always assessed the results on strict criteria, few mucositis rating scales have been tested for validity, and the many mucositis scales that exist deny good comparisons of products.

Special attention should be directed to oral infections in neutropenic ($<0.5\times10^9$/L) patients in whom oral micro-organisms are the leading cause of bacteraemia. Invasive fungal infections of the oral cavity can be associated with systemic fungal infection and are indications for the use of liposomal amphotericin B. However, antimicrobial approaches have met with conflicting results, little effect being seen with chlorhexidine and systemic antimicrobials in the prevention of mucositis in radiation patients. In patients with HSCT and patients with leukaemia, chlorhexidine may not be effective in preventing mucositis, although there may be reduction in oral colonization by Candida. Initial studies of topical antimicrobials that affect the Gram-negative oral flora have shown reductions in ulcerative mucositis during radiation therapy but have not been assessed in leukaemia/HSCT.

Biologic response modifiers offer the potential for prevention and for acceleration of healing. Various cytokines will enter clinical trials in the near future; these offer the potential for reduction of epithelial cell sensitivity to the toxic effects of cancer therapy or for stimulation of repair of the damaged tissue.

Prophylaxis of mucositis

- Monitor microbal colonization
- Antiviral prophylaxis
- Antifungal prophylaxis
- Gastrointestinal prophylaxis
- Biological response modifiers
- Specific cytokines

Radiation mucositis

The acute oral mucosal response to radiotherapy is a result of mitotic death of epithelial cells. The threshold for mucositis appears to be about 20 Gy of fractionated radiotherapy. The cell cycle time of the basal keratinocytes is about 4 days and, as the epithelium is at least 3 or 4 cells thick, radiation changes begin to appear clinically at about 12 days after the start of irradiation. Clinically, the oral mucosa may initially turn whitish, followed by erythema, and then after a few days is covered by a patchy fibrinous exudate. If a high dose of radiation is given over a short time, ulceration may supervene early on, with a thick fibrinous membrane covering the ulcers. Surviving keratinocytes respond to radiation damage by dividing more rapidly, so that spontaneous complete healing can be anticipated within 3 weeks of the end of radiation. The degree of mucositis experienced is determined by the treatment dose, radiation field size, and fractionation schedules prescribed for individual patients, and appears to be modified by saliva volume, total epidermal growth factor (EGF) level, and the concentration of EGF in the oral environment. Healing is impaired by high dose radiotherapy and by tobacco smoking.

Oral mucositis is a frequent side effect of combined myeloablative chemo- and radiotherapy preceding haemopoietic stem cell transplantation (HSCT). Mucositis causes pain, poor food intake, is a port of entry for infection, and is typically severe and prolonged with ulceration. Strong opiate analgesia is needed for a median of 6 days in up to 50 per cent of patients. Mucositis typically begins around 5 days post HSCT and persists for a similar period. By around 9–14 days post-HSCT, basal cell regeneration occurs and the mucositis resolves.

Prevention

Parotid-sparing irradiation

Sparing at least one parotid gland during irradiation of patients with head and neck cancer will preserve parotid function and reduce xerostomia. Mucositis can be reduced by protecting the mucosa with midline mucosa-sparing blocks, or by modifying the radiation treatment. One study, to assess the benefit of parotid-sparing irradiation, compared the body weights of patients irradiated with parotid-sparing technique versus those irradiated with bilateral opposed photon beams, where both parotid glands were included in the radiation fields. Patients treated with parotid-sparing techniques were better able to maintain their oral nutrition and body weight, compared with patients who had both parotid glands irradiated.

Salivary gland function protection with medical agents

Amifostine and its active metabolite, WR-1065, given intravenously before radiation treatment accumulate in high concentrations in the salivary glands and seem to result in a distinct reduction of short-term toxicity of radiotherapy or combined radio-chemotherapy. Amifostine reduced acute and chronic xerostomia but not mucositis. Antitumour treatment efficacy was preserved; nausea, vomiting, hypotension, and allergic reactions were the most common adverse effects.

Coumarin/Troxerutine (Venalot Depot) have shown favourable effects in the treatment of radiogenic sialadenitis and mucositis in prospective, randomized placebo-controlled double-blind studies.

Anti-inflammatory agents

Clinical and histopathological demonstration of reduction in oral mucositis with sucralfate suggests that sucralfate might be recommended in the prevention of radiation-induced mucositis (Etiz *et al.* 2000). Proteolytic enzymes such as trypsin, papain, and chymotrypsin can be beneficial (Gujral *et al.* 2001).

Benzydamine was evaluated in patients with head and neck carcinoma for treatment of radiation-induced oral mucositis (Epstein *et al.* 2001) when it reduced erythema and ulceration by about 30 per cent compared with a placebo; greater than 33 per cent of benzydamine subjects remained ulcer free compared with 18 per cent of placebo subjects, and benzydamine significantly delayed the use of systemic analgesics compared with a placebo. Benzydamine was not effective, however, in those receiving accelerated radiotherapy doses of more than 22 Gy/day.

Anti-infective regimens

Radiotherapy is associated with a marked increase in oral Gram-negative enterobacteria and pseudomonads, which may not only contribute to the mucositis but release endotoxins which can cause adverse systemic effects. If Gram-negative bacilli do have a role in the aetiology of irradiation mucositis, then it should be possible to prevent, treat, or ameliorate mucositis by abolishing the Gram-negative flora. Indeed, clinical trials using polymyxin E and tobramycin applied topically four times daily have given promising results. This regimen has yet to be fully evaluated for the management of irradiation mucositis, and has not been shown effective in the mucositis associated with chemotherapy. Furthermore, in patients receiving HSCT, systemic antibiotic coverage is routinely used in most centres, yet oral mucositis remains a severe and common problem. Many institutions have adopted combinations such as gentamicin, vancomycin, and nystatin as an oral decontaminating rinse for prophylactic use, but further study is needed to evaluate this bacterial hypothesis of mucositis.

Lasers

Use of the low-energy helium–neon laser therapy is capable of reducing the severity and duration of oral mucositis associated with radiation therapy.

Prevention of radiation-induced mucositis

- Parotid sparing radiation
- Salivary gland protection with medical agents
- Anti-inflammatory agents
- Anti-infective agents
- Laser therapy

Chemotherapy-induced mucositis

The oral mucosal reaction to chemotherapy is due to a non-specific inhibitory effect of the agent on the mitosis of proliferating cells including those in the basal epithelium, causing a reduced renewal rate and thus atrophy and, eventually, ulceration. Frank oral ulceration is, therefore, a particular problem for those on chemotherapy. Up to 20 per cent of patients on chemotherapy suffer oral ulceration, especially following administration of cytarabine, doxorubicin, bleomycin, etoposide, 5-fluorouracil, mercaptopurine, and methotrexate. Up to 75 per cent receiving 5-fluorouracil develop mucositis. Mucositis can cause pain and may be a portal for infection and septicaemia. The mucositis typically persists symptomatically for up to 12 days.

Prevention

Ice chips

There is some evidence that ice chips used for 30 minutes before 5-fluorouracil (5FU) administration prevent mucositis. Thirty-eight reports of chemotherapy trials were initially included in a recent Cochrane review; two were duplicate reports and nine were excluded as there was no useable information. Of the 27 useable studies, 14 had data for mucositis on 945 randomized patients and 15 included data on oral candidiasis for 1164 randomized patients. None of the prophylactic agents included in the Cochrane review prevented mucositis, with the exception of ice chips.

Anti-infective agents

Chlorhexidine is no more effective than water at reducing mucositis. Salt and soda mouthwash is cheaper than and as effective as, chlorhexidine or a mouthwash containing lidocaine, Maalox and Benadryl (Dodd *et al.* 2000). A daily preventive protocol in leukaemia consisting of: (1) elimination of bacterial plaque; (2) application of a mouthwash with a non-alcoholic solution of chlorhexidine 0.12 per cent and (3) topical application of iodopovidone, followed by 'swish and swallow' with nystatin 500,000 units results in a significant improvement in oral hygiene and a significant decrease in the incidence of mucositis and oral candidiasis (Levy-Polack *et al.* 1998). There is evidence that prophylactic use of antifungal agents, which are absorbed or partially absorbed from the gastrointestinal tract, reduce the clinical signs of oral candidiasis, and the partially absorbed drugs may be more effective (Clarkson and Worthington 2000).

Drug-induced lesions

Gingival hyperplasia is a recognized complication of phenytoin, ciclosporin, nifedipine, and some other calcium-channel blockers and has been recognized for years. Space precludes full discussion but some are discussed below under specific lesions.

Prevention of chemotherapy-induced mucositis

- Pre-treatment use of ice chips
- Anti-infective agents—topical
  —systemic

Preventing mucosal disease through nutrition

Nutritional deficiencies can impair oral mucosa health and oral immune defences, and components of some diets may be harmful to the mucosa or, indeed, carcinogenic. Conversely, oral disease can interfere with feeding and nutrition as a consequence of compromised mastication and swallowing, pain, or discomfort. For example, daily intake of non-starch polysaccharides, protein, calcium, non-haem iron, niacin, vitamin C, and intrinsic and milk sugars are significantly lower in edentate older people, and plasma ascorbate and retinol levels are significantly lower in the edentate than dentate persons (Sheiham and Steele 2001). The same workers found plasma ascorbate levels to be significantly related to the number of teeth and posterior contacting pairs of teeth.

Effects on the oral mucosa of specific deficiencies

Proteins

Protein is the source of the 20 amino acids; only eight (isoleucine, leucine, lysine, methionine, phenylalanine, threonine, tryptophan, and valine) are essential; though histidine and arginine are also necessary for growing infants. Protein-energy deficiency may, in children, vary in its effects from mild growth retardation to marasmus (general malnutrition) and kwashiorkor (protein malnutrition). Oral mucosal lesions in marasmus have not been clearly recorded or defined. However, protein malnutrition decreases collagen synthesis in rodent oral mucosa and oral lesions have been described in kwashiorkor. These include oedema of the tongue and papillary atrophy. Angular stomatitis and hypopigmentation circumorally have been recorded. Interestingly, tolerance of dentures appears to be increased if the dietary protein intake is improved in edentulous patients.

Acinar atrophy has been reported in the submandibular salivary glands of protein-deficient rodents and secretory IgA may be decreased. This has been related to oral infections such as noma. There is also evidence that bacterial adherence to oral epithelium is increased in protein malnutrition. Xerostomia is a feature of kwashiorkor.

Fat and fatty acids

Epidemiological evidence links a high intake of saturated animal fats with oral and pharyngeal cancer, at least in males. Though fatty acids can be essential dietary components, there appear to be no reports on the effects of fatty acid deficiency on the oral mucosa.

Vitamins

Vitamins are essential organic dietary factors incapable of being synthesized within the body. Vitamins are classified as water or fat soluble (Table 11.2). They are required in only small amounts; absence can result in a disease state (Table 11.3) and sometimes vitamin excess can cause disease.

Vitamin A (retinol)

Vitamin A is fat-soluble and is found in animal fats, milk, and liver. Vitamin A can also be derived from precursors (carotenes or carotenoids) found in plants, particularly green leafy vegetables. Vitamin A is stored in the liver: reserves can last about 1 year. Natural derivatives of vitamin A, and synthetic analogues of vitamin A, known as retinoids, can modulate epithelial cell differentiation, possibly by regulating gene expression.

Hypervitaminosis A

In hypervitaminosis A there is alopecia, peeling of the skin, coarsening of the hair, and bone pain. Oral features have only rarely been recorded but vitamin A and some analogues such as etretinate may cause cheilitis.

Vitamin A deficiency

Vitamin A deficiency is usually dietary in origin. In vitamin A deficiency, the eyes are first affected; night blindness, xerophthalmia, and conjunctival ulceration appear. The skin becomes dry and scaly (follicular hyperkeratosis) and the oral mucosa becomes hyperkeratinized, with non-keratinized mucosa changing into keratinized mucosa. Salivary secretory ductal epithelium undergoes metaplasia and there is also a direct effect on the taste buds. Hypovitaminosis A may be found in some patients with

Table 11.2 Classification of vitamins

Fat-soluble	Water-soluble
Vitamin A	Vitamin B1 (Thiamin)
Vitamin D	Vitamin B2 (Riboflavin)
Vitamin E	Vitamin B6 (Pyridoxine)
Vitamin K	Vitamin B12
	Vitamin C (Ascorbic acid)
	Folic acid
	Pantothenic acid
	Biotin
	Nicotinic acid (Niacin)

mucocutaneous candidiasis, and therapy with vitamin A may produce some improvement. Hypovitaminosis A also increases the susceptibility of rodents to infection with *Candida albicans*.

There has been considerable interest in the role of vitamin A in cancers, particularly those of epithelial origin. Both natural precursors (carotenoids) and synthetic analogues (retinoids) may have some protective effect against cancers.

Vitamin B

There are several B vitamins (Tables 11.2 and 11.3): all are water-soluble. Deficiencies may be diet-related or have other causes: oral ulceration and other conditions noted below, may follow.

Vitamin B12 deficiency

The most widely recognized deficiencies are of vitamin B12. This vitamin is found mainly in liver, eggs, meat, and milk: liver stores of this last up to 3 years, and thus deficiency is rarely of dietary origin—except in vegans. Vitamin B12 deficiency is typically seen in pernicious anaemia, where there is deficiency of the gastric intrinsic factor required for the absorption of vitamin B12.

Glossitis and stomatitis may result from vitamin B12 deficiency. The tongue tip reddens in the early stages of deficiency, and this eventually spreads with fissuring—the so-called beef tongue—and with papillary atrophy. Angular stomatitis, aphthae, and erosive lesions may also be seen. Some patients may have Burning Mouth syndrome, even in the absence of recognizable mucosal disease. Oral hyperpigmentation may also be seen. Mucosal changes respond rapidly to replacement therapy.

Vitamin B1 (thiamine, aneurine) deficiency

Vitamin B1 is widely distributed in foods. It is necessary in the formation of the coenzyme thiamine pyrophosphate required for oxidative decarboxylation of pyruvate and a-ketoglutarate, and utilization of pentoses. There is, therefore, in B1 deficiency, a build-up of lactate and pyruvate, interfering with carbohydrate metabolism. Deficiency of vitamin B1 is common in alcoholism and leads to Beriberi, characterized by polyneuritis, muscular weakness, cardiac failure, mental changes and, in children, growth retardation. A role for vitamin B in Burning Mouth syndrome has been proposed, though these findings have not been confirmed by others. Thiamine deficiency may also shorten the tumour induction time in experimental oral carcinogenesis.

Vitamin B2 (riboflavin) deficiency

Riboflavin is found in leafy vegetables, meat, milk, and fish. It acts in the formation of two coenzymes, flavin adenine dinucleotide and flavin mononucleotide, involved in oxidative metabolism. Deficiency of vitamin B2 is commonly dietary, is especially seen in alcoholics, and leads to seborrhoeic dermatitis, corneal vascularization, and anaemia, and oral mucosal manifestations similar to those of vitamin B12 deficiency. Angular stomatitis, glossitis and oral ulceration have been recorded in vitamin B2 deficiency.

Vitamin B6 (pyridoxine) deficiency

Vitamin B6 is found in meat and vegetables and is involved in the formation of pyridoxal phosphate and pyridoxamine phosphate, coenzymes in amino acid metabolism. Vitamin B6 deficiency is particularly found in alcoholism, pregnancy, and the use of some drugs; e.g. isoniazid. Deficiency of vitamin B6 leads to dermatitis and peripheral neuropathy and oral mucosal manifestations similar to those of vitamin B12 deficiency—with angular stomatitis and generalized stomatitis and sometimes ulceration.

Pantothenic acid deficiency

Pantothenic acid is needed for the synthesis of coenzyme A, necessary for several metabolic pathways. There is a report of glossitis in possible pantothenic acid deficiency.

Nicotinic acid (niacin: nicotinamide) deficiency

Wheat, nuts, meat, and fish are rich sources of nicotinic acid. The active derivative of nicotinic acid, nicotinamide, is necessary for the production of NAD and NADP for oxidative metabolism. Deficiency of nicotinic acid is seen mainly in the West in alcoholics, and causes pellagra (dermatitis and neurological disturbances), oral mucosal erythema, and papillary atrophy of the tongue. There may be a burning sensation in the tongue, and hypersalivation and angular stomatitis.

Vitamin C (ascorbic acid)

Vitamin C is water soluble and found especially in fresh fruits (mainly in citrus fruits) and vegetables: potatoes are a common source in the West. Deficiency is because of dietary lack of vitamin C.

Vitamin C is involved in the hydroxylation of proline in collagen synthesis, and deficiency leads to defective collagen with capillary fragility, a haemorrhagic state, anaemia, and follicular hyperkeratosis and gingival changes. Vitamin C deficiency can also occasionally predispose to angular stomatitis and oral ulceration. There is a tenuous association between vitamin C and a protective effect against oral, pharyngeal, and oesophageal cancers.

Vitamin D

Vitamin D is the general name for a group of fat-soluble sterols. Vitamin D is found in fish, eggs, and milk products, and ultraviolet light converts the skin precursor 7-dehydro-cholesterol to vitamin D. Cholecalciferol from dietary sources is converted into 25-hydroxycholecalciferol in the liver and this is converted in the kidneys to the active form 1,25-dihydroxycholecalciferol. Vitamin D affects calcium and phosphate metabolism. Oral mucosal effects have not been described but vitamin D may affect parotid function.

Vitamin E

Vitamin E is the general name for a group of fat-soluble tocopherols. Prematurely born, low birth weight infants are generally considered to be marginally vitamin E-deficient. However, although subclinical or biochemical vitamin E deficiency was seen in plasma and buccal mucosal cells in healthy, premature infants in the first 6 weeks of life, the other cells showed no such deficiency during the study and the authors concluded that these infants do not need routine vitamin E supplementation (Kaempf and Linderkamp 1998).

No oral mucosal disorders appear to have been recorded in vitamin E deficiency. However, there may be a relationship to

TABLE 11.3 Aspects of vitamin and mineral intake

Vitamin/Mineral	Source	Active form	Mode of action	Deficiency state—general	Deficiency state—oral	Cause of deficiency	Outcome of Excess
Vitamin A	Animal fats, milk, Liver (Leafy green vegetables)	Derived from caretonoids	Modulates epithelial cell differentiation	Night blindness Xeropthalmia Dry, scaly skin	Affects on taste buds	Malabsorption Inadequate diet	Headache, convulsions hepatotoxicity, teratogenicity, skin peeling coarse hair
Vitamins Vitamin B1 (Thiamine)	Fortified flours and cereals; milk, eggs, yeast extract, fruit	Thiamine diphosphate/ pyrophosphate	Formation of coenzyme to facilitate carbohydrate metabolism	Beri-beri-polyneuritis, muscle weakness, cardiac failure, mental changes Growth retardation in young people	Role in Burning Mouth syndrome	Alcoholism Inadequate diet	Not known
Vitamin B2 (Riboflavine)	Milk, cheese, eggs, fish, fortified cereals, liver, kidney, whole grains, leafy vegetables	Riboflavine	Metabolism of coenzymes in oxidative metabolism	Seborrhoeic dematitis, corneal vascularisation, anaemia	Angular stomatitis; glossitis, oral ulceration	Alcoholism Inadequate diet Drugs	Not known
Vitamin B6 (Pyridoxine)	Liver, meat, fish, whole grain cereals, milk,. Peanuts	Pyridoxal phosphate	Formation of coenzymes in amino acid metabolism	Dermatitis, neuropathy	Angular stomatitis, ulceration	Alcoholism, pregnancy, drugs	Peripheral neuropathy
Vitamin B12 (Cobalamin)	Liver, eggs, meat, milk	Requires gastric intrinsic factor for absorption	Affects development of rapidly dividing cells – oral mucosa, blood cells	Macrocytic anaemia; villus atrophy; glossitis, stomatitis	Papillary atrophy Apthae; Burning Mouth syndrome; oral hyper-pigmentation	Vegan diet Inadequate diet	Not known
Pantothenic acid			Synthesis of co-enzyme A in metabolic pathways		Glossitis		
Nicotinic acid (Niacin)	Wheat, nuts, meat, fish, dairy products, yeast extracts, instant coffee	Nicotinamide	Production of NAD and NADP for oxidative metabolism	Pellagra—dermatitis and neurological disturbances	Oral mucosal erythema, papillary atrophy of tongue, hypersalivation, angular stomatitis	Alcoholism (In the West)	Vasodilatation

Vitamin C (Ascorbic acid)	Oranges, lemons, green vegetables, potatoes, fortified fruit drinks	Ascorbic acid	Role in collagen synthesis	Capillary fragility, anaemia, haemorrhagic state, follicular hyperkeratosis	Angular stomatitis, oral ulcers	Inadequate diets	Increased urinary oxalate
Vitamin D (Sterols)	Fatty fish, eggs, liver	1.25 dihydrocholecalciferol	Converts skin precursor to active form of Vitamin D	Affects calcium and phosphate metabolism, rickets, osteomalacia	Affects parotid function	Inadequate exposure to sunlight Malabsorption	Hypercalcaemia, renal failure
Vitamin E (Tocopherols)	Vegetable oils, wholegrain cereal, eggs, margarine	Tocopherol	Antioxidant			Inadequate diet	Nausea
Vitamin K	Green vegetables, liver	Naphthaquinone derivative	Carboxylation of glutamic acid residues on factors II, VII, IX, and X, as well as proteins C and S, all involved in blood clotting	Hypoprothrombinaemia, bleeding	Gingival bleeding Post-extraction haemorrhage	Malabsorption, parenteral nutrition, anticoagulants	Hyperbilirubinaemia
Folic acid (Pteroylglutamic acid)	Green vegetables, liver, yeast	Tetra-hydrofolate	Synthesis of purine and pyrimidine bases	Megaloblastic changes in haemopoietic and other cells Villus atrophy	Chronic hyperplastic/ atrophic candidiasis mucosal lesions	Poor intake, malabsorption increased demands, drugs	Not known
Iron	Meat	Transported as transferrin	Oxygen transport, intra-cellular respiration	Hypochromic, microcytic anaemia Plummer—Vinson syndrome	Glossitis, angular stomatitis, Burning Mouth syndrome, sore tongue, apthae, candidiasis	Poor diet, malabsorption, blood loss	None known
Zinc	Meat Cheese Wheat		Essential in some enzyme systems	Skin lesions Alopecia Weight loss Poor appetite	None known	Inadequate diet acrodermatitis enteropathica	Lethargy

carcinogenesis, since vitamin E, like α-carotene, is antioxidant and appears to inhibit experimental oral carcinogenesis and, in humans, higher serum vitamin E levels appear associated with a decreased risk of oral cancer.

Vitamin K

Vitamin K is a fat-soluble naphthaquinone derivative found in green vegetables. Malabsorption, parenteral nutrition, and anticoagulants cause deficiency.

The oral mucosal manifestations of vitamin K deficiency can include gingival bleeding and post-extraction haemorrhage.

Folic acid

Folic acid (pteroylglutamic acid) is biologically inactive: folates are the active water-soluble forms. Dietary folate, present in green vegetables, liver, and yeast, is converted to the active tetrahydrofolate, which is involved in synthesis of purine and pyrimidine bases, after absorption in the small intestine. Folate deficiency is typically because of a diet deficient in green vegetables, and can arise within a relatively short period of time, since body stores last less than 3 months. Alcoholism and some cytotoxic drugs and phenytoin are other relatively common causes of deficiency of folate at the cellular level.

Folate deficiency leads to impaired synthesis and repair of DNA with megaloblastic change in haemopoietic and other cells. Buccal epithelial cells show changes similar to those in vitamin B12 deficiency.

Some patients with chronic hyperplastic candidiasis may be folate deficient. Folate-deficient individuals may also suffer from chronic atrophic candidiasis but the restoration of serum folate to normal levels rarely has any beneficial effect indicating that folate deficiency in itself may not be an aetiological factor.

The oral manifestations of vitamin deficiencies are summarized in Table 11.3.

Iron

Dietary iron is found mainly in meat. Iron is vital to oxygen transport and intracellular respiration, being inherent in some enzymes. Most iron is present in haemoglobin; some is stored in macrophages in the liver and spleen as ferritin and haemosiderin. Iron is transported as transferrin.

Deficiency can arise from dietary or absorptive causes, but usually is a consequence of chronic blood loss—typically because of menorrhagia (Table 11.4). Iron deficiency affects rapidly dividing cells such as bone marrow and oral mucosa. A hypochromic microcytic anaemia results. The serum iron and serum ferritin levels are low.

Oral mucosal manifestations of iron deficiency are common and include glossitis, angular stomatitis, and Burning Mouth syndrome. Atrophic glossitis is found in up to 40 per cent of iron deficient patients and angular stomatitis in 15 per cent. About one third of patients have a sore tongue. Manifestations respond within a few weeks to replacement therapy. Aphthae may be seen. Iron deficiency may play a role in the oral carriage of Candida species and may be one reason why oral candidal carriage is more prevalent in females than males.

There is a possible role for iron deficiency in carcinogenesis in view of the premalignant potential of the Plummer–Vinson syndrome. This syndrome, consisting of iron deficiency, dysphagia and post-cricoid oesophageal stricture may be accompanied by glossitis and angular stomatitis, and may be associated, in up to 15 per cent, with carcinomas of the post-cricoid pharynx, oesophagus, stomach, and occasionally mouth. However, any significant role for iron deficiency in oral carcinogenesis has yet to be established and, in animal models, iron deficiency has had only equivocal effects on chemical oral carcinogenesis.

Zinc

Zinc is involved in several enzyme reactions. Deficiency of zinc is usually dietary, or due to the inherited disorder acrodermatitis enteropathica. It can have many general effects (Table 11.5) but, as far as the oral mucosa is concerned, zinc deficiency does not cause atrophy—at least in animals.

Nutritional defects causing Oral Mucosal Disease

- Protein deficiency
- Excess fat and fatty acids intake
- Vitamin A deficiency
- Hypervitaminosis A
- Vitamin B1, B2, B6, B12 deficiency
- Vitamin C, D, E, K deficiency
- Folic acid deficiency
- Iron deficiency

Table 11.4 Main causes of iron deficiency

1.	Poor intake	Poverty
		Old age
2.	Malabsorption	Achlorhydria
3.	Blood loss	Haemorrhage from genitourinary or gastrointestinal tract

Table 11.5 General effects of zinc deficiency

Mild/moderate	Severe
Weight loss	Alopecia
Growth retardation	Bullous-pustular dermatitis
Rough skin	Intercurrent infections
Poor appetite	Diarrhoea
Mental lethargy .	Emotional disorders
Delayed wound healing	Hypogonadism
Oligospermia	
Taste abnormalities	

Other metals

The relevance of these is summarized in Table 11.6. There is some evidence that selenium deficiency may predispose to oral cancer.

Common oral mucosal manifestations of nutritional defects

There is evidence that malnutrition does predispose to occasional oral infections including candidiasis, to sepsis post-operatively and to the spread of acute necrotizing gingivitis to produce cancrum oris or noma as well as to non-specific stomatitis, and lingual papillary atrophy.

Oral mucosal symptoms are especially common in deficiencies of folic acid and vitamin B12: including burning mouth syndrome, glossitis, angular stomatitis, and ulcers.

Burning Mouth syndrome

Burning Mouth 'syndrome' (BMS) is the term used when symptoms described usually as a burning sensation exist in the absence of identifiable organic aetiological factors: it is often a medically unexplained symptom.

- No precipitating cause for BMS can be identified in over 50 per cent of the patients

- A psychogenic cause such as anxiety, depression or cancerophobia can be identified in about 20 per cent.

- In the others, BMS appears to follow either a dental intervention or an upper respiratory tract infection.

- Defined clinical conditions must be excluded since they can also present with burning. Organic problems with no detectable clinical lesions that can cause symptoms similar to BMS include a haematological deficiency state (deficiencies in iron, folic acid, or vitamin B) in about 30 per cent, restricted tongue space from poor denture construction, parafunction such as nocturnal bruxism or tongue-thrusting and neuropathy—such as follows damage to the chorda tympani nerve.

Glossitis

Atrophic tongue (glossitis) is common in elderly people and a marker for malnutrition.

Angular stomatitis

Angular stomatitis is predisposed by

- denture-wearing and disorders that predispose to candidiasis
- dry mouth
- tobacco smoking
- deficiency states such as iron deficiency, hypo-vitaminoses (especially B2, B6, malabsorption states (e.g. Crohn's disease).
- defects in immunity such as in Down syndrome, HIV infection, diabetes, cancer
- disorders where the lips are enlarged, such as orofacial granulomatosis, Crohn's disease and Down syndrome.

Nutritional deficiency: Oral manifestations

- Candidiasis
- Oral ulceration
- Glossitis
- Angular stomatitis
- Burning Mouth syndrome
- Gingival bleeding
- Post-extraction haemorrhage

Preventing immunologically-mediated and other disorders

Recurrent aphthous stomatitis

The aetiology of recurrent aphthous stomatitis (RAS) is in most cases unclear, but there may be a genetic basis and possibly an infective agent, as yet unidentified, and other factors may be at play. These include

- *Trauma*: minor traumatic incidents can provoke ulcers in people with RAS.
- *Stress*: emotional disturbance or stress can provoke episodes of RAS.
- *Microbial factors*: it has been suggested that RAS is caused by reactivation of a latent herpes simplex virus, but although viruses such as HSV, varicella zoster, adeno-viruses have been implicated, no viruses have been directly isolated from RAS lesions or found using cytology or electron microscopy.

Table 11.6 Relevance and deficiency features of trace metals

Metal	Relevance	Deficiency state
Selenium	Incorporated in glutathione peroxidases, thioredoxin reductase and thyroid hormone deiodinases	Cardiomyopathy
Copper	Incorporated in metalloenzymes involved in oxidative phosphorylation, synthesis of neurotransmitters and cross-linkage of collagen and elastin	Failure to thrive in babies Oedema Anaemia Impaired immunity Hair changes Skeletal and neurological abnormalities
Manganese	Incorporated in metalloenzymes	?Ataxia ?Growth retardation
Molybdenum	Cofactor in enzymes involved in metabolism of purines and pyrimidines	Developmental abnormalities

- Bacteria, mainly the L-form streptococcal bacteria, *Streptococcus sanguis* and *Strep. mitis*, could have a possible link but *Strep. sanguis* is unlikely to be the aetiological agent of RAS. *Helicobacter pylori* has been considered as a possible cause for RAS, but this possibility has not been supported by antibody studies. RAS rarely respond to antimicrobials.

- *Foods*: Certain foods are, in some patients with RAS, related to ulceration; these are chocolate, coffee, peanuts, cereals, almonds, strawberries, cheese, tomatoes, and wheat flour (containing gluten). The main allergenic substances are benzoic acid and/or cinnamonaldehyde.

- *Drug reaction*: Non-steroidal anti-inflammatory drugs and other drugs such as nicorandil may produce aphthous-like ulcers. Sodium lauryl sulphate in dentifrices may precipitate aphthae.

- *Immune defects*: Aphthous-like ulcers are found in 60 per cent of non-HIV infected patients with immunodeficiencies, mild neutropenia, myelodysplastic syndromes and other forms of neutropenia.

- *Hormonal imbalance*: A possible association between the menstrual cycle and the onset of RAS and an increase in RAS during the 7-day post-ovulation period preceding onset have been suggested but epidemiologic studies have shown no association between RAS and the menstrual cycle. However, there are patients whose RAS remits with oral estrogen contraceptives or during pregnancy and some undergo complete or partial remission during pregnancy.

- *Smoking habits*: Patients with RAS are usually non-smokers (Tuzun *et al*. 2000) and there is a much lower prevalence and severity of RAS in heavy compared to moderate smokers. Some patients report an onset of RAS parallel to smoking cessation, while others report control of RAS on re-initiation of smoking. The use of smokeless tobacco (chewing tobacco and snuff) is also associated with a significantly lower prevalence of RAS. Since the mucosal keratinization in smokeless tobacco users is generally limited locally, it is suggested that nicotine itself, or other systemically absorbed substances, may provide some additional protective role.

- *Hematinic deficiency*: Deficiency of vitamin B1, B2, or B6 has been found in around 28 per cent of RAS compared to 8 per cent in healthy individuals. Deficiency of Vitamin B12, folic acid, or iron was found in 17.7 per cent of RAS patients compared to 8.5 per cent in controls. Complete remission of ulceration was achieved in 65 per cent of those patients who were on replacement therapy and the remaining 35 per cent experienced some improvement.

- *Gastrointestinal diseases*: The chronic malabsorption associated with coeliac disease and gluten-sensitive enteropathy (GSE), can lead to deficiency of B vitamins and folate, which may play a role in the aetiology of RAS in some patients.

- *Inflammatory bowel disease (IBD)*: Crohn's disease and ulcerative colitis, may be accompanied by RAS.

Possible factors associated with RAS

• Genetic	• Immune defects
• Infective agents	• Hormone imbalance
• Trauma	• Smoking
• Stress	• Vitamin deficiencies
• Food/drugs	• Gastro-intestinal disorders

Lichen planus and lichenoid reactions

The aetiology of lichen planus remains obscure in most cases. However, a wide range of drugs have been implicated, most commonly the non-steroidal anti-inflammatory agents, antihypertensive agents, antidiabetic drugs, and antimalarials (Table 11.7). Oral lichen planus may also appear in close relationship to dental restorative materials, especially amalgam. Recent studies, however, have found little reliable evidence of hypersensitivity and the appearance of lichenoid reactions to some composite restorations should dampen the enthusiasm for the wholesale replacement of amalgams.

Orofacial granulomatosis

The group of disorders variously described as oral Crohn's disease or orofacial granulomatosis (OFG), and the related Melkersson–Rosenthal syndrome and Miescher's cheilitis (cheilitis granulomatosa) may sometimes be precipitated by identifiable agents.

There is no doubt that classic Crohn's disease can be complicated by oral lesions—especially oral ulceration and this may also be seen when gastrointestinal symptoms are absent. However, the constellation of manifestations that may be seen in any combination, including orofacial swelling, mucosal tags, gingival hyperplasia, mucosal cobblestoning, ulcers, and angular stomatitis, may also be seen in the total absence of detectable gastrointestinal disease, and the alternative term orofacial granulomatosis has,

Table 11.7 Drugs most commonly implicated in the aetiology of lichenoid reactions

Antimalarials
Beta-Adrenergic blockers
Sulphonylureas
Captopril
Methyldopa
NSAIDs
Para-salicylate
Penicillamine
Phenytoin
Procainamide
Sulphonamides
Tocainide

therefore, been suggested. This may be helpful to avoid the stigma of the term 'Crohn's disease'.

In some there may be an allergic basis to OFG and patients may respond to dietary manipulation and avoidance of putative precipitants such as various flavourings and other additives. In some patients there appear to be specific food intolerances, such as to cinnamaldehyde, carvone, piperitone, cocoa, carmosine, sunset yellow, or monosodium glutamate; micro-organisms such as *Mycobacterium paratuberculosis* may play a role.

Allergic reactions

Proven allergic reactions in the mouth are extremely rare, but it is likely that some manifestations have been overlooked and that food intolerances will, in the future, be recognized to be of greater importance than hitherto supposed. There have, for example, been clear examples of reactions to various dentifrices and other materials.

Erythema multiforme

The aetiology of erythema multiforme (EM) is unclear in most patients, but appears to be an immunological hypersensitivity reaction with the appearance of cytotoxic effector cells, CD8+ T lymphocytes, in epithelium, inducing apoptosis of scattered keratinocytes and leading to satellite cell necrosis. The reaction is triggered by:

- *immune conditions* such as BCG or hepatitis B immunization, sarcoidosis, graft vs. host disease, inflammatory bowel disease, polyarteritis nodosa or systemic lupus erythematosus

- *food additives or chemicals* such as benzoates, nitrobenzene, perfumes, terpenes

- *drugs* such as sulphonamides (e.g. co-trimoxazole), cephalosporins, aminopenicillins, quinolones, chlormezanone, barbiturates, oxicam non-steroidal anti-inflammatory drugs, anticonvulsants, protease inhibitors, allopurinol or even corticosteroids, and many others may trigger severe EM or toxic epidermal necrolysis in particular (Table 11.8).

Recurrences of drug-induced erythema multiforme are rare—unless the drug is readministered.

Plasma cell gingivitis

Gingival lesions that have been termed allergic gingivostomatitis or plasma cell gingivitis have been recognized for many years. Allergic reactions producing cheilitis and gingival changes have been described with tartar-control and some other dentifrices. Tetrasodium and/or tetrapotassium pyrophosphate (Ppi) is the anticalculus component of most tartar control dentifrices. While pyrophosphates alone are not responsible for hypersensitivity reactions, several modifications, which may lead to adverse oral manifestations may occur when pyrophosphates are added to a dentifrice. First, tetrasodium pyrophosphate in a dentifrice forms a slightly alkaline solution upon oral use, which could irritate oral membranes. Second, increased concentrations of flavoring agents, known to be sensitizers, are needed to mask the strong bitter taste

Table 11.8 Some factors precipitating erythema multiforme

Infections
Herpes simplex virus
Epstein-Barr virus
Influenza
Adenovirus
Mycoplasma pneumoniae
Many others
Drugs
Allopurinol
Aminopenicillins
Antimalarials
Barbiturates
Busulfan
Carbamazepine
C ephalosporins
Chlorpropamide
Codeine
Digitalis
Gold salts
Hydralazine
Iodides
Mercurials
Oxicam non-steroidal anti-inflammatory drugs
Penicillins
Phenothiazines
Phenytoin
Phenylbutazone
Piroxicam
Protease inhibitors
Quinolones
Salicylates
Streptomycin
Sulphonamides
Vitamin E
Others
Radiotherapy
Acute alcoholism
Hepatitis vaccination
Menstrually related hormonal (progesterone) changes

of pyrophosphates. Third, increased concentrations of detergents, capable of producing hypersensitivity reactions, are necessary to allow the pyrophosphates to become soluble in the dentifrice. Fourth, a pre-existing condition of reduced salivary flow may augment hypersensitivity to tartar control toothpastes. While pyrophosphates have been approved as additives in dentifrices, these compounds, along with the increased concentrations of flavorings and detergents and their higher intraoral alkalinity, are strongly implicated as the causative factor in certain hypersensitivity reactions.

Contact stomatitis

Contact stomatitis may result from antibiotics such as streptomycin, neomycin, and bacitracin, oils of casia and cloves, mercury, gold, vulcanite, flavouring agents such as cinnamon in toothpaste, epoxy resins, acrylic, eugenol, polyether impression material, and karaya gum. Nickel-containing and stainless-steel wire can give rise to contact allergies. Contact cheilitis has occurred with the fluorescein stains in some lipsticks, carmine, oleyl alcohol, methyl heptine carbamate, peppermint, carvone, spearmint, pineapple, mangoes, asparagus, and cinnamon oil.

Angioedema

Angioedema can result from a range of agents, for example, angioedema in response to rubber dam and to ethylene imine (in 'Scutan') has been reported.

Hypersensitivity to local anaesthetics

Hypersensitivity to local anaesthetics is uncommon. Allergies to lignocaine are rare. The parabens preservatives of local anaesthetic solutions accounted for some allergic responses, and the introduction of preservative-free preparations has minimized the hazard.

Hypersensitivity to methylmethacrylate

Methylmethacrylate sensitivity is recognized but rare.

Immunologically-mediated and other disorders

- Recurrent aphthous stomatitis
- Lichen planus and lichenoid reactions
- Orofacial granulomatosis
- Erythema multiforme
- Plasma cell gingivitis
- Contact stomatitis
- Angioedema
- Hypersensitivity

Conclusions

- The prevention of oral cancer is best achieved by reducing risk factors known to cause cancer in the mouth and elsewhere in the body. Tobacco, excessive alcohol consumption, betel use, and prolonged exposure to sunlight, are four of the most important risk factors implicated in the aetiology of oral cancer.
- The same risk factors are also implicated in the development of potentially malignant lesions.

- In addition, improving the diet by increasing intake of fruit and vegetables, treating possible infections, such as candidosis or syphilis, and improving oral hygiene, may reduce the prevalence of pre-malignant lesions.
- Denture-induced stomatitis can be prevented if dentures are not worn at night, plaque is removed by brushing, and the dentures disinfected.
- Apart from high standards of hygiene, and the avoidance of contact with those with communicable diseases, or their tissues, little can be done to prevent primary infections with viruses that can cause mucosal lesions.
- Oral infections in the immunocompromised person may be prevented by prophylactic therapy, particularly with antifungal and antiviral agents.
- Chlorhexidine gluconate aqueous mouth rinses may have an effect in the management of RAS, possibly by reducing secondary infection.
- Proven allergic reactions in the mouth can be prevented by identifying and avoiding the cause.

References

Armstrong, W.B., Kennedy, A.R., Wan, X.S., Atiba, J., McLaren, C.E., and Meyskens, F.L., Jr. (2000). Single-dose administration of Bowman-Birk inhibitor concentrate in patients with oral leukoplakia. *Cancer Epidemiol. Biomarkers Prev.*, 9(1), 43–7.

Clarkson, J.E., Worthington, H.V., and Eden, O.B. (2000). Prevention of oral mucositis or oral candidiasis for patients with cancer receiving chemotherapy (excluding head and neck cancer). *Cochrane Database Syst. Rev.*, (2), CD000978.

Dodd, M.J., Dibble, S.L., Miaskowski, C., MacPhail, L., Greenspan, D., Paul, S.M., Shiba, G., and Larson, P. (2000). Randomized clinical trial of the effectiveness of 3 commonly used mouthwashes to treat chemotherapy-induced mucositis. *Oral Surg. Oral Med. Oral Pathol. Oral Radiol. Endod.*, 90(1), 39–47.

Epstein, J.B., Silverman, S. Jr, Paggiarino, D.A., Crockett, S., Schubert, M.M., Senzer, N.N., Lockhart, P.B., Gallagher, M.J., Peterson, D.E., and Leveque, F.G. (2001). Benzydamine HCl for prophylaxis of radiation-induced oral mucositis: results from a multicenter, randomized, double-blind, placebo-controlled clinical trial. *Cancer*, 92(4), 875–85.

Etiz, D., Erkal, H.S., Serin, M., Kucuk, B., Hepari, A., Elhan, A.H., Tulunay, O., and Cakmak, A. (2000). Clinical and histopathological evaluation of sucralfate in prevention of oral mucositis induced by radiation therapy in patients with head and neck malignancies. *Oral Oncol.*, 36(1), 116–20.

Gujral, M.S., Patnaik, P.M., Kaul, R., Parikh, H.K., Conradt, C., Tamhankar, C.P., and Daftary, G.V. (2001). Efficacy of hydrolytic enzymes in preventing radiation therapy-induced side effects in patients with head and neck cancers. *Cancer Chemother. Pharmacol.*, 47 (Suppl.), S23–8.

Harris, C., Warnakulasuriya, K.A., Gelbier, S., and Johnson, N.W., Peters, T.J. (1997). Oral and dental health in alcohol misusing patients. *Alcohol. Clin. Exp. Res.*, 21(9), 1707–9.

Kaempf, D.E., and Linderkamp, O. (1998). Do healthy premature infants fed breast milk need vitamin E supplementation; alpha- and gamma-tocopherol levels in blood components and buccal mucosal cells. *Pediatr. Res.*, 44(1), 54–9.

Levy-Polack, M.P., Sebelli, P., and Polack, N.L. (1998). Incidence of oral complications and application of a preventive protocol in children with acute leukemia. *Spec. Care Dentist*, 18(5), 189–93.

Negri, E., Franceschi, S., Bosetti, C., Levi, F., Conti, E., Parpinel, M., and La Vecchia, C. (2000). Selected micronutrients and oral and pharyngeal cancer. *Int. J. Cancer*, 86(1), 122–7.

Scully, C. (2002). Oral ulceration: a new and unusual complication. *Br. Dent. J.*, 192(3), 139–40.

Scully, C., Epstein, J.B., and Saris, S. (2003). Oral Mucositis. *Head and Neck*, (in press).

Sheiham, A., and Steele, J. (2001). Does the condition of the mouth and teeth affect the ability to eat certain foods, nutrient and dietary intake and nutritional status amongst older people? *Public Health Nutr.*, 4(3), 797–803.

Tuzun, B., Wolf, R., Tuzun, Y., and Serdaroglu, S. (2000). Recurrent aphthous stomatitis and smoking. *Int. J. Dermatol.*, 39(5), 358–60.

Wan, X.S., Meyskens, F.L., Jr. Armstrong, W.B., Taylor, T.H., and Kennedy, A.R. (1999). Relationship between protease activity and *neu* oncogene expression in patients with oral leukoplakia treated with the Bowman Birk Inhibitor. *Cancer Epidemiol. Biomarkers Prev.*, 8(7), 601–8.

12

Prevention in the ageing dentition

Prevention in the ageing dentition

James Steele and Angus Walls

Introduction: What is old age and what are the oral health issues?

Dental disease and tooth loss are not an inevitable consequence of increasing age, but both are almost universal and both are irreversible. Eventually, if a person lives long enough, disability through the functional impairment resulting from tooth loss will take its toll, to a greater or lesser degree. As age increases, the emphasis of dental care often moves away from preventing and managing every diseased tooth, towards a wider strategy aimed at the prevention of a more general condition: functional limitation and dental disability, which usually result from tooth loss. Preventive dentistry for older people, whether aimed at the individual or the whole population, is generally best viewed from this perspective. Preventing or minimizing this disability involves primary prevention (preventing disease, for example by fluoride use or oral hygiene), secondary prevention (preventing disease progression, for example by early detection) or tertiary prevention (preventing the impairment and disability resulting from disease, for example by treatment planning strategies and tooth replacement).

The proportion of the population who are elderly is increasing globally. As we will see, the proportion of this increasing number of elderly people who are dentate is also rising, at least in most of the developed world. In the medium term, this will add up to a lot of dental care for a lot of older people.

Some diseases and management problems such as dry mouth and root caries, are fairly specific to older adults, so there need to be specific preventive approaches tailored to suit these. However, many of the differences between the elderly and the rest of the population are simply of degree, so the broad strategies available for the prevention of such diseases are similar to those used for any adult at risk. What is very different for the elderly is the context in which the prevention takes place. Disease prevention is an essential step by which oral disability can be prevented, but it is not the only consideration. Difficult questions often have to be asked about the most efficient use of resources, because the complexity (and so the cost) of care has the potential to rise while the benefits may diminish. A number of other peripheral issues may determine what preventive strategies are most appropriate and whether they are effective. These include individual variations in the risk of dental disease and limitations on the ability to receive care as a result of medical, social, or economic constraints. Prevention of disease in every case is rarely an appropriate philosophy, and the concept of prioritizing different items of care becomes increasingly important with increasing age.

One further point should be made. Just as there is no age at which someone becomes officially elderly, any change in the emphasis of dental care is not sudden, occurring at some predetermined stage of life, but is gradual and dictated by individual considerations. One definition of elderly is anyone who is ten years older than you are yourself (this is a definition particularly prevalent amongst dental students and grandparents). Old age can last a long time. Normal retirement age is in the early sixties and in most Western countries, life expectancy for women is over 80 years, while many individuals survive for considerably longer. As age increases, so does life expectancy. Prevention of dental disability is required for the rest of a person's life. Our objective should be to extend the oral health span to match the life span of our patients. Table 12.1 shows life expectancy for adults at different ages in the UK and illustrates that the average years of life remaining, even for 70-year-olds (12 years for men, 15 years for women), is often considerably longer than the median survival of a conventional restoration. Furthermore, the potential for discrepancy between biological and chronological age is well known and applies to oral health as much as to any other aspect of health.

How does the oral environment change with age?

Ageing is associated with some pathological and physiological changes that can affect both oral health care and disease patterns. These affect both hard and soft tissues.

Table 12.1 Life expectancy at different ages in the United Kingdom in 1999

	50 years	60 years	70 years	80 years
Men	27.7	19.2	12.1	6.9
Women	31.7	22.8	14.9	8.6

Changes to the dental hard tissues occur throughout life. There is a continued surface maturation of enamel and of exposed dentine, with increased crystal growth, altered orientation, and incorporation of other minerals into the tooth surface. These changes result in the surface enamel and dentine being more resistant to demineralization. Dentine undergoes an increase in peritubular dentine formation and in secondary dentine deposition, giving a more highly mineralized tissue. The vascularity and the volume of the pulp is reduced with an increase in pulpal fibrous tissue, areas of ectopic calcification, and a reduced number of odontoblasts. The net effect of these changes are teeth that are more mineralized and with smaller and less vascular pulps in older people.

There are a number of other age changes that affect the soft tissues of the oral cavity, but that have no bearing upon the dentition. They comprise:

- Thinning of the oral epithelium with reduced density and depth of the rete peg apparatus, impairing epithelial attachment to the sub-mucosa.

- Reduction in the quantity of connective tissue with increased collagen density and a reduced rate of collagen turnover.

- Reduction in the elasticity of elastin giving diminished tissue flexibility.

These changes are usually of limited clinical significance in terms of maintaining oral health.

It is in the salivary glands that some of the most clinically significant changes take place. There are marked changes in the structure of the salivary glands, with a reduced number of secretory units, and an increase in fibrous and fatty tissue within the gland that are potentially of more direct relevance to oral health. Studies on the alteration of salivary flow with age are complicated by the involvement of the salivary glands in systemic disease, and the influence of a wide variety of medications upon salivary function. However, if these variables are controlled for, it is now accepted that there is little alteration in salivary flow from the major glands with increasing age, either in terms of stimulated or resting flow rates. There is, however, some diminution in flow from minor salivary glands, which may have important implications in terms of mucosal immunity. Table 12.2 shows the findings for a range of studies on the relationship between salivary flow and age.

The profound structural changes that can be observed with age do not appear to fit with this apparent lack of functional impact. One explanation is the suggestion that there is a significant "functional reserve" within the salivary glands, and the reduction in secretory capacity with age is insufficient to interfere with normal functional flow. However, should any further challenge to the secretion occur, then a reduction in flow is more likely in older individuals than in the young (Fig. 12.1) (Baum et al. 1992). This hypothesis is supported by the finding that older people experience a more profound reduction in salivary flow with a given anticholinergic challenge than the young (Fig. 12.2). This is an important consideration in an age group where drugs with the capacity to reduce salivary flow are frequently prescribed.

There are also some alterations in salivary composition with increasing age, with reduced protein and IgA, alteration in the pattern of salivary mucins, and reduced sodium content. These changes will have some influence on the functional characteristics of this important oral fluid, although the nature of these effects has yet to be determined.

There are also age associated medical changes that can influence the prevention of disease. These include:

- Increased use of prescription medicines to counteract disease;

- Reduced visual acuity from presbyopia and cataracts;

- Reduced muscle bulk leading to fatigue during oral hygiene;

- Forgetfulness.

Although these may seem to be rather detached from oral health, they can have a profound effect on the oral environment, related to difficulty cleaning, the potential for dietary change, and (in the case of medications) salivary effects.

In summary, there are relatively few true age-changes that directly affect the dentition, although some (such as the changes to the dental pulp) can make dental treatment more complex. However, because of the increasing risk of systemic disease and its treatment with age, there can be quite a substantial alteration in both the risk and the implications of oral disease.

Age related changes

- Age related changes in tooth structure include increased mineralisation and reduced pulpal vascularity

- Structural changes in the salivary glands reduces their functional capacity

- Salivary flow rates are relatively unaffected by structural changes in the absence of additional challenges to salivary flow

- Age related changes in general health can also affect oral health

Population trends in the oral health of older people: the rise of the dentate older adult

The oral health of a population is not static: conditions come and go, and diseases and conditions affect various demographic groups in different ways at different times in history. Dental caries is an excellent example; secular trends in dental caries are described in Chapter 16, with rates of disease reducing markedly over recent decades in the industrialized nations. More subtle changes also occur though. In the middle of the last millennium caries was a disease of the wealthy, in the twentieth century it became a disease of everybody, while now, the pendulum has tended to swing just a little the other way, with the highest levels of caries associated with relative deprivation in industrialized countries. Such trends are important if preventive philosophies are to be

Table 12.2 Variation in salivary flow rates comparing old and young populations in healthy unmedicated individuals

Author	Whole		Parotid		Submandibular		Minor	
	Unstimulated	Stimulated	Unstimulated	Stimulated	Unstimulated	Stimulated	Unstimulated	Stimulated
Baum				Same				
Ben-Aryeh	Reduced	Same						
Ben-Aryeh	Same	Same		Same				
Bertram	Reduced							
Chauncey			Same	Same				
Gandara	Same	Same		Same				Reduced
Ghezzi				Same				
Gutman	Reduced							
Heft			Same	Same				
Navazesh	Reduced	Increase	Increase					
Niedermeier							Same	
Parvinen			Same					
Pedersen					Reduced	Reduced		
Ship			Same	Same				
Ship					Same	Same		
Smith				Same				Reduced
Tylenda				Same	Same	Same		

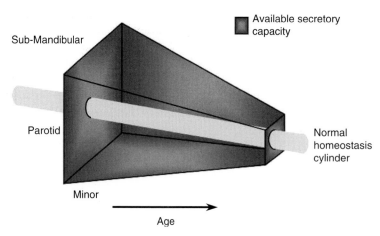

Figure 12.1 The functional capacity of the salivary glands

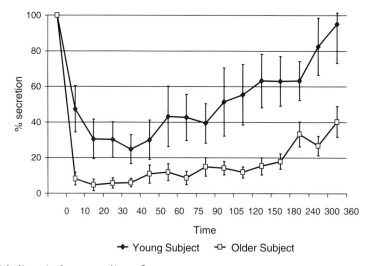

Figure 12.2 The effect of anticholinergic drugs on salivary flow

developed for different groups. The oral health of older people has undergone transformation in recent decades and the changes we have seen are probably more dramatic than for any other population group. What is more, changes will continue. The preventive needs for the elderly now are quite different from those of forty years ago, and in another forty years we are likely to be faced with a new set of problems again. This section describes what has happened, what will happen, and how this affects preventive dentistry for the older person.

Trends in oral health in the last fifty years

Recent decades have seen some remarkable changes. Fifty years ago the concept of prevention in the elderly would have been seen as quite absurd in many countries, not least in the UK where, in 1968, over 80% of people of pensionable age were edentulous Gray *et al.* 1970. Many of the remainder were so far down the road towards total tooth loss that prevention for this population would have

seemed like a complete waste of resources. How times change. Figure 12.3 shows the rapid reduction of the proportion of people edentulous between 1968 and 1998 in the United Kingdom (Kelly *et al.* 2000). In this regard, the UK may be little different from many similar countries, but because there has been a comparable survey conducted every decade since 1968, the trends in oral health have been easy to track. There is evidence that in other countries, the starting point was probably better with lower levels of edentulousness (WHO 1986), but the trend has been similar in most of those countries where national surveys have been conducted, with the exception of those where rates of edentulism were already low.

Knowing how a population has behaved over a period of time is invaluable, as it allows us to make predictions of how it may continue to change in future years. Figure 12.3 also shows the predicted trends for total tooth loss over the next three decades in the UK. Total tooth loss is predicted to reduce to very low levels indeed by 2028, even among people aged 75 or more. However, the reduction in prevalence of total tooth loss is partly to do with older, largely edentulous generations dying out and being replaced with cohorts of ageing adults who have retained their teeth. There is evidence that even amongst these groups there is a slight reduction in the incidence of edentulousness (i.e. the number of new cases), but this reduction is small and looks unlikely to disappear completely. What is more, the incidence is highest in the late middle aged and elderly. In other words, there will always be a few people who, for whatever reason, lose their natural teeth at some stage. As tooth loss is cumulative, most of the edentulous are likely to be old. This was probably not always the case. At one time there was a relatively high incidence in the young and middle aged, but less so in the old. The data from the UK in 1998 suggest that the decennial incidence was about 2–4 per cent per decade for people aged between 45 and 74. The incidence is quite difficult to calculate for people aged over 75 years, but may be a little higher. Facing a denture for the first time is not easy when you are old, and the oral disability that can result is better prevented by careful planning and targeted prevention.

The reason for such a dramatic change in oral health fortunes, particularly among middle aged and older adults has little to do with the reduction in rates of dental caries observed in younger generations. The explanation for much of the change can be found in Figure 12.4. This shows the number of restored teeth per 100 people in the population for each age group in each year that a national survey was conducted. The effect is of a wave of restorations moving across the page from left to right, with the peak (the largest concentration of fillings) being among those born between 1944 and 1963. This was a time when caries rates were high, before widespread fluoridation of toothpastes or water supplies and when restorative dental care was becoming comfortable and widely accessible, not least through an increase in the number of dentists and their willingness to undertake restorative procedures. In the UK this came about with the availability of relatively inexpensive National Health Service dentistry, but in other countries alternative systems were available which made dentistry more accessible. When allied with social changes, this saw restorative care becoming more desirable.

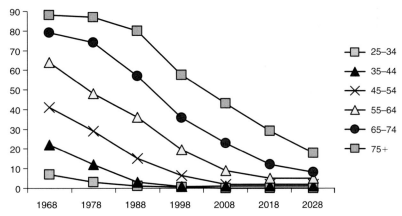

Figure 12.3 The percentage of the UK dentate by age, 1968–1998, with projections to 2028, based on data from the UK Adult Dental Health Surveys (Kelly *et al.* 2000).

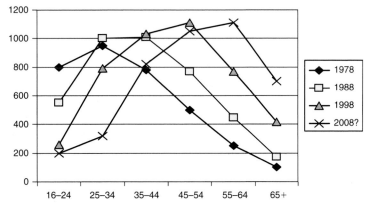

Figure 12.4 The number of restored teeth by age from 1978 to 1998, based on data from the UK Adult Dental Health Surveys (Kelly *et al.* 2000).

The legacy of all of this is an important and interesting one, if we hope to prevent oral disability in older people. Not being edentulous is not enough to ensure a functional dentition. Many older adults have some teeth, but are dependent on prosthetic replacements of those that have been lost in order for them to function. Even among those with something approaching a full set of natural teeth, Figure 12.4 shows that these are likely to be present by virtue of restoration, and repeated restoration. A typical dentate adult aged 70 years of age in the UK would have around 18 teeth, with about half of them filled, would have about a 40 per cent chance of having an artificial full coverage crown, but if they had a crown would have around 2 or 3 on average. Restorations such as large fillings and crowns are rarely permanent, and usually need servicing and replacement from time to time if the tooth underneath is to survive. Preventive strategies for the elderly have to be seen in this context, and designed around maximizing the functional possibilities that this new found general improvement in oral health allows.

Trends in oral health of older people

- The rapid increase in the number of older people with natural teeth will continue for several decades in many industrialized countries
- Older people who have natural dentitions will tend to have a high proportion of their teeth restored
- Preventive strategies for the elderly need to be seen in this context

What could be achieved with older adults' oral health?

Cohen (Cohen and Henderson 1991) has described the concepts of 'perfect health' and 'optimum health', and the distinction between the two is useful when trying to identify goals for the elderly. From a biological perspective, 'perfect health' has been defined as 'the state in which every cell is functioning at optimum capacity and in perfect harmony with each other cell' (Twaddle 1974). An often quoted 1958 World Health Organization definition of health takes a much wider, less biological approach and describes health as 'a state of complete physical and mental well being' (WHO 1958). While these definitions cover health in its widest sense, they could just as easily be applied to the narrower area of oral health. 'Perfect oral health' is not difficult to understand, but in itself, it is not a particularly useful concept. According to the strictly biological definition, it would require 32 sound teeth in a mouth that harbours no disease and where the occlusion is ideal. To set this as an objective for older adults would be meaningless. It is unachievable by all but a tiny minority, and even should it be possible, the cost of achieving and maintaining it would usually be prohibitive. The concept of 'optimum oral health' is useful though. 'Optimum health' has been defined as 'that state where the cost of any improvement outweighs the value attached to the improvement' (Cohen and Henderson 1991). The terms 'cost' and 'value' may be interpreted purely in terms of economics, but could just as readily be applied to quality of life or any other major parameter by which health is assessed. 'Optimum oral health' can apply to any age group, but changes occur in both the cost and the value of care with increasing age, so the balance tends to shift. This is a particularly useful concept when evaluating the dental needs of older adults.

Optimum oral health: what is a "functional dentition"?

At the beginning of the twenty-first century, there can be almost no elderly population anywhere in the world where 32, or for that matter even 28 natural teeth is the norm. Substantial loss of individual teeth with increasing age is almost universal, and in the United Kingdom, the mean number of teeth among dentate people aged 75 and over in 1998 was 15.4. Older people do not appear to be universally affected by their impairment, and clearly most people suffer no ill effects from partial tooth loss. On the other side of the coin, complete loss of teeth can be associated with functional and nutritional deficiencies (Sheiham et al. 2001). It would be convenient if somewhere in between, a minimum dentition could be defined; a point above which we could be confident of good function. For both the individual and for populations this could act as a minimum target; preventing functional limitation and dental disability would be built around maintaining a dentition above this level by preventing dental disease and tooth loss.

Some years ago, the WHO attempted to define such a minimum dentition, consistent with general health and function (WHO 1982). The functional dentition was set at 20 teeth, this being the number which was seen as being able to provide sufficient function without the need for any removable prostheses. The figure was used on the limited evidence available at the time.

If such a concept is to be valid, it is important to be clear about what 'functional' might actually mean. Teeth have a range of roles, but in biological terms, the most important is related to mastication and eating. A glance at comparative dental anatomy illustrates the close relationship between the dentition, diet, and evolution. Classic studies as long ago as the 1950s though showed that chewing is not entirely necessary for digestion of most foods, at least in healthy young adults. This does not mean that they are irrelevant to good nutrition as the absence of teeth may alter foods choice or the efficiency with which nutrients can be extracted, but complete digestion of many foods can occur without first being chewed.

Natural teeth and nutrition

There is no question that natural teeth are mechanically much more efficient than complete dentures. There is also evidence that the number of teeth affects the ability to bite and chew specific foods and that this can alter diet and nutrition. The evidence comes from quite a large number of relatively small scale studies (for example, Chauncey et al. 1984, Carlson 1984, Moynihan 1995, Joshipura 1996, Krall et al. 1998) and some national surveys conducted more recently. Both the British National Diet and Nutrition Survey (Steele *et al.* 1998) and the third National Health and Nutrition Survey in the USA showed that people without teeth had difficulty eating a range of foods or could not eat them at all. This relationship held even after correcting for the effects of age and gender. The problem foods included a number of commonly eaten fresh fruit and vegetables, particularly in their raw state. Furthermore, the probability of being able to eat these foods increased as the number of teeth increased. Almost everyone with 20 or more teeth had complete dietary freedom.

Just because there is dietary freedom, it does not automatically follow that the diet is entirely satisfactory and nutrition is good. However, data from both UK and US studies suggest that there is a strong trend in this direction. Intakes of key dietary components and nutrients such as dietary fibre and various vitamins and minerals were much higher in the dentate than in the edentulous, while for fibre and vitamin C there was also a measurable increase in intakes with an increasing number of teeth. People with 20 or more teeth had the highest intakes of all key nutrients and, generally, the highest blood values for these as well (Sheiham *et al.* 2001). Table 12.3 shows the values from the British survey, and illustrates the relationship between dental state and nutrition after correcting for the confounding effects of age, gender, and social class.

Generally, nutrition is best where there are more teeth. Given that having more than 20 teeth is associated with being able to eat even the most challenging foods, such as apples, nuts, and raw carrots, and that this is supported by additional material on intakes and blood values of key nutrients, the existing diet and nutrition data would broadly support the 20 tooth concept.

Natural teeth and other concepts of health

The function of teeth extends to more than just eating. The role of natural teeth includes communication and social functioning. The appearance of a person's teeth is important for social functioning, and the number of teeth can be an important variable in their appearance. Concepts of a minimum dentition required for satisfactory appearance are not really valid though, as the position, colour, and shape of the teeth are also important factors. The same argument might apply to speech. However, there is clear evidence that there is a sharp reduction in the proportion of people who wear dentures where there are more than about 20 teeth (see Fig. 12.5). Broadly speaking, having 20 or more teeth is associated with being able to function, at all levels, without dentures. Even where there are missing teeth anteriorly, the more teeth that are present and in good health, the more diverse the

Table 12.3 Dietary intake values and plasma values for selected key nutritional components in older adults, by number of teeth, after correction for the influence of age, gender, social class, and partial denture status (from Sheiham *et al.* 2001)

	Edentulous	1–10 teeth	11–20 teeth	21+ teeth
Intake of non-starch Polysaccharides (dietary fibre) (g)	11	13	13	15
Intake of intrinsic/milk sugars (from natural sources such as fruit) (g)	34	41	40	47
Intake of vitamin C (mg)	60	82	78	84
Intake of calcium (mg)	722	825	804	884
Plasma ascorbate (mmol/l)	40	46	49	53
Plasma retinal (m/mol/l)	2.1	2.3	2.3	2.2

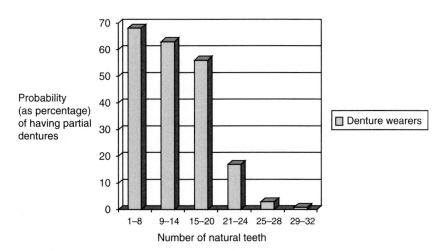

Figure 12.5 The proportion of the population with dentures according to the number of teeth they have (From Kelly *et al.* 2000).

restorative options for filling the spaces with something other than dentures. Some work suggests that the benefits extend well beyond eating function, as retention of 20 or more teeth has been shown to be associated with reduced mental and physical impairment in old age, and even lower mortality (Shimazaki *et al.* 2001).

Modern concepts of oral health have extended beyond disease and function. Locker's model of oral health recognizes that while impairment and functional limitations are important, disability and handicap can occur, perhaps even where physical functional limitation does not. Measuring oral health based on the person's oral health related quality of life suggests that the number of teeth is also related to this, as well as simply to function. The evidence that there is any sort of threshold at 20 teeth is less clear though, and quality of life issues include the presence of discomfort and pain, satisfaction with the dentition and also the expectation that a person has of their own dentition. The evidence is limited, but studies from several countries, including the UK, Greece, and Australia suggest that there is some cultural variation within this and that more teeth generally means better oral health related quality of life, up to and indeed beyond the 20 tooth threshold.

The number of teeth may correlate with dietary potential and nutritional outcome, but it is a crude measure and does not take into account the way that the teeth meet, or for that matter their condition. To some extent the way that teeth are lost or the pattern of retained teeth would appear to be simple chance; dependent on the location of disease. However, treatment planning strategies have been suggested that alter the way that disease is managed, and therefore, over a period of time, the distribution of teeth that emerges. Foremost among these is the concept of the 'shortened dental arch' (SDA). This is a simple philosophy, first developed by Käyser (1981) that can be applied to any dentition so long as there are sufficient teeth. As resources are almost always limited when dealing with older people (whether they be financial, time, specialist skills, or the ability to receive care) then treatment will often need to be prioritized. SDA theory would argue that the anterior teeth take the highest priority, as they are aesthetically and mechanically important, but also because they are accessible for cleaning and for dental care. In short, they are a good bet. Premolar teeth are also a good bet, being accessible, but are also generally single or double rooted and therefore are easy to treat, and also easy to access and clean; particularly important in the elderly. Molars though are less accessible, have two or three roots with furcations between them and complex canal systems. Maintenance is difficult and treatment is often time consuming and expensive. Although these may often be treated, they should take a low priority, only receiving care when the priority teeth further forward have received the care they need to secure their future. If resources are exhausted and these teeth need complex treatment, they can be extracted or even left untreated.

SDA is an attractive concept and very appropriate for older patients, but in many cases may not be appropriate because the distribution of teeth precludes it. Nevertheless, the principle of prioritization of key teeth is an important one and increases the efficiency of the teeth that are there. Careful planning and prioritization may help to prevent oral disability, even when the 20 teeth threshold is approached. Where more teeth are lost, there is still a place for strategic planning as a means of preventing disability. Targeting resources to key teeth for maximum prosthetic benefit and managing the process of becoming edentulous can both make a useful contribution towards preventing oral disability.

In summary, the target of 20 natural teeth initially suggested by the WHO, is probably a reasonable working rule, and would seem to be associated with the potential for comfortable and efficient eating, and for dietary and nutritional freedom. The precise number is not critical. Eighteen well-aligned teeth may occasionally be more functional than 22 that fail to make posterior contact, but a threshold value of around 20 teeth is valid. At a public health level, preventing oral disability in most of the population could be achieved by maintaining 20 or more healthy and functional natural teeth. At an individual level there will always be people who cannot function with lots of teeth and others who can eat a challenging meal with nothing but two ill fitting pieces of acrylic to help. However, even when dealing with individuals, strategic treatment planning around securing this minimum can help to ensure a level of function consistent with health and help to prevent severe oral disability.

Functional dentition

- Loss of natural teeth is associated with significant disability and may be associated with altered nutrition

- Around 20 or more natural teeth allows good function and nutritional freedom

- Quality of life and general health benefits from natural tooth retention have also been identified

- A functional natural dentition of around 20 or more natural teeth for life is a reasonable long-term population goal

- Prevention in older adults is as much about preventing oral disability resulting from tooth loss by good planning as it is about preventing disease

What will limit the ability to achieve a functional natural dentition for life?

Missed targets

It is all very well, having a target to aim at for the population or for your patient, but it has to be something that is achievable. Despite the increase in the retention of natural teeth in the older population that has been described, we are still some way off 20 natural teeth being a universal possibility. Once again, the most recent data comes from the UK, where in 1998 just over one-fifth of all adults aged 65 years and over actually had 21 or more natural teeth. The remainder have already missed the target and preventing disability for them will be dependent on careful planning and management of what is left. However, even 20% is a great deal better than the situation 20 years ago where a functional dentition in older adults was a genuine rarity. If we look at the future generations of older adults, for example at the 45–54 year olds of 1998, the potential to maintain a functioning natural dentition is considerable; over 80% had 21 or more teeth, 10% more than 10 years previously. This generation could be strategically managed, could have disease prevented or slowed and a high proportion could continue into old age with the potential for a complete diet and good nutrition. These trends can be modelled to see where we are likely to be in the future, though much less accurately than for total tooth loss. Nevertheless, using crude modelling techniques, by 2018 61% of 65–74 year olds (45–54 year olds in 1998) are predicted to have 21 or more natural teeth. There does seem to be the real potential to prevent the disability resulting from tooth loss in older age for the majority of people. To do this though we need to address the barriers to achieving this. These include social, economic, and attitudinal barriers, as well as preventing dental disease and the consequences of dental treatment.

Factors limiting the ability to receive care

Dental non-attendance

Not everybody goes to the dentist for check-ups. This is not a profound intellectual statement that will come as a surprise to anybody reading it, but dental attendance may be one of the major limiting factors in the ability to retain teeth. Despite the unnecessary tooth tissue removal that has undoubtedly been undertaken in the name of good dentistry over the years, the impact of dental attendance does seem, on balance, to be associated with better oral health in the form of more teeth over a lifetime than non-attendance. This is not to say that it is the attendance that has necessarily resulted in more teeth being retained, but there is a clear association. Figure 12.6 shows clearly the difference in the

number of teeth between attenders and non-attenders based on data from the 1998 UK Adult Dental Health Survey. Although these data are cross-sectional the implication is that dental attendance does result in tooth retention. This is supported by data showing much higher levels of untreated disease in non-attenders. In the UK, around 60 per cent of dentate people aged 75 years and older said they were regular attenders. In the next generations (55–74) the proportion is even higher at 68 per cent, and generally the proportions of dentate people attending for treatment is slowly increasing. Nevertheless, around 20–30 per cent of older people only attend when they suffer pain or problems. If strategic planning is to have any chance of preventing oral disability, then that 20–30 per cent of the population, and their successors in younger generations will need to be brought into some kind of dental care. Furthermore, those charged with providing the care will need to be well briefed in the concepts of strategic planning, and will need to be working in an environment where this is encouraged.

The reasons why people do not attend the dentist are many and varied, but include fear, anxiety, and cost. In older adults, there are also data to suggest that a feeling that there is no need for treatment is also an important consideration, perhaps reflecting changed priorities with increasing age. Recent data suggest that the proportion of people for whom fear and anxiety is a barrier is reducing. Nevertheless, fear does appear to be a major factor in non-attendance amongst older adults, but cost may be a more important variable in determining whether treatment is actually received.

It is impossible and unwise to make bold statements about the importance of cost as a barrier to receiving care in older people, just as it is inappropriate to make bold statements about the role of wealth. The willingness to receive care depends in large part on the value placed by the individual on oral health as well as their ability to pay for it. Imbalances are common. The role of the dental practitioner is to keep in sight the ultimate objective of care, i.e., is the long-term prevention of disability, discomfort,

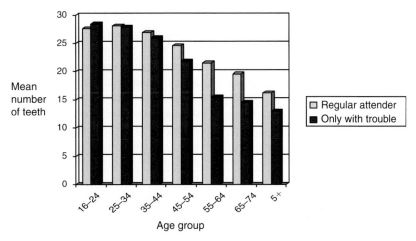

Figure 12.6 Tooth retention of dental attenders compared with non-attenders at different ages (Kelly *et al.* 2000).

and dissatisfaction. It is then the job of the professional to find a programme of prevention and treatment that can be managed within both the financial, physiological, and psychological limitations that prevail, but that still meet the key objective. Management concepts such as the shortened dental arch (see above) can encompass preventive principles and take account of economic limitations as well as the limitations imposed by fear and anxiety.

Limitations related to disability and illness

When planning oral care in older people, the dentist has to draw on a number of resources. At the top of the list of resources are financial resources, in other words the ability for the costs of care to be met. Sometimes, that is met by the state, sometimes by insurance or sometimes directly by the patient. However, there are other resources that may limit the ability of the elderly to receive care. The dentist has to have the skills, the equipment, and the time to deal with some of the complex problems he or she faces. The patient also has to have the time, and in the case of the elderly, the ability to receive care. The ability to get to the surgery, to sit for long enough in a chair so that treatment can be provided, and the dexterity to maintain a clean and healthy mouth are all key resources that can limit the ability to prevent oral disability.

Despite the column inches in dental journals devoted to the provision of dental care to old people unable to leave home or to tolerate intervention, most older adults (over the age of retirement 65, for the sake of argument) are mobile and relatively self-reliant. Mild disability is common in older adults, but both the frequency of disability and its severity tend to increase with age, particularly over the age of 80 years. The range of disabilities is wide, but difficulties with locomotion and personal care are the most common forms; and both might have some bearing on the ability to maintain a reasonable standard of oral health.

Oral health problems may be complicated because of an inability to obtain care as a result of disability, for example, where a subject is housebound and unable to reach a dentist. Severe disability, to a level that limits people to their own home is not uncommon, though it affects a minority of older people, even of over 75 year olds. It is reasonable to assume that a large majority of adults beyond retirement age would be able to visit the dentist's surgery. However, while the subject may be able to reach a dentist, treatment might still be compromised in other ways by general health. For example, the dentist may have difficulty providing good-quality care because of the involuntary movements of Parkinson's disease, or where the patient cannot be treated supine due to musculoskeletal or cardiovascular problems. The scale of such problems in the community as a whole is unknown but all become more likely with increasing age, and may be a significant impediment to maintaining oral health.

In other circumstances, it may be possible for the professional to provide, and the patient to receive quality treatment, but this may be compromised by the patient's inability to maintain the dentition in good condition because of difficulties with oral hygiene. A wide range of specific conditions may be responsible, for example, severe chronic arthritis, any neurological disturbances of motor function (e.g. stroke and neuromuscular diseases), and perhaps also painful oral mucosal conditions. However, among even the most severely disabled adults, epidemiological data suggest that a majority are able to wash their hands and face and could perhaps be expected to perform the most basic oral preventive measures, such as fluoride mouth rinsing, even if brushing is not possible. A range of alternatives to conventional toothbrushes are available that may help to offset the hygiene problems that result from disability and illness. The provision of domiciliary care from a hygienist may also be a cost-effective way of providing this. Education of carers is definitely a priority for dependent elderly.

Medical conditions and their resultant disabilities can lead to an impaired ability to achieve oral health in one other way. Where medical problems are severe, or a chronic debilitating illness exists, there may be a tendency for oral health to seem trivial and 'not worth the effort'. In many circumstances this is understandable. On the other hand, if subjects reach this stage with a reasonable dentition, the effort required to maintain at least one aspect of their own well-being in good condition may not be great. Where older adults can be empowered (by proper instruction and education) to take care of their own oral health, the benefits in terms of self-esteem and general well-being, may extend well beyond the teeth themselves.

The effects of dental disease and of dental care

Older people are at greater risk of specific diseases, notably caries of the exposed root surfaces, which can be very damaging and a risk to the survival of the tooth. Treatment for clinical conditions that are common in younger life is also more difficult, altering our ability to manage dental disease. This particularly applies to pulp and periodontal diseases. Specific preventive methods for the conditions of most relevance to older people are discussed in detail in the next section.

Preventing dental disease in older people is an essential step in preventing the disability that can result from uncontrolled tooth loss, so oral disease is certainly a threat to our ability to prevent oral disability; but the treatment of that disease is equally a problem. Dental treatment can contribute to accelerate dental disability, through iatrogenic tooth tissue destruction or through inappropriate planning.

Traditional restorative solutions for the management of dental disease, particularly dental caries, have the potential to be very damaging to the structure of the tooth. Modern techniques now allow the removal of the minimum of healthy tissue in order to access caries, but careless or thoughtless use of a bur can still result in extensive loss of valuable tooth tissue, and shorten the life of the tooth. Thoughtless planning is probably more of a problem. Full coverage crowns, often used to improve the appearance of a tooth, generally require extensive removal of sound tooth tissue inevitably weakening the structure of the tooth and potentially threatening the pulp. Most dentists will be familiar with the downward spiral of a tooth that has a crown placed to improve its appearance, and then loses vitality. The tooth then requires endodontic treatment followed by post placement and a new crown only to then end up with a root fracture, extraction, and then preparation of the teeth either side as bridge abutments, as the whole cycle starts again. The problems of prevention are generally exacerbated in people with extensively restored mouths as all restorations have margins that are subject to breakdown and will harbour plaque, acting as a focus for disease progression.

Technology has provided some solutions to these problems with materials and techniques that reduce the need for removal of large amounts of tooth tissue, but bad planning will always be a barrier to good treatment.

Limiting factors

- Despite the increase in tooth retention, a majority of older people will need some kind of removable prostheses for some years to come
- Dental non-attendance through fear and financial restraints may limit the ability to achieve a functional natural dentition in many people
- Poor general health and poor planning and delivery of dental treatment will also limit the ability to achieve a functional natural dentition in old age

Preventing dental disease in the elderly: root caries

In most cases, the prevention of specific dental diseases in this group conforms to the same basic rules as for younger adults. The changes in the oral environment may alter the emphasis a little, but the strategies are similar. This section deals with the conditions where there are specific additional issues related to age. The most important of these is root caries, a form of dental caries that

is rare in the population under 50 years of age, but probably the biggest threat to the viability of natural teeth in old age. Because of the cumulative effects of damage over a lifetime two other diseases/conditions are worthy of discussion in the context of the elderly: periodontal disease and tooth wear. Both are covered in detail elsewhere in this book, so these will be discussed only in the context of increasing age.

Root caries: prevalence, incidence and distribution of lesions

There is wide variation in the reported prevalence of root caries, from as low as 7.3 per cent in a fluoridated community to 100 per cent in patients attending a gerontology clinic. This range represents natural variation in prevalence and differences in the diagnostic criteria and examination methods used by the research workers. One significant source of variation is the way that data on restored root surfaces are handled. It is not possible to decide why any given restoration has been placed, so restorations placed because of cervical wear inflate the 'filled' component of a root surface DMF score. For example, data from the UK suggest that only 45 per cent of restorations placed on root surfaces are to manage caries. This problem has been discussed in detail by de Paola et al. (1989). One further confounding problem is that restorations placed to restore cervical wear can subsequently undergo marginal breakdown and develop recurrent decay. It is possible such root surfaces would have developed decay had they not been restored to manage the wear; alternatively, it is also possible that the only reason they developed decay was because of the presence of a restoration margin.

One thing that is clear is that the prevalence of root caries in a population increases with increasing age. Table 12.4 shows the variation in the number of lesions per person affected, depending upon the age and nature of the population studied, and demonstrates much higher levels of root caries in an institutional compared to a free-living population. These figures are useful, but

Table 12.4 Mean number of vulnerable roots, root lesions, and RCI in a UK older adult population, by age for free-living adults and for those older adults living in an institution (from Steele et al. 1998).

	65–74 free-living	75–84 free-living	85+ free-living	All free-living	Institution
All vulnerable roots	13.7	12.8	9.6	13.3	9.3
Gross decay	0.3	0.4	0.6	0.3	0.7
New decay	0.8	0.8	1.3	0.8	1.7
Unsound restoration	0.2	0.1	0.2	0.2	0.3
All unsound roots	1.3	1.3	2.1	1.3	2.7
Mean RCI[a]	25%	28%	38%	26%	46%
Mean RCI (d)[b]	12%	15%	25%	13%	39%
Prevalence of unsound roots				50%	79%
Mean number of unsound roots in affected people				2.6	3.5

[a]RCI, the root caries index, or the proportion of of roots that are exposed in the mouth that were recorded as being decayed, or restored, or restored and decayed.

[b]RCI (d), the root caries index for decay, or the proportion of of roots that are exposed in the mouth that were recorded as being decayed, or restored and decayed.

they do not give any idea of the likelihood that any given individual will develop root caries. If caries is to occur on the root, it is first necessary that the root surface is exposed in the oral cavity by loss of periodontal attachment. Without taking into account the amount of root exposure it is impossible to assess the real level of risk. The root caries index (RCI) gives an 'attack rate', relating to the number of surfaces at risk (Katz 1984). RCI is given in Table 12.4. Once again, there is a trend for an increase in RCI with age, up to 38 per cent by the age of 85 years. In the case of the data presented, restorations are counted within the RCI score so the values indicate disease history rather than active disease. An alternative calculation for decay only is given, RCI(d) which shows a similar trend. Furthermore, there is an uneven distribution of root caries/restorations within the population such that 80 per cent of new lesions occur in about 20% of the population, and only about 50 per cent of the free-living older population have root caries at all, although up to 80 per cent show carious lesions or a pattern of restorations that suggest a history of caries on the root surfaces. This concentration occurs despite the almost universal presence of root surface exposure in older individuals.

The limited data available on annual incidence in a variety of populations suggests about two new carious surfaces per hundred surfaces at risk per year. The exception to this is data for chronically ill subjects, among whom caries rates are much higher. Once again, most studies found that these new lesions occurred in a minority of the population.

There is a characteristic distribution for root caries lesions within the oral cavity, with an increased prevalence in mandibular molar teeth, followed by maxillary anterior teeth, and maxillary posteriors. Mandibular anteriors seem to be the least susceptible to root caries. In addition, the buccal and interproximal surfaces are more susceptible to attack than the palatal or lingual aspects of vulnerable teeth. This pattern of caries susceptibility has a marked similarity to the pattern of oral sugar clearance reported by Dawes and Macpherson (1993). Where sugar clearance is slowest, caries rates are raised. However, this perceived pattern of attack may be distorted by the characteristic pattern of tooth loss amongst the elderly, and also by the inclusion of restored cervical wear lesions. Once again it is very difficult to pick apart.

Root caries: risk factors

There have been a large number of variables associated with the development of root caries from both prevalence and incidence studies. Beck et al. (1987) proposed a multifactor model that illustrates the intricate web of aetiological variables that may be associated with either the severity or the progression of the disease (Fig. 12.7). As would be expected, subjects with periodontal disease have an increased level of root caries because they have more exposed root, but the attack rate is greater for those with untreated periodontal disease compared with subjects after periodontal care. This perhaps reflects better hygiene in these subjects (older individuals who demonstrate a good standard of oral hygiene have few root caries lesions).

There is now a large number of studies investigating risk factors for root caries, and it can be difficult to disentangle the real risk factors from their co-variables. Chronological age is probably of little significance per se in determining root caries activity, but increased biological age, with associated medical/physical deterioration and disability may be of much greater importance. For example, high levels of root caries have been reported in the chronically ill, institutionalized older adults, drug addicts, and in individuals with altered salivary function as a result of disease or its treatment. There is also a strong relationship between past root caries experience and the development of new lesions, and a weaker association between coronal decay experience and root caries. Higher prevalence rates are seen in men compared with women and there are a number of social attitudinal variables that are associated in both a positive and a negative manner with root caries. The numbers of remaining teeth and active social participation are both negative predictors for root caries. Negative life events, low educational attainment, low income, recurrent chronic illness, infrequent oral hygiene, irregular attendance, and smoking are all positive predictors of the level of disease activity.

Caries though needs sugar, plaque, and a suitable environment if it is to develop, and root caries is no different. Realistically, these are the areas at which a preventive strategy can be targeted. Epidemiological studies have shown that root caries is strongly related to the frequency of sugars intake. Dentine has a higher pH for demineralization than enamel, so reductions in pH that occur with sugars intake will be maintained below the demineralizing threshold for longer on a dentine surface (Fig 12.8). Poor or infrequent hygiene is also associated with an increased risk of disease, while a number of studies have shown that wearing a partial denture may also be important, perhaps more than doubling the risk of root decay being present.

Root caries: microbiology and histology

Decay is a process of microbial origin. *Streptococcus mutans* is of prime importance in initiating coronal caries, although other species may be of greater significance in extension of the carious lesion into dentine. There remains however, some debate concerning the species of bacteria that are responsible for root lesions. As a consequence of the elevated critical pH for demineralization of dentine, bacteria of lesser acidogenicity could contribute to demineralization of root lesions. The organisms most commonly cultured from plaque overlying root caries lesions or from the dentine itself are *Actinomyces* species (*viscosus, naeslundii*, and *Israelii), Streptococcus mutans*, Lactobacilli and Candida species.

The detection of *S. mutans* and Lactobacilli in plaque samples, even at very low levels, has been related to the development of root caries within that individual. This pattern holds true for the mouth as a whole, but detection in plaque at a specific site did not necessarily mean that caries was also present at that site. Beighton and Lynch (1993) used a novel sampling technique to remove small quantities of carious dentine from root lesions with varying degrees of clinical 'activity'. Microbiological culture of these

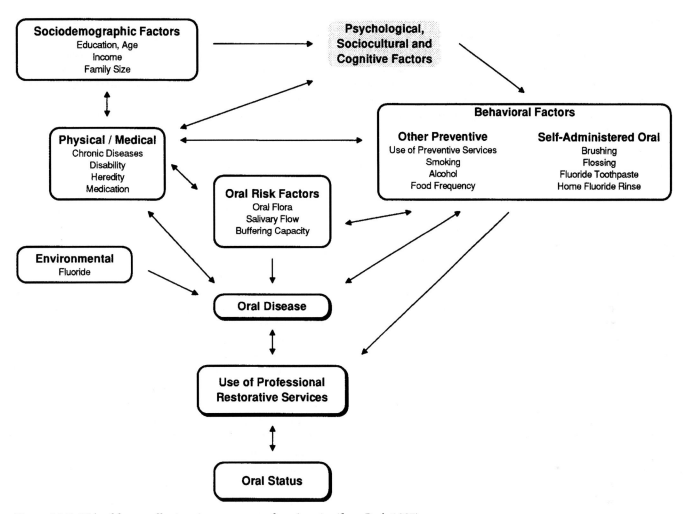

Figure 12.7 Web of factors affecting the occurrence of tooth caries (from Beck 1987)

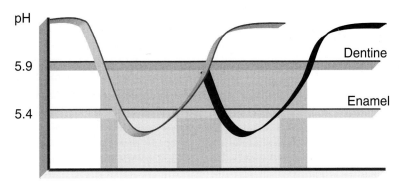

Figure 12.8 pH threshold for decay in dentine

dentine samples has demonstrated a strong positive relationship between caries activity (assessed on clinical criteria) and the frequency of isolation of both *S. mutans* and candida species. *S. mutans* were isolated more frequently from soft lesions, larger lesions, and those closest to the gingival margin. The candida species, while isolated more frequently at similar sites, were present in low numbers. Their presence was thought to be linked to their suitability for the environment rather than their acidogenicity, although candida do produce collagenase enzymes that may facilitate the spread of caries in dentine.

The macroscopic and microscopic appearance of root surface lesions will depend upon the stage of progression of the disease.

A root surface that is exposed in the mouth will take up mineral from oral fluids forming a hypermineralized surface layer that is not present on root surfaces that have not been exposed in the oral cavity. The early root caries lesion is characterized by demineralization beneath this hypermineralized surface. Dissolution of apatite crystals and splitting of the collagen bundles within the dentine matrix accompany demineralization. Clinically detectable softening of the root surface occurs at a relatively early stage of the lesion, with surface breakdown at a number of discrete, localized sites. Bacterial penetration into the demineralized surface occurs quite quickly after the onset of decay, but the rate of progression of the lesion can be slow, resulting in a clinical picture of extensive, but shallow, carious lesions on the root surface. Obviously, such lesions can progress towards the pulp of the tooth, and will lead eventually to pulpal exposure.

The diagnosis of caries activity in dentine is dependent on detecting the texture of a lesion rather than its colour. However, pushing a sharp probe into a shallow lesion that has the potential to remineralize may produce a surface defect that cannot be cleansed resulting in localized caries progression. The texture of the lesion should be assessed using a scraping action with either a probe or an excavator, rather than by pushing the probe tip into the dentine surface.

Root caries: prevention

Strategies to prevent or control root caries can be targeted at the any of the key factors in its development: the root surface and its environment (for example using fluorides or sialogogues), plaque control, diet control or combined strategies where all of these are applied.

The root surface and the oral environment

Lifelong exposure to water-containing optimum levels (1 ppm or pro rata for the climatic conditions) of fluoride reduces the prevalence of root caries. The magnitude of the reduction is not as great as that for coronal lesions. The effect is 'dose related'. The attack rate for a population with 3.5 mg/L fluoride in their water was significantly less than that for subjects exposed to 0.7 mg/L (Burt *et al.* 1986). Fluoride also has a beneficial effect in adults who drink fluoridated water but did not do so when their teeth were developing, with reduction both in caries prevalence and incidence. (Whelton *et al.* 1993; Brustman 1996). These data are independent of the acknowledged preventive benefits from using a fluoride containing dentifrice (Jensen 1988). Topical application of fluoride either as in a dentifrice, or as a rinse or gel assists in preventing decay. However, there is little information available about optimal delivery systems for fluoride when trying to prevent root caries. The variation in critical pH for dentine, when compared to enamel, and the relatively greater uptake of fluoride by dentine, when compared to enamel, must affect the dose/response gradient for fluoride and the method of fluoride delivery (neutral/ acidulated, solution/gel/foam). New toothpastes with high fluoride concentrations of fluoride (up to 5000 ppm) are now available to facilitate this process.

A variety of regimes have been described for the prevention and remineralization of root caries in individuals with reduced salivary flow. All include the use of topical fluorides, either as a mouth rinse, or in gel form, with or without custom-filled polyvinyl guards. In addition, a supersaturated calcium phosphate mouthwash can be used to enhance remineralization. All of these treatment modalities are of benefit in the xerostomic patient giving a reduction in caries prevalence. They have also been shown to be beneficial in subjects with a high caries incidence and normal salivary flow. Many of these treatments act by reducing the *S. mutans* colonization of the root surface as well as enhancing remineralization.

Prevention in people with xerostomia should also include some form of stimulus for substitute for saliva (Fig. 12.9). Salivary flow can be enhanced using taste (although care needs to be taken in patients with teeth not to use acidic or sugar-containing agents), pharmacological, or mechanical stimuli. The drugs used to enhance salivary flow must be cholinergic agonists, and hence have the potential for causing systemic side-effects. Nevertheless, there are reports of good short-term success in enhancing oral wetness with oral pilocarpine hydrochloride and Cimevidine® used in low doses. Recently it has been established that chewing sugar-free gum stimulates salivary flow and enhances the rate of increase in pH of plaque after a cariogenic challenge, and does benefit xerostomic subjects. Chewing gums are available which contain fluoride to maximize the preventive effect and chlorhexidine to assist in bacterial control.

There are a number of commercially available salivary substitutes for use where the patient has a dry mouth. In many cases these will have little impact on root caries, but those containing fluoride have been shown to be effective remineralizing media for enamel *in vitro*. Some artificial salivas attempt to increase salivary flow by incorporating an acid taste stimulus. These substances can cause demineralization of tooth tissue in their own right and may be counterproductive in the prevention of root caries.

Plaque and microbiological control

It has been demonstrated that the development of new carious lesions can be prevented, during the maintenance phase of periodontal treatment, by vigorous and regular individual and professional tooth cleaning, but such vigorous oral hygiene may lead to iatrogenic problems of its own. Nevertheless, effective hygiene is of fundamental importance in preventing root caries.

Chlorhexidine gluconate is a bis-biguanide antiseptic that can be used to reduce oral colonization with *S. mutans*, and hence assist in reducing caries activity. It has been used to some benefit either as a stand-alone rinse or gel, or in association with fluoride in preventing decay. Longer-term use is associated with staining of the dentition and changes in taste, but the gel preparations are less likely to be associated with these problems. Chlorhexidine can also be applied to the root surface in a varnish where it remains active for between 3 and 6 months. It has also been used as a component of chewing gum. Regular use of this gum has

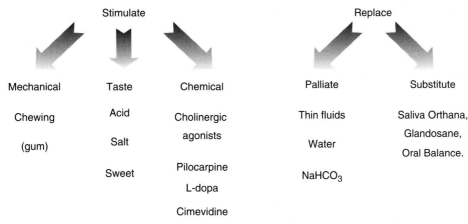

Figure 12.9 Saliva substitutes

been shown to reduce plaque and caries levels and increase salivary flow in debilitated older people, and this may prove to be a very useful adjunct to other methods of caries protection.

Dietary control

The relationship between sugars in the diet and caries, described elsewhere in this book, is well established and extends to root caries. Prevention by managing diet though requires a substantial behavioural change and in the context of the older patient, altering dietary habits developed over a lifetime is not easy. It is the frequency of sugars intake that is critical. Data from the UK National Diet and Nutrition survey demonstrated that the risk of root caries being present was approximately doubled where the frequency of sugars intake exceeded nine episodes per day. In practical terms, high frequencies of sugars intake are often the result of sugar in tea and coffee, biscuit eating, or sometimes sucking sweets, perhaps to alleviate the effects of a dry mouth, the latter scenario can be quite devastating to the dentition. Patients will often be prepared to replace sugar with saccharine in hot drinks, and to alter their dietary habits when the strategic importance is fully explained.

The dietary problem is particularly acute in the institutional setting where food is mass produced, and the diet often tailored to the lowest level of masticatory function, resulting in a high carbohydrate diet, often with frequent sugar intakes. Probably largely because of this, rates of root caries in institutions are much higher than in free-living older people. Altering dietary practice in such circumstances is exceptionally difficult.

Root caries: managing lesions to prevent disease progression

Root caries can be a difficult treatment problem, especially if the decay extends sub-gingivally, interproximally, or into the furcation region of periodontally involved molar teeth. There are three possible treatment strategies.

1. Chemotherapeutic treatment leading to remineralization. Remineralization of shallow carious root surface lesions is practical, but the remineralized tissue takes on the appearance of an arrested carious lesion. The surface is dark brown or black with a leathery texture initially, and will eventually harden to give a polished highly mineralized surface. Some patients may not be prepared to tolerate this discolouration of the root surface. Such remineralized surfaces are reported to be more resistant to further carious attack than adjacent, otherwise sound, dentine.

2. Surface recontouring. The earliest form of operative management simply comprises removal of the softened surface dentine with a disc or large bur, followed by recontouring of the root architecture to give a smooth, cleansable surface that is then managed chemotherapeutically. This approach is only applicable for shallow lesions, where excellent results have been reported.

3. Restoration of the defect. Once frank cavitation has occurred or where access for cleaning is simply not practical even after recontouring, carious dentine should be removed and the defect restored conventionally. A plethora of tooth-coloured materials are now available and are the usual materials of choice, ranging from glass ionomer cements to composite resins, with a range of products combining the components of both.

Where restoration is required, the restorative material itself can potentially have a preventive role. Both Glass Ionomer Cement (GIC) and compomers release fluoride, although at different rates. In addition, GICs have the capacity to act as a fluoride sponge taking up fluoride ions when the local ionic concentration is high (e.g. when exposed to a fluoride-containing dentifrice or rinse), and subsequently releasing it. There is extensive evidence from both *in vitro* and *in situ* studies that this fluoride release prevents demineralization and enhances remineralization around restorations. However, this does not extend to being able to observe a long-term anti-caries effect as there is no clinical evidence of caries inhibition from currently available trials data (Randal and Wilson 1999). The reasons for this disparity are unclear, but could be related to there being insufficient fluoride to show a clinically significant benefit, or it may simply reflect the types of lesions used in trials and their duration.

Root caries lesions can be inaccessible to conventional instrumentation. In such circumstances, the chemo-mechanical removal of carious dentine using a hypochlorite agent to disrupt damaged collagen fibres may be a viable alternative to classical cavity preparation techniques using burs. This is virtually pain free and can be very useful, particularly in a domiciliary setting.

Preventing root caries

- Root caries is a significant oral health problem for the elderly
- The distribution of disease is not even across the population and a small proportion of people are at much higher risk than the rest
- Strategies for prevention of root caries in individual patients include hygiene, dietary management and avoidance of removable dentures, and use of fluorides and other specific chemo-therapeutic techniques
- Intensive preventive regimes may be appropriate for patients at highest risk

Preventing dental disease in the elderly: periodontal disease

Loss of periodontal attachment is virtually universal and increases with age, but the relationship between age and attachment loss is a result of long-term exposure to plaque rather than to any age-changes within the periodontium. The rate of progression of periodontal disease is influenced by the body's immune response that alters with age resulting in modified patterns of disease. Shallow pockets are at reduced risk of progression in older populations when compared to deep pockets. Periodontal disease may be the principal reason for tooth loss in people aged above 35, but it is not for oldest adults. This may be a reflection of an innate resistance to periodontal destruction amongst older adults who retain some teeth, or simply that the teeth most likely to be lost as a consequence of periodontal destruction have already been extracted in the older cohorts. In other words, the teeth left with shallow pockets are the survivors, those at lower risk from periodontal damage.

Combined with professional scaling and root planing (older individuals respond just as well as the young to non-surgical management techniques, see Fig. 12.10), oral hygiene remains the mainstay for prevention of further loss of attachment, and an essential pre-requisite of successful management. Unfortunately, oral hygiene in older patients is complicated by the alterations in gingival architecture that result from disease and is made more difficult by the exposure of root surfaces, and the involvement of root furcations. This does not prevent effective oral hygiene, but can make it much more difficult for the patient to achieve.

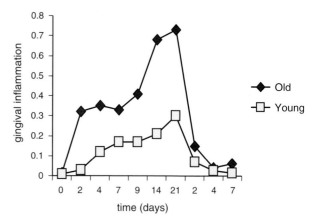

Figure 12.10 Surgical versus non-surgical treatment of periodontal diseases at different ages (Reproduced from Holm-Pedersen *et al.* (1975) with permission from the editor of J. Clin. Perio.).

It is often necessary to help older patients adapt their oral hygiene techniques, and to introduce aids such as wood points and bottle brushes to facilitate interproximal cleaning. Care needs to be taken to ensure that this education process is self-paced rather than forced, and that the genuine problems of undertaking a task that is far from straightforward are fully acknowledged. Reduced manual dexterity, poorer vision, and changing priorities mean that there will often come a time when an older person can no longer cope with their own oral hygiene. When this occurs the help of a carer is essential, but teaching and enthusing a carer in the skills required to brush somebody else's teeth is often more difficult than helping a patient develop their own skills. Introducing an electric toothbrush and/or chemical plaque control can help in these difficult circumstances, but minimizing the ongoing loss of attachment through good hygiene depends on excellent communication and a large helping of empathy.

Preventing periodontal disease

- Preventing the progression of periodontal disease in older adults is dependent on good plaque control
- Good plaque control may be more difficult to achieve in older adults

Preventing dental disease in the elderly: tooth wear

Wear occurs as a natural phenomenon on all teeth with use, so is technically not a disease at all. As it is irreversible, the severity of wear will increase with age though, so, for certain individuals, wear in excess of this physiological norm will occur, and may occasionally become unacceptable, warranting intervention to prevent further damage. Tooth wear is universal in older people with exposure of both primary and secondary dentine being commonplace. With increasing age, it becomes difficult to define the line between acceptable and unacceptable levels of wear, and in the end this is often decided on the basis of the patient's own assessment. Tooth wear is described in detail in Chapter 7. This section deals with the issues specific to older adults.

Prevalence

Data on the prevalence of tooth wear in older adults are fairly sparse. There are some data concerning the prevalence of cervical wear. Wear around the necks of the teeth is almost universally present in older populations and the prevalence increases with age. Premolars are the most frequently involved teeth, followed by incisors in all age groups. Data from national surveys that have attempted to measure wear suggest that while mild to moderate wear is universal, severe coronal wear in the elderly, at a level that might require intervention, is probably quite uncommon. People who are at risk from the most severe forms of wear will often have had this treated before they reach old age. Their needs may be more related to maintenance of restorations rather than treatment of wear.

Aetiology

Tooth wear occurs throughout a lifetime as a result of normal function and is a product of all three mechanisms of wear. These are:

- Erosion (the progressive loss of hard tooth substance by chemical dissolution, not involving bacterial action).

- Attrition (the progressive loss of hard tooth substance caused by direct contact between occluding and proximal surfaces of the teeth).

- Abrasion (the progressive loss of hard tooth substance caused by mechanical factors other than mastication or tooth to tooth contacts).

Attrition and abrasion will occur, to a limited extent, with sound tooth tissue. These two mechanical effects will be potentiated by the damage caused by erosion, as the softened surface produced after acid attack will be more readily removed by mechanical trauma. Excessive wear is normally the product of an exacerbation of one of the mechanisms responsible for 'physiological wear'. This tends to result in a pattern of tooth tissue loss that may be of use in helping to determine the cause of wear in a particular clinical situation. Wear is commonly a product of more than one aetiological variable. For example, cupping of the tooth surface is thought to result from a combination of acid softening of the dentine and then preferential wear during parafunction or when chewing.

Prevention and management

The treatment of an older patient presenting with a worn dentition that requires operative intervention can be very complex indeed and is beyond the scope of this chapter. However, prevention is appropriate in all cases, whether or not operative intervention is used. There are a number of steps that can be taken, once diagnosis

of excessive wear has been made, to prevent the condition from getting any worse. These procedures are all designed to negate the aetiological factor that has become dominant in the wear process.

It is obvious that removal of the decalcifying agents in erosive wear will help to arrest its progress. It should be relatively easy to perform dietary counselling for a subject whose erosion was of dietary origin. This should arrest the rapid progress of the tissue loss, if the dietary advice is followed. A number of medications with low pH have also been reported as producing erosive damage (abnormal use of aspirin, chewable Vitamin C, 'iron tonic'), and in the elderly, this may be of relevance. As with diet, modifying the habitual pattern of use, or changing the form of medication may be required.

Erosion as a result of gastric regurgitation may present a more complex problem. Any preventative measures should begin with eliminating the aetiology if at all possible. Regurgitation as a result of incompetence of the cardiac sphincter at the base of the oesophagus can cause severe erosion, and because reflux is more common when the patient is supine, and salivary secretion (and hence protection) is at its lowest at night, medical/surgical advice should be sought. Asymptomatic gastro-oesophageal reflux disease has been implicated in patients with erosive pattern wear in whom no overt aetiology could be identified. There are also a number of drugs which may cause nausea or vomiting as a side effect. Once again, the patient's physician could be consulted to see if an alternative therapeutic agent is available. If there is an obvious time during which reflux or regurgitation occurs, then it may be possible to protect the dentition using a soft splint. This should extend well onto the palatal mucosal in the upper arch, and it may be of benefit to place a fluoride gel or antacid preparation inside the splint before use.

There is some evidence that topical fluoride therapy is of benefit in the control of erosive tooth tissue loss. A management regime similar to that for patients with xerostomia may be of benefit during the care of patients in whom an aetiological factor cannot be eliminated. This is particularly important if salivary change is contributing to the problem in the first place.

Mechanical wear as a result of normal masticatory function cannot be eliminated completely and is part of normal ageing. The most difficult problem when faced with attrition and abrasion is deciding when the perceived wear is in excess of the physiological 'norm' and thus requires treatment.

Attrition is most likely to occur in the presence of bruxism, and the management of bruxism is a complex subject. Secondary preventive regimes might include, occlusal splint therapy, (hard or soft), occlusal adjustment, psychotropic medication, and sometimes psychological counselling. On an empirical basis, the provision of some form of occlusal splint should act as a mechanical buffer, preventing tooth-to-tooth contact and ensuring that damage is to the splint and not the teeth; but there is no evidence to support the efficacy of any of these treatments.

A problem worthy of specific mention in relation to older people is the potential for damage from porcelain restorations.

Porcelain is a very hard material and can have an abrasive surface if it is poorly glazed or if it has been adjusted and not re-glazed. Regular contact with opposing natural tooth tissue will result in very rapid wear of the natural tooth producing a very complicated management problem. Even in the absence of a bruxist habit, unglazed porcelain can cause substantial damage. It is always desirable to produce tooth to artificial crown contacts on a metallic surface or, if this is not practicable for aesthetic reasons, on a highly glazed porcelain surface. Awareness of the potential for damage can prevent a more serious problem from developing.

Generally, wear in the older population may not be the problem it seems. The most problematic wear occurs when the loss of tooth tissue is rapid, and rapid wear usually presents as a problem earlier in life and this often needs complex treatment. In older adults a rather conservative treatment approach built around preventing excessive wear is usually appropriate.

Preventing tooth wear

- Tooth wear is a normal physiological process, but irreversible, so the teeth of older adults become progressively worn with age
- Complete prevention of wear is impossible, but simple steps to address underlying disease processes or to provide direct protection of the teeth from damage may be appropriate for older people with rapidly progressing wear

Conclusions

The trend towards the retention of natural teeth into old age offers the distant prospect of a functional natural dentition for everyone for life. The potential benefits of this in terms of nutrition, health, and general well-being for older people are considerable. However, this is only a prospect and is still some way from reality.

Achieving a functional natural dentition depends on the ability to prevent the functional limitations of uncontrolled tooth loss, and the potential disability and handicap that might result. Impaired oral function can occur at any stage in life, but is generally greater where more teeth have been lost, so it is the oldest in the community who suffer the greatest limitations. Thoughtful treatment planning around the concept of a minimum functional dentition might help to prevent this, but in turn will depend on prevention of specific diseases including periodontal disease and caries, particularly root caries. Furthermore, disease prevention and the delivery of well planned and executed treatment need to be provided in an oral environment that presents its own problems. The impact of age changes, financial and attitudinal barriers, and an accumulating burden of systemic illness can combine to make the process much more difficult than it is for much of the rest of the population.

The retention of a functional and natural dentition for life is now a realistic goal for most individuals currently in middle age and even for many people in older age groups. Preventing disease and

functional impairment is an essential step by which this could be achieved and is relevant to everyone, but success depends on a recognition that increasing age presents unique problems requiring imaginative and, often individual, solutions.

References

Baum, B.J., Ship, J.A., and Wu, A.J. (1992). Salivary gland function and ageing: a model for studying the interaction of aging and systemic disease. *Critical Reviews in Oral Biology and Medicine*, 4, 53–64.

Beck, J.D., Kohout, F.J., Hunt, R.J., and Heckert, D.A. (1987). Root Caries: physical, medical and psychosocial correlates in an elderly population. *Gerodontics*, 3, 242–247.

Beighton, D., and Lynch, E.J.R. (1983). Relationships between yeasts and primary root caries lesions. *Gerodontology*, 10, 105–108.

Brustman, B.A. (1986). Impact of exposure to fluoride-adequate water on root surface caries in elderly. *Gerodontics*, 2, 203–207.

Burt, B.A., Ismail, A.I., and Eklund, S.A. (1986). Root caries in an optimally fluoridated and high-fluoride community. *Journal of Dental Research*, 65, 1154–1158.

Carlson, G.E. (1984). The effect of age, the loss of teeth and prosthetic rehabilitation. *International Dental Journal*, 34, 93–97.

Chauncey, H.H., Muench, M.E., Kapur, K.K., and Wayler, A.H. (1984). The effect of the loss of teeth on diet and nutrition. *International Dental Journal*, 34, 98–104.

Cohen, D.R., and Henderson, J.B. (1991). *Health, Prevention and Economics*. Oxford University Press, Oxford.

Dawes, C., and MacPherson, L.M.D. (1993). The distribution of saliva and sucrose around the mouth during the use of chewing gum and the implications for the site specificity of caries and calculus deposition. *Journal of Dental Research*, 72, 852–858.

De Paola, M.S., Soparkar, P.M., and Kent, R.L. (1989). Methodological Issues relative to the quantification of root surface caries. *Gerodontology*, 8, 3–8.

Gray, P.G., Todd, J.E., Slack, G.L., and Bulman, J.S. (1970). *Adult Dental Health in England and Wales in 1968*. London HMSO.

Jensen, M. (1988). The effect of a fluoridated dentifrice on root and coronal caries in an older adult population. *Journal of the American Dental Association*, 117, 829–832.

Joshipura, K.J., Willett, W.E., and Douglass, C.W. (1996). The impact of edentulousness on food and nutrient intake. *Journal of the American Dental Association*, 127, 459–467.

Katz, R.V. (1984). Development for an index for the prevalence of root caries. *Journal of Dental Research*, 63, 814–818.

Käyser, A.F. (1981). Shortened dental arches and oral function. *Journal Oral Rehabilitation*, 8, 457–462.

Kelly, M., Steele, J., Nuttall, N., Bradnock, G., Morris, J., Nunn, J., Pine, C., Pitts, N., Treasure, E., and White, D. (2000). *Adult Dental Health Survey: Oral Health in the United Kingdom in 1998*. London. TSO.

Krall, E., Hayes, C., and Garcia, R. (1998). How dentition status and masticatory function affect nutrient intake. *Journal of the American Dental Association*, **129**, 1261–1269.

Locker, D. (1988). Measuring oral health: a conceptual framework. *Community Dental Health*, **5**, 5–13.

Moynihan, P.J. (1995). The relationship between diet, nutrition and dental health: an overview and update for the 90s. *Nutrition Research Reviews*, **8**, 193–224.

Randall, R.C., and Wilson, N.H. (1999). Glass-ionomer restoratives: a systematic review of a secondary caries treatment. *Journal of Dental Research*, **78**, 628–637.

Sheiham, A., Steele, J.G., Marcenes, W., Bates, C.J., Prentice, A., Lowe, C., Finch, S., and Walls, A.W.G. (2001). The relationship between dental status and haematological and biochemical measures of nutritional status among older people. A national survey of older people in Great Britain. *Journal of Dental Research*, **80**(2), 408–413.

Shimazaki, Y., Soh, I., Saito, T., Yamashita, Y., Koga, T., Miyazaki, H., and Takehara, T. (2001). Influence of dentition status on physical disability, mental impairment and mortality in institutionalised elderly people. *Journal of Dental Research*, **80**, 340–345.

Steele, J.G., Sheiham, A., Walls, A.W.G., and Marcenes, W. (1998). *The National Diet and Nutrition Survey: Adults aged 65 years and over. Oral Health Survey*. London, TSO.

Twaddle, A.C. (1974). The concept of health states. *Soc. Sci. Med.*, **8**, 29–83.

Whelton, H.P., Holland, T.J., and O'Mullane, D.M. (1993). The prevalence of root surface caries among Irish adults. *Gerodontology*, **10**, 72–75.

WHO (World Health Organization) (1958). Constitution of the World Health Organization. Annex 1. *The First Ten Years of the World Health Organization*. WHO, Geneva.

WHO (1982). *A Review of Current Recommendations for the Organization and Administration of Oral Health Services in Northern and Western Europe*. WHO regional office for Europe, Copenhagen.

WHO (1986). *Country Profiles on Oral Health in Europe 1986*. WHO regional office for Europe, Copenhagen.

13

Impairment–preventing a disability

Impairment–preventing a disability

June Nunn

Introduction

The last five years have seen significant changes in the whole issue of disability; the reasons for this will be discussed in this chapter. It is important that we define what is meant by impairment, disability, and handicap before proceeding further.

In the early nineties the term 'handicapped' was still in use in many countries and indeed, remains so today in places like Japan and Hong Kong. Pressure from the wider disability movement, and from advocates of people with disabilities persuaded those in health and social care, as well as a wider audience, that this term stigmatized people who were different. There has been a gradual move away from this medical model—describing people as 'handicapped'—to the social model where the emphasis is more on the environment imposing disability on a person with impairment (Hutchison 1995).

Medical and Social Models of Disability

- Medical Model:
  - Impairment
  - Organic dysfunction
  - Disability
  - Lack of physical capacity
  - Handicap
  - Disadvantage. Social role restriction
- Social Model:
  - Impairment
  - Organic dysfunction
  - Disability
  - Relationship between people with impairments and society

The trend now is away from attaching a label to a person and by implication, what they cannot do, towards an enabling culture of how the society we live in can empower people, anybody, by removing some of the barriers to self-fulfilment in those who are seen as different (Watson 2000).

As an example of this stance, think about yourself; you may well be short sighted, so you have an impairment. Whether it disables you depends on a number of things: text may be too small to read or you cannot get close enough to see things; you prevent it becoming a disability by substituting with artificial lenses. In other words, you do not allow the impairment to disable you.

While society is more aware of its role in this, there is still inappropriate discrimination; people with disabilities do not have equity of access to general health care, let alone dental care. There is still confusion over terminology and an out-of-date approach to being inclusive: witness the classic 'disabled toilets', frequently accompanied by a wheelchair logo. What a mental picture this conjures up!

So, while most people with impairments have to coexist alongside some degree of disablement, the extent to which this occurs will depend on their impairment(s), and the society's response. We mistakenly talk about 'special needs' when all it means is ordinary needs not ordinarily being met. Special Care is perhaps more apposite since it implies that it is the approach that is special or different and not the individual. And in essence that is what should separate out the care and services for people who have impairment since, in most instances, the oral and/or dental needs are routine, but it is the approach which is required that demands special attentionl; for example, a young person who has seizures of unknown origin, a questionable history of a heart murmur, and moderate learning disability, but needs to have a tooth extracted.

Impairment—general and dental

Two broad areas are emerging here. There is the disability consequent or not, upon a generalized impairment like, for example, cerebral palsy, and the disability suffered as a consequence of dental impairment.

To consider the latter first, the most recent national dental survey of UK adults looked at the way in which people's actual and perceived dental status impacted upon their quality of life. For the first time in 1998, the UK national oral health survey inquired into peoples' perceptions of the way in which their oral status affected aspects of daily living. This was based on the use of the Oral Health Impact Profile (OHIP), as developed by Slade and Spencer. The latter authors adapted the World Health Organization's classification of impairment, disability, and handicap into seven domains that impact on oral status of an individual: functional limitations, physical pain, psychological discomfort, physical disability, psychological disability, social disability, and

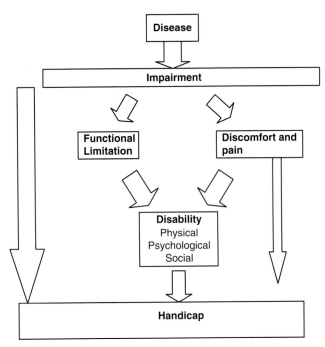

Figure 13.1 The seven domains of the Oral Health Impact Profile (After Slade and Spencer).

handicap (Slade 1997). (Figure 13.1) The survey reported that over half of the adults studied (*n* = 5281) had experienced problems in one or more of these domains in the year prior to the survey. For 7 per cent of the adults, these problems occurred very often. Problems that were most commonly reported related to physical pain in 40 per cent of the respondents, and feeling tense and self-conscious in 27 per cent. Nineteen per cent of people reported that they occasionally or often found it difficult to relax or were embarrassed by their oral state. The characteristics of people who reported problems were that they were more often from unskilled manual backgrounds and attended a dentist only when they had problems. Dentally, these people were reliant on a mix of natural teeth and dentures, had more actively decayed teeth and fewer sound teeth (Nuttall *et al.* 2000).

The former scenario, of disability consequent on a general impairment, like cerebral palsy, is more familiar. The issues that surround this will be explored in the succeeding paragraphs.

Size of the problem

Putting an exact figure on the number of people with impairments in the UK is difficult because it depends on the definition used. A figure of around 10 per cent of the population may not be unrealistic. What is more certain are that the group of people who will come within the remit of special care dentistry will widen (Waldman *et al.* 1999).

The survival of low birth weight babies with impairments improves all the time. However, this survival is not without consequence. The very act of keeping such high-risk babies alive can

in itself produce impairment. Neonatal care in many centres is now so sophisticated that babies born barely within the definition of viability survive, but at a cost. To offset this potential increase in numbers of disabled children born annually is the possibility, afforded by genetic screening and testing, of identifying high-risk pregnancies with the possibility of termination of severely affected foetuses (Edwards 2001).

The ethics of disability are emotive, tortuous and this is not the forum to air these. Screening allows for the detection of foetal abnormality but the question is: can others legitimately decide the fate of an individual? In an ideal world we would wish for no impairment; this is not a reality and the best we can hope for is that Society does not sit in judgement on who survives, but merely provides for those who do; the mark of any civilized society must be how well it cares for those who cannot look after themselves. So, while many children with impairments who, ten or fifteen years ago, would not have survived now do so and into adolescence and beyond. The burgeoning group of those in middle life who, for example, have intellectual impairments, but who have outgrown and even outlived the care and attention of their parents are those who find themselves in community care. While many of these challenged adults would, in decades past, have been accommodated in long-stay institutions, these have closed their doors under the 'normalization' policy of the 1980s. Many such adults are now to be found in small communities living in shared homes with carers, 24 hours of the day. While this is desirable for all sorts of reasons, the philosophy is not without its problems, particularly where dental care is concerned.

A recent advertisement from a drug company, with a picture of a number of older people dancing, ran a headline that announced: 'by 2008 the number of heavy drug users will double'. Old age does not come alone; many older people acquire impairments as they age, and in fact, the majority of all disabled people are elderly. In the UK there are 6.5 million disabled people, that is, one in eight of the population of whom 60 per cent are greater than 65 years. Increasingly, these older adults will have more natural teeth and will expect their dentist to go on providing care for them into late old age. So, more older people, with impairments and more of them with teeth. A challenge for the profession in ensuring that not only do clinicians of the future have the very varied skills necessary to provide the continuing care that these adults will demand, but also the flexibility to provide care in a setting appropriate for that individual, which may nor be in a dental surgery.

From the foregoing, we can assume that there is likely to be an ever larger burden for dental services, from an increasing proportion of the population with some form of impairment that may or may not justify special dental care.

Dental status

We acknowledge that the number of people with impairments may well increase, and that more of them will have higher expectations of dental services than might currently be the case. What of their dental state? Most reports on people with impairments will show one depressing fact. While oral health may for the most part be little different between those with impairments and so-called normal peers, the way in which that dental disease is managed is different. Historically, people with impairments have tended to have more teeth extracted and fewer teeth restored. Dental care is often generated as an emergency (Persson *et al.* 2000). With few exceptions, preventive care has not been emphasized in the way it should.

In part, this is a reflection of awareness; the awareness of the dental profession, awareness on the part of patients and of carers. The other aspect is of barriers. These take many forms but the obvious ones are attitudes which are stigmatizing, aspects of the environment that prevent ease of movement, and lack of knowledge about disability that prevents health care workers providing optimal care.

Why is dental care so important? For many people with disabilities, the presence of oral/dental disease or the need for dental care, can be life threatening; for example, a person with muscular dystrophy and extensive dental needs, and for whom a general anaesthetic almost certainly means a period of weeks in an intensive care unit.

Many patients have to cope with the side-effects of their impairment or its treatment: the person with spina bifida who has a latex allergy as a consequence of the type of shunt they have had; the organ transplant patient whose compliance with their anti-rejection medication is poor because of their drug-related gingival overgrowth. Renal transplant patients also have a dental impairment, bearing as they do the hallmarks of long-standing renal disease with discoloured and hypoplastic teeth. Although difficult to quantify, many people with learning disabilities, unable to articulate their pain, not only eat and sleep better and, as a consequence put on weight, but their behaviour also improves once they have received dental care.

Issues surrounding optimal oral health for people with disabilities

In the 1970s there was a movement, started in Sweden, to 'normalize' the lives of people with impairments, particularly intellectual impairments. In the UK this resulted in the scaling down of many long-stay institutions and the setting up of small group homes in scattered communities, in order to more closely integrate people with disabilities into society. What were the consequences of this, on the whole, desirable move? In many of the traditional long-stay hospitals, salaried personnel working on-site for the residents had provided dental care. This was in many ways an enviable service, because it meant that residents got comprehensive care in an environment that was familiar and secure—a bonus in terms of achieving a successful outcome for some challenging patients for whom care in the community has compromised their dental care (Tiller *et al.* 2001).

While the changes to the Community Dental Service in the UK enabled oral care to be provided for patients with disabilities, the restriction on resources, including the lack of training opportunities for staff have militated against an optimal service being available. The move towards a delivery of care based on the Personal Dental Services model has the potential to detract further from the comprehensive preventive and curative dental care that such people need.

Issues surrounding the delivery of care to people with impairments

- Normalization
- Lack of funding for training in the Community Dental Service
- The development of Personal Dental Services
- Cost of specialist services and facilities
- Unwillingness of some general dental practitioners to provide dental services to some groups in the community
- Consent and restraint

Compounding this are the attitudes of the carers and advocates of people with disabilities. Carers often feel that their clients should be treated 'normally', which means not forcing the issue of mouth cleaning. In most cases their charges are unable to undertake mouth care adequately on their own.

This is an issue also for economics; undertaking comprehensive care under general anaesthesia is expensive, the costing depending on the unit from which such treatment is provided, up to £1000 per patient treated. If there is not an aggressive programme of prevention to accompany such procedures post-operatively, then the waste of resources is tangible; patients return for repeat treatment under general anaesthesia, for repair of repair and in most instances, more extractions. General anaesthesia is not without associated morbidity and even mortality. The dental profession needs to decide, on the basis of evidence, what level and sophistication of care should be offered under such circumstances, particularly if aftercare is unreliable.

Aside from economics, the wish on the part of carers and advocates for their clients to avail of 'normal' dental services means that they get no care at all, such is the reluctance of many general dental practitioners to offer the dental care required. The reasons for this are numerous but centre around lack of experience and training and the perception that dentistry for people with impairments is both time consuming and requires special facilities. Surveys show, however, that the latter is only true for a minority of people. The lack of any additional fees in the general dental services, as exists for children with impairments, means that adults potentially lose out.

Consent and restraint are related issues in delivering oral and dental care for people with disabilities. There is, not unnaturally, a resistance among health care workers to restrain a patient, even for something like tooth brushing. It becomes a bigger issue for the safe delivery of care for adult patients with intellectual impairments who do not have the capacity to consent to care and for whom no other adult may legally consent to treatment on their behalf. Current guidance in England would suggest that dental care should proceed, provided the dental care envisaged has the agreement of parents or guardians, and is in the best interest of the patient. Good practice dictates that, where feasible, agreement on the treatment plan by a second, experienced clinician is advisable. The legislation in Scotland governing this issue for adults who do not have the mental capacity to consent is more restrictive in that it requires a dentist to obtain a certificate of incapacity from the patient's general medical practitioner for each course of treatment (Department of Health 2001, Lyons 2001).

Preventing oral disease, optimizing care—general principles

There are general ways to promote the oral health of people with disabilities before consideration of specific techniques and modalities of dental care.

Care needs to be accessible and to that end, people with disabilities themselves ought to be involved in the planning of services. The most basic way to promote this is, of course, to have an advocate—someone to ensure that the individual concerned receives the care they need if they are not in a position to demand it themselves (Goodley 1998). This relies on carers being aware of potential needs, the need for regular check-ups and the absolute necessity of daily mouth-cleaning routines.

Simple things like physical access to buildings and adequate car parking are integral issues (Fig. 13.2). Ensuring that financial barriers to dental care are removed is vital and this includes the hidden costs of having to travel unnecessarily long distances for so-called special care, as well as taking time off work and school. Services themselves need to be offered flexibly, for example, with domiciliary care more generally available.

The British Society for Disability and Oral Health has Guidelines on the standards for oral care for people with physical impairments, and the basic requirements as for impairment are listed below.

BSDH Guidelines on standards of oral care for people with physical impairments

- Oral assessment criteria to identify risk factors for oral health
- Development of individual oral care plans
- Appropriate oral hygiene facilities and aids
- Custom designed preventive and palliative measures
- Identification of need for, and access to, dental care
- Dental input to multi-professional teams
- Support and continuing education for health care personnel and carers

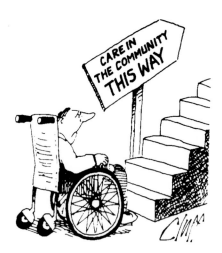

Figure 13.2 A cartoon depicting architectural barriers to community integration.

Recent legislation will protect people with impairments when it comes to accessing services; the Disability Discrimination Act of 1995 and the Human Rights Act of 1998 in the UK both have far-reaching implications for access to and opportunities for, oral and dental care. General dental practitioners, as owners of small businesses, must make reasonable alterations to their practices to enable people with impairments to access their premises. It is illegal to refuse to offer care to a patient on the grounds of their impairment alone.

It is invidious to talk about preventing oral and dental disease in the context of people with disabilities as a group apart because each one is an individual with individual needs. In the same way as other chapters have applied current and even novel principles to aspects of the promotion of oral health for individuals, the same applies to people who have an impairment — only more so, if we are to prevent dentistry, or the lack of it, disabling them.

There are though, specific aspects of oral health care and prevention of disease for people with impairments that need to be considered differently, and these will be dealt with in the following paragraphs.

Preventing oral disease—practical aspects

Behaviour management

People with limitations of movement as a consequence of their impairment need special considerations for the safe delivery of care. There are a number of options but, as with other aspects of dentistry, the least invasive, in terms of optimizing care and minimizing the need for restraint should be utilized. This will in some instances involve particular behaviour management techniques involving safe and effective positioning and may extend to the use of conscious sedation or even general anaesthesia as an adjunct to care (Klingberg et al. 2000) (Fig. 13.3).

Tooth tissue

Dental caries

The overall prevalence of dental caries in people with profound disabilities tends to be similar to that found in people without impairments. Where it differs is in the components of the caries experience index; people with poor cooperation or challenging behaviour as well as limited access to dental services for whatever reason, often tend to have more untreated decay, more missing teeth, and fewer restorations (Fig. 13.4)

However, where preventive and treatment services are targeted at particular groups, the evidence is that oral health can be maintained at a high level.

Topical fluoride applications are indicated in this patient group who may be at higher risk for the development of carious lesions. Administration of such agents can be difficult in a severely intellectually impaired person, although Duraphat® varnish is quick to apply and is very tolerant of moisture so that ensuring a dry field for a protracted period, as is required with

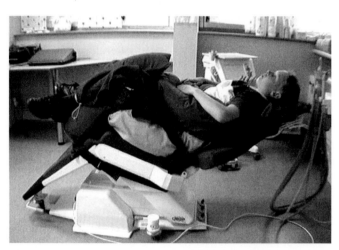

Figure 13.3 Treatment cushions in use with a disabled patient

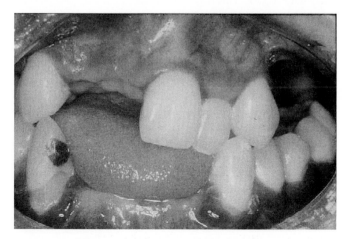

Figure 13.4 Oral status of patient with haemophilia

other topical fluoride agents, is not vital. There is a new, high-fluoride toothpaste (2800 ppm F) available on the market. While it may have a place in the prophylaxis against rampant caries in, for example, radiotherapy patients, its use in patients who cannot expectorate is to be cautioned against.

Conventional dental treatment may not be appropriate for all patients. For some, the only means to deliver successful treatment safely is with the aid of general anaesthesia. This implies radical treatment planning, since the opportunity to provide aftercare will be severely limited. Accompanying this approach must be very intensive preventive care, if costly resources are not to be wasted. For other patients, a compromise may need to be reached and recourse made to the use of an alternative approach to managing carious lesions, for example, using Carisolv® in combination with glass ionomer restorative materials or a simple atraumatic restorative technique (ART).

Risk factors and management strategies for dental caries

- Dietary constituents and form
- Liquid oral medicines
- Poor oral clearance/stagnation
- Resistance to mouth cleaning
- Infrequent attendance
- Attitude of carers
- Toothpaste alternatives—fluoride mouthwash
- High dose topical fluorides
- Radical treatment planning
- Chlorhexidene—gel, varnish
- Carisolv® and ART
- Ozone therapy
- Close liaison with dieticians

Others are exploring the use of ozone for the control of carious lesions in this group of patients for whom conventional dental care is not practicable. The use of ozone renders the carious lesion inactive without the need for dental drills or the use of local anaesthesia. Neither is there an absolute necessity to place a restoration in the cavity, if patient management is difficult. For patients in whom unpredictable movements are common or where the attention span is short, this is a useful method of rendering a tooth free of active caries in a short space of time. Clinical trials are now being conducted on this method of treatment. (Baysan *et al.* 2000).

Dietary considerations for people with impairments may need to be different. For people with very profound impairments, food is often liquidized or fed in semi-solid state after mashing. Food thus needs to be in a form that can be broken down easily and this tends to be foods high in NMES. Related to this is the move towards increased independence following on normalization, for people with milder intellectual impairments. Clients in adult training centres are encouraged to budget using their pocket money and buying foodstuffs, usually confectionery, to aid this. In addition, some very disabled children and adults need to take high calorie supplements in order to maintain their nutritional status. Liquid oral medicines taken on a regular basis can be devastating for the dentition and in chronic users, as with those on long-term nutritional supplements. The dental team need to work closely with the prescribing physician and dieticians to ensure that the least dentally harmful drug regime is adopted.

For patients who have potentially damaging diets, carers and others involved need to be made aware of this additional risk, and together with the dental team, to undertake aggressive preventive care. This will include regular mouth cleaning using fluoride toothpaste where possible. If the patient will not tolerate the use of toothpaste, then a toothbrush dipped in fluoride mouthwash (0.2% sodium fluoride) as part of the mouth cleaning routine, will deliver an equivalent amount of fluoride but in a vehicle that the patient may find more acceptable.

Tooth wear

A significant number of people with neurological impairment carry out habitual tooth clenching or grinding. This form of attrition can be devastating to the dentition, particularly in combination with erosion. For a significant proportion of people with cerebral palsy, gastroeosophageal reflux disease (GORD) may be an issue. This causes considerable pain and is seen in those patients who are orally fed as well as in people fed via a percutaneous endoscopic gastrostomy (PEG) and can result in gagging as well as frank vomiting. If this becomes chronic then the potential for aspiration of gastric contents becomes a reality and respiratory infections occur more frequently.

Tooth wear of this nature is linked with erosion, especially on the palatal surfaces of maxillary teeth, and the occlusal and buccal surfaces of lower molar teeth. It may be that the dental team are the first to notice any such disorder and have been instrumental in such a patient being investigated for GORD. In a patient who cannot tolerate extensive, rehabilitative dental care then it may be necessary to remove badly worn and sensitive teeth. For a more cooperative patient who can cope with procedures under sedation or one who is sufficiently fit for a general anaesthetic, full coverage of affected molar teeth with pre-formed metal crowns, may alleviate symptoms and prevent further tooth tissue loss (Shaw et al. 1998).

Professional staff in hospitals, in particular those looking after bedridden patients, need to be made aware of the potential for the constituents of proprietary mouth cleaning aids to be erosive. While these commercially available swabs or mouth sponges are often used on hospital wards, a toothbrush in combination with toothpaste or fluoride mouthwash, as described above, is perfectly satisfactory.

Abrasion is also seen in people who practice bizarre oral habits and it is in these patients that the crowns of teeth may be worn to such an extent that extraction is the only alternative.

Soft tissues

Gingivitis

The gingival status in many people with impairments, and the periodontal health of some, are going to be affected by the relatively poor levels of oral hygiene that prevail in this population. That notwithstanding, there are few data on the actual periodontal status of people with impairments. Recent studies indicate that periodontal disease is ubiquitous but then, that is the case also in the general population. This issue needs to be kept in perspective; while severe gingivitis may progress to periodontitis and thus tooth loss, small amounts of plaque are not incompatible with life, and so there is little point in mounting costly intervention programmes based on professional care if there is not a good chance that these efforts can be maintained at home. This is not a cost-effective approach.

For certain subgroups, like people with Down syndrome, periodontal disease and early tooth loss has been noted to be more prevalent, perhaps due to a combination of poorly controlled plaque levels and an alteration in the phagocytic activities of neutrophils. With this in mind, carers and others need to be vigilant in helping to maintain really good oral hygiene in individuals with Down syndrome.

Mouth cleaning is a difficult area for carers; the dental hygienist or dentist needs to work through a custom-made programme for people who cannot maintain their own oral hygiene. This protocol must be incorporated into the patients' Care Plans so that all staff involved in their care or relatives, know what needs to be done and how.

There are a number of ways in which toothbrushes can be modified to make them easier to manipulate. For patients who have difficulty grasping a conventional, slim-handled brush, as for example, the person who has arthritis or muscular dystrophy, a larger handle can make mouth cleaning a feasible proposition. Many such modifications resemble a bicycle grip and are made in rubber or plastic to fit over the toothbrush handle.

For patients who are resistant to mouth cleaning, carers need to carry out this task. This may be facilitated by the use of a powered brush although some severely intellectually impaired patients are startled by the noise and vibration, and resist attempts at introducing a brush into their mouths. A 'Superbrush' has merit in that the three sets of opposing bristles allow cleaning of three surfaces—buccal, occlusal and lingual—with one brush stroke. When access is limited or brief, this brush is reported to be efficient at removing plaque. Likewise for patients who have a sore mouth but in whom excellent plaque control is vital, the patient with mucositis induced by chemotherapy or radiotherapy for example, then a soft bristled brush is helpful: one such brush is the 'Ultrasuave', which is available from the US and limited outlets in the UK and Sweden (Ahlborg 2000).

Patients who are either too ill or extremely challenging in their behaviour need a different approach. For those unable to swallow, the patient in ITU or those with life-limiting illness, mouth care needs to be carried out for the patient in bed by a nurse or other carer, aided with an aspirating toothbrush. Instructions on the routine to follow must be kept with each patient so that changeovers in staff do not lead to a lack of oral hygiene maintenance. The nurse or carer may need to use a mouth prop to gain access. Toothpaste or the brush dipped into fluoride mouthwash as described above may be used around all tooth surfaces. If gingival health is poor, chlorhexidene gel can be swabbed around the mouth either on a brush or using some gel smeared onto a gauze wrapped finger. It is important to remember that the foaming agents in toothpaste inactivate chlorhexidene so that the two should not be used at the same time. Carers need also to be aware of the potential interaction between antifungals and chlorhexidene and to avoid their concurrent use.

Alternatively, chlorhexidene can be inserted into the gingival sulcus area in a varnish form, thus leaving a reservoir in this area. Evidence, currently available, suggests that the antimicrobial benefit from this is sustained for up to six months.

The challenging patient who either cannot or will not allow anybody to clean their mouths presents more of a problem; some patients prevent carers cleaning by positive resistance—something that carers will often not confront. Some carers have a philosophical view that they should not be restraining clients in order to accomplish routines of normal daily living, like tooth brushing. This needs to be discussed and a relevant analogy made; for example, with care of an ulcer elsewhere in the body; would carers not clean and dress a leg ulcer? In essence, periodontal disease can be likened to the same process and carers help enlisted in mouth cleaning as part of their duty of care.

Some patients may resist cleaning by adopting different behavioural strategies, like retching or gagging when a toothbrush is introduced or even when their mouths are touched. A conventional approach to this problem, relying as it does on a high degree of cognitive functioning to bring about acclimatization, is not suitable. Alternatives, utilizing a combination approach of behaviour modification and neurodevelopmental theory have achieved success in desensitization sufficient to accomplish oral hygiene, and dental care without recourse to general anaesthesia (Reid *et al.* 2000).

Self-inflicted Trauma

Infection of gingival tissues is an almost intractable problem in some individuals with severe learning disabilities. However, a more profound problem for a minority, because of its acute nature, is self-mutilation involving oral tissues. In people with specific syndromes, like for example, Lesch–Nyhan syndrome, self-mutilation is an integral part of the condition. For others, a trigger that can be something like teething is sufficient to set off a vicious circle, when inadvertent biting of lips or tongue can produce pain and swelling that perpetuates the cycle of trauma. This can result in dehydration necessitating hospitalization as the individual's mouth becomes too sore to eat or drink. Prevention lies in minimizing the worst effects either by extracting the offending tooth or teeth, if they are in the primary dentition; or more usually,

fitting soft PVAC-PE splints to prevent further soft tissue trauma and allow the area to heal. Occasionally the trauma is a consequence of malocclusion and orthodontic treatment can prevent recurrences, provided sufficient cooperation can be achieved for the adjustment of arch wires, often under conscious sedation. Band and bracket placement, any orthodontic extractions, and debonding will usually need to take place under general anaesthesia.

Saliva

Hypersalivation

The use of oral appliances can also be useful in another problem found in people with impairments, that of excessive drooling. This is seen in those with poor neuromuscular control, as found in cerebral palsy or in those who have had a cerebro-vascular accident. This can be an unpleasant habit for all concerned. In the young, toys become covered with saliva, the child often requires frequent changes of bibs or other clothes during the day, and in winter the circumoral soft tissues become excoriated. In children with impairments, there have been three broad approaches to the prevention of such a problem: surgical, pharmacological or with palatal training aids. Each has its advocates, and the pros and cons are listed in Table 13.1.

Currently, the evidence supporting each is anecdotal and further research is required to ascertain whether the benefits of the less invasive approach using the palatal training plates is as cost-effective as, for example, the use of hyoscine patches. The latter self-adhesive dermal patches contain hyoscine hydrobromide, which is gradually released over a 72-hour period, acting as an antagonist to parasympathomimetic activities, in this case drooling. However, the drug is costly and prevention requires regular, sustained use. Surgery on the other hand, involving as it does the re-routeing of salivary gland ducts and on occasions gland ablation, is immediate; although, there is evidence of a paradoxical return of function post-surgery in some cases. However, as in patients for whom radiotherapy has removed most if not all salivary gland function, the resultant rise in rampant caries, in previously caries-resistant teeth like lower incisors, is dramatic. What is less clear objectively, is how successful the palatal training plates are and whether the benefits attributed to their use are sustained.

There is a link between GORD and hypersalivation. Patients in whom hypersalivation is a observed, should be investigated for the distressing condition of GORD. The dental team may be the first to notice the dental erosive sequelae of chronic regurgitation (Nunn 1999).

Xerostomia

This is an impairment that is more devastating than excessive salivation for a larger number of people. Both the quality and quantity of saliva change with age, but added to this are the effects on saliva of disease and its treatment.

Ageing brings with it impairment and chronic conditions, like for example, Sjogrens disease, which is accompanied by symptoms

Table 13.1 Pros and Cons of different approaches to the prevention of drooling

Method	Advantages	Disadvantages
Behaviour modification and bio-feedback	Simple	Labour intensive; Need for equipment; Patient has to be at least 8 years, motivated; only suitable for moderate drooling problem
Radiotherapy	Immediate effect	Variable dose required to produce gland atrophy; Recovery possible; Residual saliva quality changes unfavourably; Possibility of sarcomas, osteoradionecrosis and caries
Speech therapy	Not invasive	Time consuming; Continuous maintenance
Oral motor therapy	Conservative	Benefits variable and not sustained
Drug therapy	Not invasive	Expensive; Side effects; Tolerance
Orofacial regulation therapy	Possibility of sustained benefit when therapy withdrawn	Intensive and time consuming for carers; No objective evidence of benefits
Surgery	Usually has a profound effect Choice of techniques—with varying outcomes	Possibility of relapse; Perforation and loss of taste; Xerostomia and caries; Alterations in quality of saliva Patients need to be hospitalized, treated under general anaesthesia

of a dry mouth. It is estimated that by the end of this decade, the number of elderly people on medication will double. One of the side effects of many of these medicines is that they produce a dry mouth. This exposes older people, far more of whom now have natural teeth, to dental caries and for those who are edentate, the difficulties of managing dentures without adequate reserves of saliva.

For a proportion of people, treatment for malignant disease with radiotherapy induces changes in salivary gland tissue such that the secretion of saliva is drastically altered. With careful planning, some of the deleterious effects of this approach can be minimized, if not prevented, by careful construction of stents to shield the salivary gland tissue from the radiation beam.

It is essential that a dentist be a part of the oncology planning team, so that patients who are scheduled to have irradiation to the head and neck region are provided with the necessary pre-operative dental care to avoid extractions, and thus minimize the risk of osteoradionecrosis post-operatively. Peri-operatively, a prosthodontist should be available for the construction of stents to shield dental tissues in the line of the beam. In addition, a prosthodontist will be needed to construct obturators for such patients to prevent the worst of the dental disability that can accrue from radical, reconstructive surgery.

Post-operatively, these dentate patients are at high risk of developing dental caries and must be maintained on an aggressive preventive programme with high-dose fluoride applications. Clinical trials have indicated that sodium fluoride toothpaste at a concentration of 5000 ppm was able to remineralize root surface lesions and to reduce plaque scores significantly by comparison with a conventional 1100 ppm fluoride toothpaste.

Most oncology programmes will employ a protocol that incorporates daily use of chlorhexidene mouthwash or gel to facilitate mouth cleaning and provide respite from oral ulceration. It is important that care staff administer nystatin as antifungal therapy

at a time distant, preferably one hour, from chlorhexidene to avoid inactivation of the former. Similarly, fluoride toothpaste should not be used in conjunction with chlorhexidene for the same reason.

There are a group of patients for whom practical help with saliva replacement is required. For some, stimulation of residual gland function with, for example, pilocarpine can be helpful. For others, substitutes are indicated and the plethora of solutions offered is indicative of the relative non-success of many of these.

List of saliva substitutes

- Saliva stimulation:
  - Pilocarpine
- Saliva substitution:
  - Frequent sips of water
  - Sucking ice cubes
  - 'Tooth-friendly sweets' (sugar and acid-free)
  - Artificial saliva DPF
  - Saliva Orthana
  - Glandosane
  - Luborant
  - Biotene (Mouthwash, spray, gum, toothpaste)

Patients who are dentate should be warned about the danger of using confectionery that is both cariogenic and erosive. Similarly, the pH of a number of saliva substitutes, for example, Glandosane, may be low enough to promote dental erosion (Table 13.2).

For some patients, the components of replacement saliva may be culturally unacceptable as for example with Saliva Orthana, which contains porcine gastric mucins. Others, for example, Biotene, cannot be used with detergents or other such tensioactive agents like the foaming constituents in toothpastes that inactivate

Table 13.2 The pH of some saliva substitutes

Name of product	pH
Salivace	6.9
Saliva Orthana Lozenges	6.4
Spray	5.5
Luborant	6.0
Glandosane Natural	5.2
Lemon	5.1
Peppermint	5.1
Salivix pastilles	4.5

the enzyme system integral to the product: these agents are normally marketed as a spray, mouthwash, chewing gum, and toothpaste as a complete system for patients home use. A number of the substitutes come with added fluoride, for example, Luborant and Saliva Orthana. The exact contents should be checked against the current Dental Practitioner's Formulary, so that it is appropriate for the individual patient's needs (Daniels 2001).

Conclusions

For those dentists and hygienists involved in palliative care, there will be the responsibility for a group of patients, some of whom will be bedridden and unconscious, others of whom will have life-limiting illness. While this may be a temporary stage for some, the combined effects of life support with nasal oxygen, an open mouth posture, parenteral feeding, and occasional suction of the airway will add to the sensation of a dry mouth. While oral comfort may seem to be a relatively minor consideration in such a patient, it can detract markedly from the patient's quality of life.

In conclusion, intelligent and proactive preventive dental care can do much to prevent the unwanted sequelae of dental disease as well as enhancing the quality of life for people who may not be able to demand that care themselves, but in whom a sense of positive oral well-being is just as important. This must be the imperative of any dental team.

References

Ahlborg, B. (2000). Practical prevention. In: *Disability and Oral Care* (Nunn, J, ed.) FDI World Dental Press. ISBN:0 9539261 0 9

Disability and Oral Care.(2000). (Nunn, J.H. ed.). Federation Dentaire Internationale. ISBN 0 9539261 0 9. Available from the printers: Tel: 01502 580881

Baysan, A., Whiley, R., and Lynch, E. (2000). Antimicrobial effects of a novel ozone generating device on micro-organisms associated with primary root carious lesions *in-vitro*. *Caries Res.*, 34, 498–501.

British Society for Disability and Oral Health. Guidelines. On: www.bsdh.org.uk

Department of Health (2001). Seeking consent: working with people with learning disabilities. Department of Health. www.doh.gov.uk/consent.

Daniels, T.E. (2001). Evaluation, differential diagnosis and treatment of xerostomia. J. Rheumatol. Suppl. 61, 6–10.

Edwards, S.D.(2001). Prevention of disability on grounds of suffering. *J. Med. Ethics*, 27, 380–382.

Goodley, D. (1998) Supporting people with learning difficulties in self-advocacy groups and models of disability. *Health Soc. Care Community*, 6, 438–446.

Hutchison, T. (1995). The classification of Disability. *Arch. Dis. Child*, 73, 91–99.

Klingberg, G. (2000). Behaviour management – children and adolescents. In: *Disability and Oral Health* (Nunn, J. ed.). FDI World Dental Press. ISBN:0 9539261 0 9

Lyons, D. (2001). Adults with incapacity (Scotland) Act 2000. *Health Bull*, 59, 146–149.

Nunn, J.H. (1999). Drooling. A review of the literature and proposals for management. *J. Oral. Rehab*, 27, 735–743.

Nuttall, N.M., Steele, J.G., Pine, C.M., White, D., and Pitts, N.B. (2001). The impact of oral health care on people in the UK in 1998. *Br. Dent. J.*, 190, 121–126.

Persson, R.E., Stiefel, D.J., Grifith, M.V., Truelove, E.L., and Martin, M.D. (2000). Characteristics of dental emergency clinic patients with and without disabilities. *Spec. Care Dent.*, 20, 114–120.

Reid, J.A., King, P.L., and Kilpatrick, N.M. (2000). Desentization of the gag reflex in an adult with cerebral palsy: a case report. *Special Care Dent.*, 20, 56–60.

Shaw, L., Weatherill, S., and Smith, A. (1998). Tooth wear in children: an investigation of etiological factors in children with cerebral palsy and gastroeosophageal reflux. *J. Dent. Child*, 69, 484–486.

Slade, G.D.(1997). Derivation and validation of a short-form oral health impact profile. *Community Dent. Oral Epidemiol.*, 25, 284–290.

Tiller, S., Wilson, K.I., and Gallagher, J.E. (2001). Oral health status and dental service use of adults with learning disabilities living in residential institutions and in the community. *Community Dent. Health*, 18, 167–171.

Waldman, H.B., Perlman, S.P., and Swerdloff, M. (1999). Children with disabilities: more than just numbers. *J. Dent. Child*, 65, 487–491.

Watson, N. (2000). Barriers, discrimination and prejudice. In: *Disability and Oral Care*. (Nunn, J. ed.) FDI World Dental Press. ISBN:0 9539261 0 9

14

The prevention of social inequalities in oral health

The prevention of social inequalities in oral health

Nigel Nuttall

Introduction

Evidence for the existence of social inequalities in health has existed throughout history. In fifteenth century Florence, mortality rates have been shown to be related to the size of women's dowries on marriage; women with higher dowries were found to be less likely to die within any given year than women with lower dowries. In other cases the evidence is still visible in our architectural heritage. It was fashionable among the wealthy in Victorian Glasgow to have an obelisk as a memorial, which has created an impressive array in The Glasgow Necropolis, a Victorian cemetery (Fig. 14.1). Davey Smith and colleagues have shown that these vary in height according to age at death. This has been interpreted as indicating that wealthier people (who would be more likely to afford a taller obelisk) tend to live longer. As well as showing the historical aspect of variations in mortality associated with varying degrees of wealth, these findings also raise two further significant points. The first is that in both examples the

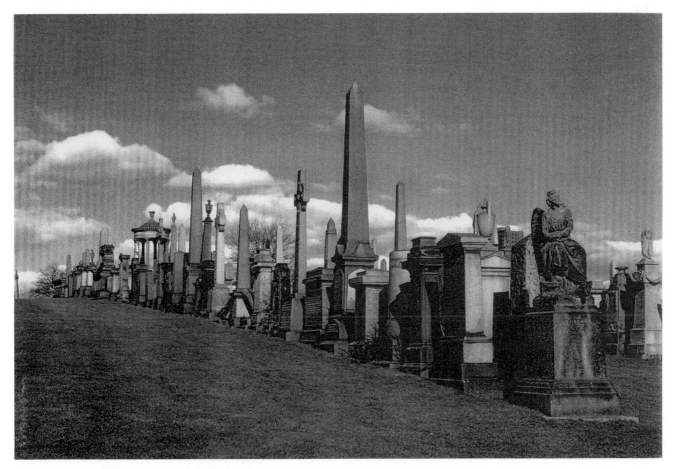

Figure 14.1 The Necropolis of Glasgow Cathedral.

social stratification of the people involved is quite a narrow band of the population as a whole. Women with dowries in the fifteenth century were the most privileged of their time, as were those interred in the Glasgow Necropolis. Yet mortality seems to have been unevenly distributed on the basis of financial wealth even within this narrow band of the privileged. The second point identified by Carroll, Davey Smith, and Bennett is that these historical findings also seem to demonstrate that explanations for inequalities based on contemporary concerns may not be sufficient to explain historical inequalities as many of the unhealthy activities we recognise today were the preserve of the affluent classes in the past.

The issue of social inequalities in health was beginning to be specifically discussed in the mid-nineteenth century. In the United Kingdom in 1842, Chadwick reported that the average age at death for gentry and professional persons was 35; for tradesmen, 22 years and for labourers and servants, 15 years. Deaths from all causes among men working in differing occupations were reported as part of the 1851 Census; and in 1887, a proposal was made for a system to classify people by 'social class' specifically to look at the issue of differences in the age of death between poor and rich people, although this was not actually done until 1911. So, before the close of the nineteenth century, there was already a widespread acceptance that class differences in life expectancy existed. However, the causes of these differences were disputed and echoes of this dispute are still rumbling on in the twenty-first century.

The dispute can be considered as another facet of the nature/nurture issue that has permeated so many debates (e.g. the nature of human intelligence). In the case of social inequalities it divided into the view that a person's position in society was derived through biologically determined inherited factors (nature) versus the view that social conditions, environment, and upbringing (nurture) were the determinants. At one extreme of these positions lay the proposition that a person's social class was a result of the process of natural selection as proposed by Darwin. This process not only determined membership of the 'lower' social classes but also explained their disadvantaged position in terms of their health and physique (nature). At the other extreme there was another damning view, exemplified by the quote below, that social inequalities between deaths in infants were largely due to their upbringing (nurture):

> The terrible heavy death rate among young children in our town is of course due to a certain extent to the relative unhealthiness of our surroundings, but that is by no means the chief cause. The factor that is of primary importance is maternal mismanagement … Every visitor in the homes of the working class knows only too well the hopeless ignorance of the majority of the mothers in regard to everything connected with the rearing of healthy offspring.

(Dr Harold Kerr, Assistant Medical Officer, Newcastle upon Tyne, 1910.)

The fact that social inequalities in health have been discussed in the United Kingdom for at least 150 years is a fairly strong clue about the lack of any clear cut agreed approach to how they ought to be tackled. There was a flurry of controversy during the 1980s on the publication of the Black Report and the later publication of The Health Divide. The controversy is detailed in the Introduction to the collection of both reports that was later issued in paperback, largely to make up for the difficulty in obtaining original copies which were produced by the UK Government in a deliberately limited print-run. The problems stemmed from the proximity of the issues involved in social inequalities and the political philosophies of the major political parties in the United Kingdom. One side of this was famously illustrated in Margaret Thatcher's pronouncement that 'there is no such thing as society' (a view which is not likely to be entirely sympathetic to considerations of 'social inequalities'). The issue was largely buried as a Government concern throughout the 1980s and 90s with what Macintyre has described as only an occasional consideration of 'variations in health'.

However, it is difficult to stifle a 150-year-old debate for long, and in 1998 the subject was revisited by a committee chaired by Sir Donald Acheson. It noted that that while average household income had grown by 40% in real terms during the previous two decades, it had grown much faster among the richest in the population. For the poorest tenth, average income increased by only 10 per cent (before housing costs) or fell by 8 per cent (after them). Furthermore, the inequalities in health between social classes in the 1990s had risen from those of the recent past; the difference in life expectancy between social class I and V rose to 9.5 years for men and 6.4 years for women. Infant mortality was found to be twice as high in Salford, one of the worst health areas, than in south Suffolk, one of the best health areas.

The Acheson Report recommended that health inequalities should be tackled on a broad front recognizing that they are the outcome of causal chains that run into and from the basic structure of society. The report uses the term 'upstream' for policies that would have their influence through societal change such as one addressing inequalities in income from 'downstream' ones with a narrower range of benefits such as free nicotine replacement therapy. The Acheson Report was also quite clear that the key to beginning the reduction in health inequalities was to concentrate on the needs of present and future mothers and their children to provide enhanced opportunities for health for the next generation.

The literature on social inequalities in health is riddled with contradictory evidence regarding many of the underlying issues. A great deal of the evidence is based on the interpretation of patterns and trends in mortality data. This opens up the possibilities of a lack of completeness in datasets, changes in definitions over time (of the measure used to classify people or of the circumstances of their death) and in some cases, perhaps, the use of value judgements and the implication of a degree of certainty that may not be entirely justified by the data quality. However, one matter is unchallenged; in Western Society socially disadvantaged people die younger and are much more likely to have babies who die in comparison with people from more privileged backgrounds. This chapter considers the comparatively less significant issue of how their social circumstances affect their oral health.

What are social inequalities in health?

Social inequalities in health are the differences in experience of illness, or death, between groups of people when classified on the basis of some social indicator. Often this is the Registrar General's classification of social class (Table 14.1). The difference in health is often referred to as a 'gradient' derived from the general pattern in graphs of a line decreasing or increasing from the more affluent or advantaged in society to the most impoverished or disadvantaged. The pattern is invariably the same: sloping from good indications of health among the socially advantaged professional group to poor indications of health among the socially disadvantaged unskilled working group. Furthermore, the magnitude of the differences can be huge; for instance, women in the most disadvantaged groups of society have been found to be nearly 20 times more likely to die from causes related to pregnancy and childbirth than women in the two highest social classes.

The term 'deprivation' is used quite commonly in the context of inequalities. Deprivation singles out the most disadvantaged in society and can take several forms although, in the past, it has been more commonly measured only in terms of a lack of the material aspects enjoyed by society as a whole. Material deprivation concerns whether people have specific goods or resources that are common within a society. Other forms of deprivation are 'social deprivation' which describes the roles and relationships, membership and social contacts in society and 'multiple deprivation' which describes the experience of several forms of deprivation concurrently, such as low income, poor housing, and unemployment. Social exclusion is also a term used in some contexts. This describes what can happen when people or areas suffer from a combination of linked problems such as unemployment, poor skills, low incomes, poor housing, bad health, family breakdown, and high crime environments. The terms deprivation and social exclusion are, therefore, similar but, perhaps, can be distinguished as differing in their coverage. Social exclusion is probably

more correctly applied to the most deprived of the deprived; those often deprived of a home; of an education; of health care and/or of social contact.

People in deprived areas are likely to have a higher exposure to negative influences on health, and to lack resources to avoid some of them or their effects, than people living in less deprived circumstances. There are other forms of exclusion as well; people with disabilities, and those of some ethnic or age groups, may also experience varying exposure to these influences on health; and in certain circumstances a person's sex may influence health opportunities (unrelated to those naturally associated with gender differences).

What effect does deprivation have?

The Black Report of 1980 presented a comprehensive review of inequalities in health and in access to healthcare between occupational classes. The central finding was that mortality and morbidity was greater among people from unskilled and partly skilled working backgrounds. The report also noted that people within these groups also used health services less frequently than other occupational groups and, in particular, services that might be considered as preventive. The report concluded that

> This pattern of unequal use is explicable not in terms of a non-rational response to sickness by working class people but of a rational weighting of the perceived costs and benefits to them of attendance and compliance with the prescribed regime. These costs and benefits differ between the social classes both on account of differences in way of life, constraints and resources, and of the fact that costs to the working class are actually increased by the lower levels and perhaps poorer quality of provision to which many have access.

Social inequalities

- Have existed throughout history
- Class differences in life expectancy
- Health inequalities should be tackled on a broad front
- Mortality and morbidity is greater among people from unskilled and partly skilled backgrounds
- People within these groups use health services less frequently than other occupational groups

What causes social inequalities in health?

The mechanism of the relationship between deprivation and ill health is a matter of intense interest and is still an issue being debated.

The Black Report considered four possible explanations for observed social inequalities in health:

- The Artefact Explanation suggests that periodic changes to the Registrar General's social class system have artificially

Table 14.1 Social class in the United Kingdom defined by the Registrar General's classification based on occupation

Social class I	Professional (e.g. lawyer, dentist, accountant)
Social class II	Intermediate (e.g. teacher, nurse, manager)
Social class IIINM	Skilled non-manual (e.g. typist, shop assistant)
Social class IIIM	Skilled manual (e.g. bus driver, cook)
Social class IV	Partly skilled (e.g. bus conductor, farm worker)
Social class V	Unskilled manual (e.g. cleaner, labourer)

inflated the inequalities in health between occupational groups. According to this explanation, the failure to reduce inequalities between occupational classes can be attributed to a re-assignment to a more affluent class of some of the poorer members of society who either are in better health, or whose health then improves, leaving a smaller but still disadvantaged group. This was largely dismissed as a process as it was felt that there was little evidence of this upward movement. It was also felt that the contraction of the size of poorer occupational groups was unsupported, although lately there has been clear evidence of the contraction of social class V. Furthermore, inequalities in health can be seen using a variety of alternative measures of deprivation, which, if anything, suggest that the Registrar General's 'social class' classification may underestimate differences between groups of people based on their level of deprivation.

- The Natural and Social Selection Explanation suggests that health itself may somehow determine socio-economic position. People in poor health would by virtue of their health disadvantage move 'down' the social classes while the healthy would have an advantage that would help them get good jobs and so move 'up' the social ladder. Evidence for this type of process has come from two sets of findings that taller women tend to move 'up' the occupational classes at marriage. This is also an explanation that would apply to people who as children had major health problems that may have excluded them from the same educational and occupational opportunities as their peers. There is now general acceptance that this process does make a limited contribution to inequalities in health and health care, but that it is far from being a complete explanation.

- The Cultural/Behavioural Explanations suggest that health-related behaviours, like cigarette smoking, poor diet, and lack of exercise, lead to the observed inequalities. In this view inequalities in health arise because people from an unskilled occupational background are more likely to adopt health-damaging behaviour and may have less interest in protecting their health than those from skilled occupational backgrounds.

- The Material or Structualist Explanations concern the role of external conditions; hazards relating to poor housing, certain dangerous occupations, pollution, unemployment, and psychosocial stress have all been associated with poorer health.

There have been challenges to whether the latter two explanations can, in fact, be regarded as distinct from each other, as behaviour cannot be separated from its social context. An example of this is evidence on childhood accidents. It is known that there is a greater likelihood of children from unskilled occupational backgrounds being involved in accidents, in comparison to children from skilled occupational backgrounds. The cultural/behavioural view may explain this as being due to greater recklessness or risk-taking behaviour and/or a lack of parental supervision. Whereas the materialist/structualist explanation may see this as being due to greater exposure to risky environments (lack of play space leading to playing on roads) and difficulty in supervising children in high-rise housing estates.

The issue of the role played by these explanations is a key to the understanding of social inequalities in health and how they might be tackled. The behavioural/cultural explanation would indicate that prevention of individual behaviours (e.g. smoking) might help reduce health inequalities. On the other hand, the materialist/structualist explanation would look to the provision of a better social and physical environment for those from deprived backgrounds as a means of improving their health.

The Black Report in the 1980s and subsequent review of the literature by Margaret Whitehead in The Health Divide in 1992 seemed to subscribe to the view that the materialist/structualist explanation was the dominant, if not exclusive, explanation for inequalities in health. Several studies were quoted to show that mortality from heart disease was explained more by social inequalities than by smoking behaviour. Other evidence was cited to show that the adoption of 'healthy behaviours' could help differentiate between the health of people in a favourable social environmental, but not between people living in deprived areas. Other work cited concerned the cultural aspect of the explanation that has looked at the role of the 'culture of poverty', which proposes that people from poorer backgrounds have more negative concepts of health, and a lack of orientation that would lead them to take an interest in preventive health behaviour. Again, the evidence cited did not support the idea that people from poorer environments actually hold such views. For example, in a study of disadvantaged mothers and daughters in Scotland, health service use in the younger generation seemed less affected by factors associated with cultural beliefs than by a lack of skill in dealing with the health care system.

Macintyre, however, has claimed that the Black Report has been widely misinterpreted as entirely supporting the materialist/structualist view. In her view people have placed too much attention on its analytical section rather than its section on recommendations that take a 'softer' line by recognizing the need for action to address issues such as disability and unhealthy behaviours in order to reduce social inequalities in health.

Work since the Black Report has unearthed more clues about how social inequalities can affect peoples' health. These tend to support the contribution of a variety of processes to health inequalities. Evidence suggests that adolescents from deprived backgrounds may be less disadvantaged by their social circumstances than young children and adults. It has also been found that people who were chronically ill in childhood tend to be severely disadvantaged by early middle age if they came from a deprived background, but not if they came from an affluent background. This has been seen by some to provide evidence for natural selection; resulting from a process whereby healthy teenagers are selected for educational and occupational opportunities from which less healthy teenagers from deprived backgrounds are excluded. The Black Report noted that inequalities in health persist even when many behavioural and biological factors are controlled for. Subsequent work has confirmed this, but also shows that differences in behavioural factors between social groups, such as smoking, can still account for around 33–50% of differences in their experience of heart disease.

Wilkinson has argued that it is poverty relative to others in a particular society that has a greater influence on mortality than absolute poverty alone. He cites three pieces of evidence: firstly, mortality is related more closely to relative income within countries than to differences in absolute income between them; secondly, national mortality rates tend to be lowest in countries that have smaller income differentials and; thirdly, most of the longer term increase in life expectancy appears to be unrelated to long-term economic growth rates. Wilkinson extended this argument to identify what he considered was an underlying cause of health inequalities. The gradients that are observed in health when examined by social class reflect both social position (where people stand in relation to others in society) and material circumstances (e.g. ability to afford housing, heating). If material standards were the main cause of inequalities, the differences in health would increase or decrease directly as material standards increased or decreased. However, the finding that relative poverty is more influential than absolute poverty suggested that it was aspects of social position that had the greater effect on health inequalities. Wilkinson believed the indirect effects of these psychosocial circumstances to include increased exposure to behavioural risks resulting from psychosocial stress including stress-related drinking, smoking, and the direct effects of the physiological effects of chronic mental and emotional stress.

However, the basis for Wilkinson's claims has been challenged. Judge has claimed that data underlying the claims lacked completeness, while Lynch and colleagues have suggested that the process advanced by Wilkinson is improbable. Lynch has advanced the neo-material interpretation as an alternative explanation. Pared down, this view states that it is the direct effects of poverty and its consequences that affect health. In modern society (increasingly perhaps) money is the key to a wide range of resources; not just to 'private' resources such as housing, private transport, food, and heating, but also indirectly to resources within the 'public domain' such as libraries and education and health. Lynch summarized the differences between his and Wilkinson's views using the metaphor of air travel.

Differences in neo-material conditions between first and economy class may produce health inequalities after a long flight. First class passengers get, among other advantages, better food and service, more space and a wider, more comfortable seat that reclines into a bed. First class passengers arrive refreshed and rested, while many in economy arrive feeling a bit rough. Under a psychosocial interpretation, these health inequalities are due to negative emotions engendered by perceptions of relative disadvantage. Under

a neo-material interpretation, people in economy have worse health because they sat in a cramped space and an uncomfortable seat, and they were not able to sleep. The fact that they can see the bigger seats as they walk off the plane is not the cause of their poorer health. Under a psychosocial interpretation, these health inequalities would be reduced by abolishing first class, or perhaps by mass psychotherapy to alter perceptions of relative disadvantage. From the neo-material viewpoint, health inequalities can be reduced by upgrading conditions in economy class.

A useful general framework for trying to understand all the factors that might conceivably affect people's health has been proposed by Dahlgren & Whitehead (Fig. 14.2). This emphasizes that at the core of the process is the individual who has particular factors that can affect his or her health such as genetics, age, and sex. These are seen as influential, but largely unchangeable. Surrounding this, like an onion, are layers of other influences; in which the layers above influence lower layers. Thus general socio-economic, cultural, and environmental conditions will affect the living and working conditions within which a person has to exist. These in turn may influence the local community environment and, finally, the lifestyle factors of an individual. The benefit of the model is in its emphasis that factors found to be significant at one layer will be influenced by the layers above. For example, registration of infants for general dental care is known to be lower among the socially disadvantaged. This may reflect difficulties in access in terms of time and cost of travel (layer 1). The position of these infants may also be worsened by the location of dental surgeries away from poorer areas and by the level of patient charges levied on NHS dental treatment and regulations for exemption from payment, that might influence their parents' attendance (layer 3). All of these are influenced by general Government policy (layer 4).

The international perspective

The Black Report also considered international evidence about social inequalities in health. They noted that the type of social stratification used in the UK was not common in other countries. In the United States, social groups are often delineated on the basis of ethnicity or wealth, whereas in European data, geographical region is often the basis for stratification. Nevertheless, the authors of the Report were interested in determining the experience of social inequalities related to health were a universal phenomenon. An analysis of mortality rates in Denmark, Finland, France, The Netherlands, Norway, Sweden, and Germany indicated that inequalities associated with wealth did also exist in other countries. In Finland, France, Germany, and The Netherlands the differences in mortality rates between occupational groups or between regions seemed similar to the differences found in the United Kingdom. However, a variety of studies have shown that Denmark, Norway, and Sweden have less marked social inequalities. Overall, international comparisons have suggested that low infant death rate is associated with per capita GDP with some additional evidence for

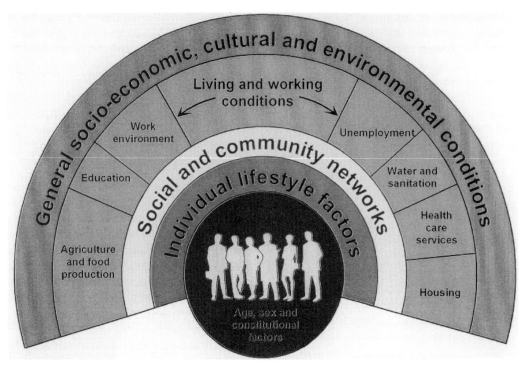

Figure 14.2 The main determinants of health. (Source: Dahlgren and Whitehead, 1991.)

an association with a more egalitarian income distribution; in other words, with wealth and its distribution.

Main determinants of health

- Age, sex, and constitutional factors
- Individual lifestyle factors
- Social and community networks
- Living and working conditions
- General socio-economic cultural and environmental conditions

How is deprivation measured?

There are a variety of measurement issues in the field of inequalities. The first is whether social inequalities are best measured in terms of social class of an individual or in terms of the characteristics of the area in which the individual lives. Some of the main measures that have been proposed and used are shown in Table 14.2.

Inequalities in health in terms of mortality rates among occupational groups have been measured by the Registrar General's definition of social class in the United Kingdom as part of the decennial reports of the Registrars General of England and Wales and of Scotland since 1911. The current measure based on five categories (with the third split) is based on the system developed for the 1921 Census that classifies people on the basis of their occupation (Table 14.1). Traditionally, men and single women are classified according

to their own occupation, whereas married women are classified according to their husband's occupation. The system is a proxy measure for material deprivation as earnings tend to decrease 'down' the social class ladder. The method continues to be used, but has been criticized on the basis that it will not always accurately classify married women and that changes to the definitions have been accused of causing problems in assessing trends. It differs from all the other measures in Table 14.2 by being based on information regarding an individual rather than a geographical area.

Most of the recent work on classifying deprivation has been in the development of area-based measures. In 1971, the Department of the Environment devised a new type of deprivation measure to identify areas with poor social and environmental conditions. The benefit of area-based measures is that there are regular decennial updates of the base information during the National Census (the last being undertaken in 2001). These measures enable a person's deprivation score to be determined without any need to gather personal information, other than their address or postcode. Some of these area-based measures (DoE and Jarman) have been criticized on the grounds of inclusion of aspects, which in themselves are not matters of deprivation (e.g. ethnicity). This has largely stemmed from their intended use. Jarman, for instance, was concerned with establishing the impact of deprivation on primary care workloads and, therefore, included any factors that might require additional time to manage (e.g. size of the retired population in an area). The DoE deprivation index includes factors such as the number of children under 14, which is not an issue that is directly associated with deprivation but one that may be useful as a measure of the need for services.

Table 14.2 Components of the major measures of material deprivation used in the United Kingdom (Adapted from Carstairs and Morris 1991)

Factor	Registrar General's Social Class	Carstairs	Indices of deprivation		
			DoE	Jarman	Townsend
Occupational group	*	*		*	
Unemployment		*	*	*	*
Overcrowding		*	*	*	*
Households without car		*			*
Not owner occupied					*
Lone pensioners			*	*	
Single parents			*	*	
New Commonwealth			*	*	
Lack of amenities			*		
Children under 5 years old				*	
Standardized Morality Ratio		*			
Population change/mobility			*		
Permanent sickness/long-term illness			*		
Introduced	1921	1983	1971	1988	1983
Weighting of factors	No	No	Yes	Yes	No

The Carstairs & Morris and Townsend systems on the other hand have more 'face validity' in what they measure, in that they concentrate on circumstances that appear directly related to deprivation. However, these too may have problems. Both include the level of car ownership in an area. The impact of car ownership, however, is likely to differ between mainly rural and mainly urban areas; in a rural area a car may be absolutely essential for personal transportation, whereas in an urban area it may be largely a drain on people with limited resources. A further point is that both measures are largely concerned with material deprivation and take no account of other types of deprivation such as social deprivation.

Area-based measures on the whole also have the problem that many people who are not deprived may live in a deprived area, and many people who are deprived may live in non-deprived areas. In England and Wales, for example, it has been estimated that as many as 55 per cent of the most deprived individuals live outside the 20 per cent of areas that are most deprived. This sort of problem makes targeting anti-deprivation schemes extremely difficult. The most serious attack on area-based deprivation measures comes from Sloggett and Joshi who looked at the mortality among 300,000 adults over 9 years. They found the usual gradient in mortality across areas categorized on the basis of deprivation, but also looked at similar indicators of individual deprivation; for example, where the area measure looked at level of car ownership in an area, the individual measure looked at whether the person had access to a car. They concluded that

deprivation was 'wholly' an individual issue rather than an environmental or geographical one; areas differed because of the proportion of deprived individuals they had living in them. Individuals living in deprived areas who were not personally disadvantaged did not experience excess risk.

The measurement of deprivation is developing all the time and new measures might be expected when the 2001 Census findings become available. Furthermore, there are now measures that are not reliant on Census data. One such measure is the Index of Multiple Deprivation developed by the Department of Environment, Transport and the Regions in 2000. The IMD uses 33 indicators of deprivation measuring 6 domains of deprivation: income, employment, health deprivation and disability, education skills and training, housing, and access to services. The system still operates on a geographical rather than individual basis and, therefore, may be prone to the same problems identified for earlier area measures that may misclassify many deprived individuals who live in non-deprived areas.

While area measures have their problems of misclassification, they do have the advantage of the ability to be linked to post codes, thereby providing a simple and non-intrusive method of classifying individuals on the basis of their likely experience of deprivation. However, United Kingdom post codes take the general form AA1 2BB which identifies a fairly small area of houses, but deprivation measures such as that of Carstairs and Morris, which have a post code breakdown available, use only the post code sector (e.g. AA1 2) which often covers an area containing several thousand people. An arduous, but ultimately more useful, measure might be one which uses the entire post code and may be the way in which future measures ultimately go, although this might be stymied by issues of privacy that ought to be afforded to individuals who may be identifiable by use of a full post code.

Deprivation and oral health

It has been shown in terms of mortality that the health of infants and children is affected by social inequalities from birth onwards. Despite the fact that dental health in children is improving, evidence presented to the Acheson Committee showed that the differential between caries in the primary dentition of 5-year-old children from poor backgrounds and those from affluent backgrounds widened enormously between 1983 and 1993. This has also been true in geographical terms; 5-year-old children in the North West of England (with extensive areas of deprivation) had almost 60 per cent more experience of caries, and 12-year-olds 75 per cent more experience compared with similarly aged children in the South (with comparatively fewer areas of deprivation).

By the age of five a social class gradient in oral health is already well established, as shown in findings from the annual Scottish Health Boards' Dental Epidemiological Programme series of biennial surveys for the primary dentition of 5-year-olds (Fig. 14.3). Only 20 per cent of children living in deprived areas of Scotland had no experience of dental caries compared with almost 60 per cent of children who lived in the most affluent areas. Figure 14.3 also shows that approximately the same level of disadvantage can be

seen in the permanent dentition at age 12 years. United Kingdom findings for the mean number of actively decayed teeth in 12- and 15-year-olds from two of the national children's dental health surveys undertaken in 1983 and 1993 are shown in Figure 14.4. These also show that, despite a fall in caries experience between 1983 and 1993 among both age groups, a social class gradient continues to be present in the findings for 12- and 15-year-olds.

Deprivation and oral health

- Social class gradient established by the age of five years
- Similar levels of disadvantage evident in the permanent dentition in 12 year old children
- Marked gradient in levels of edentulousness and social class

The 1998 Adult Dental Health survey is a trove of material for examining social inequalities in adult oral health. The survey data includes measures of social class, both individual and the more traditional 'head of household', as well as oral information related to the Jarman index of deprivation for England, and Carstairs and Morris index of deprivation for Scotland. Figures 14.5–14.10 show the relationship of three measures of deprivation to oral health in the United Kingdom. The figures show the relationship between various oral health measures with deprivation. The Jarman system used for England is based on 'quintiles' which is a division of the scores into 5 groups of approximately equal size (i.e. each group consists of approximately 20% of population). Assignments to categories in the Carstairs and Morris system are based on

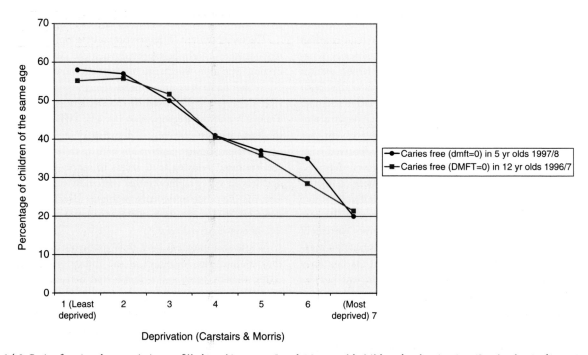

Figure 14.3 Caries free (no decay, missing or filled teeth) among 5 and 12 year old children by deprivation (Scotland, 1996/1998).

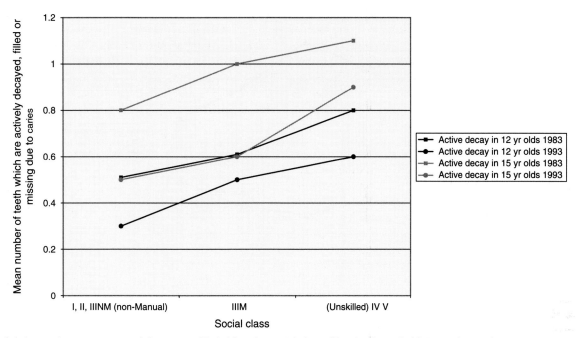

Figure 14.4 Active decay among 12 and 15 year old children by social class of head of household (United Kingdom, 1983 & 1993).

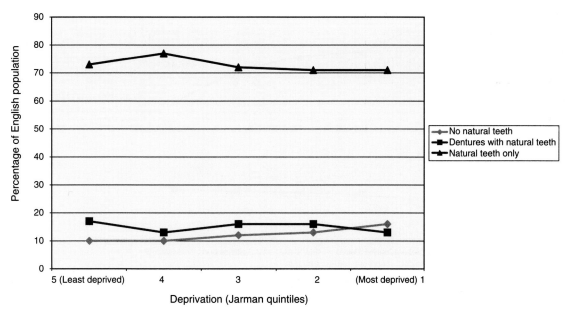

Figure 14.5 Oral status by deprivation (England, 1998).

predetermined scores. In the 1998 Adult Dental Health sample approximately 8% of the Scottish dentate population were included in the most deprived group. Direct comparison of the results between countries is not meaningful as these measures of deprivation have different components and classification methods.

There was a statistically significant but small gradient for people who had no natural teeth grouped according to the Jarman score of where they lived in England (Figure 14.5); 10 per cent of those living in the most affluent areas were found to have no natural teeth remaining compared with 16 per cent of those living in the most deprived areas. The deprivation measure used in Scotland showed a more marked difference between deprivation and oral status. A quarter of people living in the most deprived areas of Scotland had no teeth in 1998, compared with 14 per cent in the most affluent areas (Figure 14.6). There was also a very

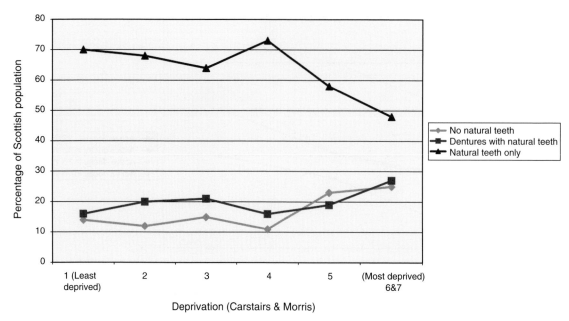

Figure 14.6 Oral status by deprivation in Scotland in 1998.

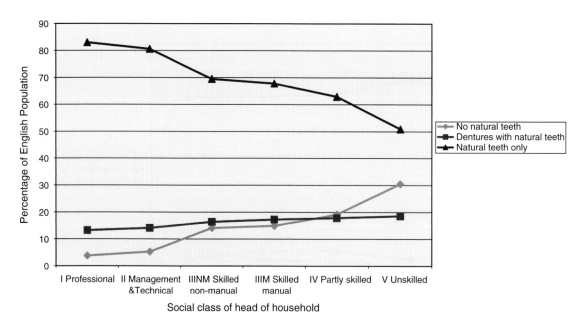

Figure 14.7 Oral status by social class of head of household (United Kingdom, 1998).

marked gradient between people living in the United Kingdom classified according to social class of head of household; only 3.8 per cent of people from professional household backgrounds had none of their own teeth left compared with over 30 per cent of those from an unskilled household background (Fig. 14.7).

There was little difference in the mean number of missing teeth and the mean number of decayed teeth among people living in different areas of deprivation in England classified by the Jarman measure (Fig. 14.8). However, the deprivation measure used in Scotland did indicate that people in deprived areas had

significantly more missing and decayed teeth than people living in affluent areas in Scotland (Fig. 14.9). Social class of head of household also revealed a gradient in the experience of missing and decayed teeth across people from professional and unskilled working backgrounds in the United Kingdom as a whole (Fig. 14.10). People from social class V (unskilled) had 50 per cent more missing teeth and twice as many decayed teeth on average than people in social class I (professional).

There is evidence from studies in general medicine that people from socially disadvantaged backgrounds are less likely to attend

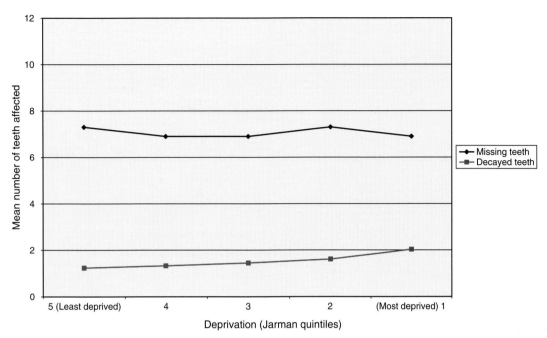

Figure 14.8 Mean number of missing and decayed teeth by deprivation (England, 1998).

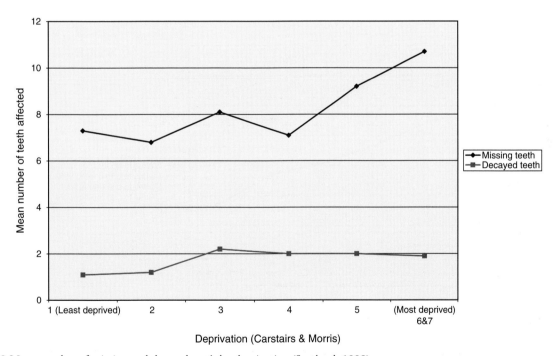

Figure 14.9 Mean number of missing and decayed teeth by deprivation (Scotland, 1998).

for preventive consultations and less likely to follow health messages. Figures 14.11–14.13 examine some issues in dentistry by using social class of head of household as an indicator of material deprivation.

There were significant differences in a variety of oral health behaviours which people were asked about in the 1998 Adult Dental Health survey. More people from a professional background

than from an unskilled working background said they tended to do the sort of things that dentists say are good for dental health: attend dental check-ups, brush teeth at least twice a day, and use an additional method for cleaning teeth (Fig. 14.11). The issue of unequal use of health services is one which has also been identified in general medicine and termed the 'inverse care law' which states that those with least need of health care use the health services

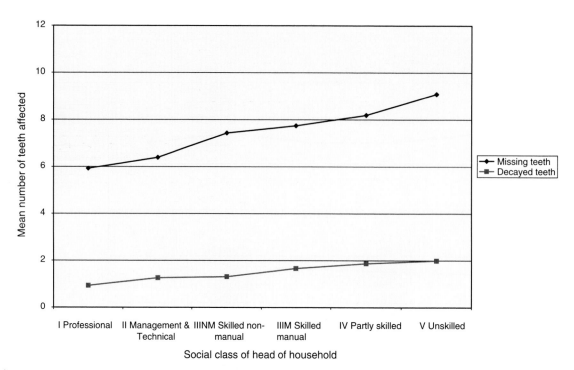

Figure 14.10 Mean number of missing and decayed teeth by social class of head of household (United Kingdom, 1998).

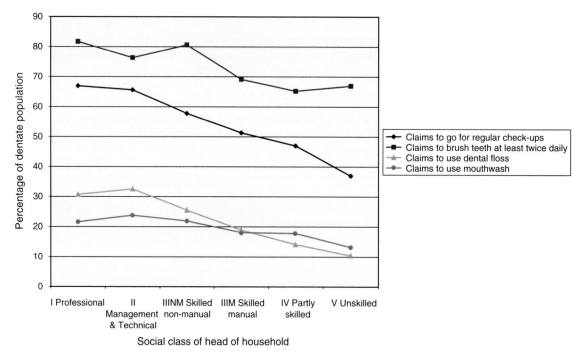

Figure 14.11 Self-reported oral health behaviour by social class of head of household (United Kingdom, 1998).

more, and more effectively, than do those with greatest need. The 'inverse care law' also applies to preventive interventions as well as treatments. Health promotion based on providing information to the population as a whole has had the greatest impact on people who are socially and economically advantaged.

People from unskilled working backgrounds were also found to be less likely to take time off work to go to a dentist than people from a professional background (Fig. 14.12). Furthermore, when asked about their last dental visit people from social class V (unskilled) were four times more likely to have had some teeth

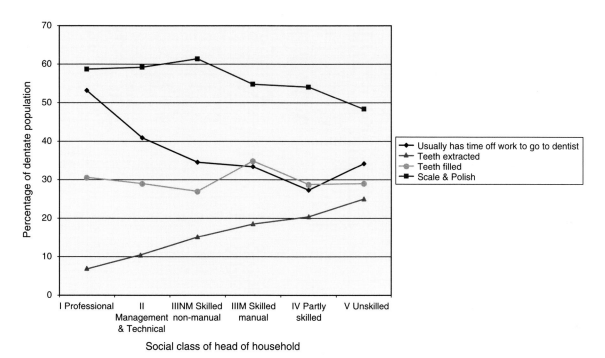

Figure 14.12 Dental treatment during last visit to dentist by social class of head of household (United Kingdom, 1998).

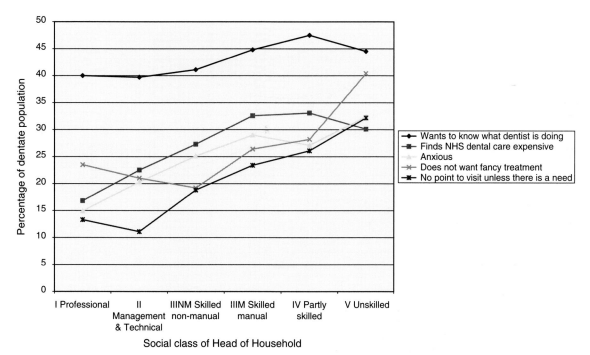

Figure 14.13 Views about dental visits by social class of head of household (United Kingdom, 1998).

extracted as those from social class I (professional). However there was no social class gradient in the experience of having teeth filled, and only a slight, but statistically significant difference in the experience of having a scale and polish.

Figure 14.13 considers some issues that have been identified as factors that put people off going to a dentist for check-ups. People

from social class I were the least likely to say they find dental treatment expensive. The gradient for this only extends to social class IV then reduces in social class V. This is likely to reflect the effect of exemption from treatment costs among many in social class V, but may also result from opting for less expensive treatments such as tooth extractions. There may also be a general lack of familiarity

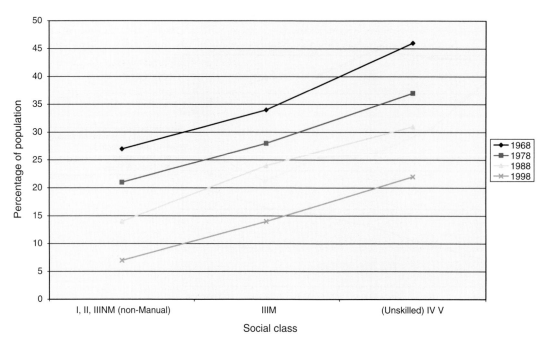

Figure 14.14 Total tooth loss by social class of head of household (Adults in England & Wales 1968–1998).

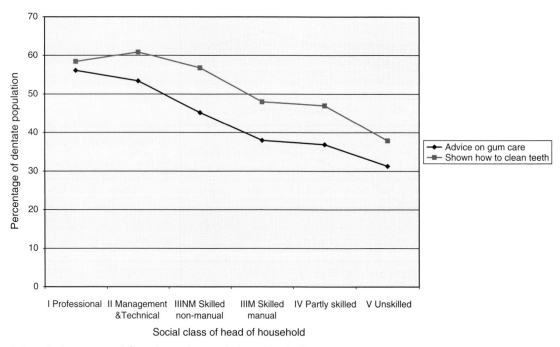

Figure 14.15 Dental advice received from dentist by social class of head of household (United Kingdom, 1998).

with the current level of dental charges among those who rarely attend. On the whole, people from social class V are almost twice as likely than people in social class I to say that they do not want 'fancy' dental treatment and believe that there is no point in attending a dentist unless they have a specific need to do so. One factor that may perhaps be less predictable is that of a gradient for dental anxiety. Dental anxiety is a major barrier to attending a dentist and presents a considerable barrier to the provision of clinical care. The survey results presented here suggest it too has a social class gradient and that people in social class V are twice as likely as those in social class I to say they feel anxious about going to a dentist.

People from a professional background are:

- More likely to attend for dental check-ups, brush teeth twice a day, use an additional method for cleaning teeth
- Less likely to have teeth extracted
- Less anxious about going to the dentist

The prevention of social inequalities in oral health

It seems that wherever there is socio-economic stratification of society, health inequalities will appear. Social disadvantage is largely inherited in the sense that it is bestowed on people from birth and its effects on the newborn are immediate, as shown by greater infant mortality among those living in deprived circumstances. Generally speaking, policies to reduce social inequalities themselves need to be directed specifically at the elements of life that differentiate between the affluent and the poor, such as wages, housing, health, and education. Tackling these is a political issue, and will depend on the philosophy of the Government in power and the approach they take. Absolute redistribution of wealth need not be the issue as Carr-Hill has pointed out; there is a difference between policies aimed at 'redistribution' to bring about equality and welfare policies aimed at raising the standards of the poor to a socially acceptable minimum.

Perhaps the most observable Government policy in the United Kingdom to reduce inequalities (although undertaken in an age when the term was not in vogue) is the National Health Service itself. Despite the difficulties the system finds itself in from time to time, it has undoubtedly presided over a general health improvement. In dental health the improvement is clear in the quite dramatic reduction of the percentage of edentulous adults in the population. This has fallen from 37 per cent to 12 per cent between 1968 to 1998 in England and Wales. However, as Figure 14.14 shows, the dental health gradient between different social classes has remained more or less unchanged over the period. More pertinently, although there is an improvement among people in each social class group, the relative dental health difference between classes has increased over the 30 year period. In 1968, 27 per cent of those from social classes I, II, & IIINM were edentulous compared with almost twice as many (46 per cent) among those from unskilled working backgrounds. By 1998, this had increased to a three-fold difference: 7 per cent of social class I, II, or IIINM were edentulous, whereas 22 per cent were edentulous among those from unskilled working backgrounds. This is a good example of the problems confronting those who want to reduce health inequalities; where a universal intervention is undertaken, it can often be the most affluent in society who gain most. Similar findings permeate general health where Carr-Hill has summarized the position regarding early death rates (those before the age of 65) as one in which the number of deaths has decreased during the National Health Service era but a greater proportion of them still occur among the most socially deprived.

There is an important lesson for reducing social inequalities in health that can be learned from this. Where the goal is to reduce health inequalities preventive methods should be targeted if economically feasible.

Macintyre and others have examined the quality of evidence of many of the submissions (including their own) to the Acheson Committee in 1998 that were proposed to enable health inequalities to be reduced. They noted that while many had evidence of the effects of social inequalities on various health issues, most lacked evidence about the effectiveness of interventions to reduce variations in health. Furthermore, this was particularly the case for macro-level interventions at the societal level (e.g. taxation policies to combat smoking), than micro-level interventions at the individual level (smoking cessation by nicotine replacement strategies). Nevertheless, Macintyre has also called for interventions planned under the initiative 'Saving lives: our healthier nation' to consider 'upstream' issues such as 'what is pushing people into the river?' (social circumstances) as well as downstream issues that are concerned with 'pulling people out of the river' (medical care).

Table 14.3 considers some plausible interventions that may reduce dental health inequalities. The evidence base for most of these as a means of reducing health inequalities does not exist to any great extent, except in the case of water fluoridation where a systematic review of the evidence to date has been undertaken by the NHS Centre for Reviews and Dissemination. These interventions should, therefore, be regarded as suggestions for consideration rather than evidence-based guidelines.

Prevention of early development of oral health inequalities

The Black Committee felt that the preventive way to attack inequalities in health lies in childhood and, in the light of massive research, the first years of life. Dentistry is perhaps fortunate to have one extremely effective method for the prevention of dental caries that has its effect during the development of the dentition: water fluoridation. It is known that population measures such as health promotion often increases health inequalities; so a concern about water fluoridation might be that it, as another form of population intervention, might also increase, rather than reduce, health inequalities. However, the reason why many health promotion interventions increase gradients in health is that the affluent are more likely to respond to these types of intervention, but there is no behavioural change component required for water fluoridation to have an effect. Furthermore, there is currently more dental caries developing in children living in deprived conditions; if fluoridation has an equal effect on all teeth then the benefit to deprived children should in theory be greater than for those from more affluent backgrounds. The Acheson Committee seemed quite content with the evidence presented to it to say health inequalities in children were

Table 14.3 The prevention of oral health inequalitites

Prevention of early development of oral health inequalities	Prevention of oral health inequalities in adulthood
Upstream	
Social policies 'favouring' the socially disadvantaged	Social policies 'favouring' the socially disadvantaged
Midstream	
Fluoridation of water supplies	Extension of coverage of free dental care for deprived groups
Action on 'hidden' sugars	Locate 'drop-in' dental surgeries in health centres
Restriction of less healthy food at school	
Attendance/Registration of infants with a General Dental Practitioner (extend/ increase or improve accuracy of current deprivation) payments	
Downstream	
Fissure sealants for children from deprived backgrounds	Effective communication Empowerment Programmes to promote smoking cessation Programmes to promote alcohol control Programmes to consider dental anxiety amongst the socially disadvantaged

reduced by fluoridation and went on to recommend fluoridation of water supplies. However, the Systematic Review of Water Fluoridation subsequently carried out by the NHS Centre for Reviews and Dissemination was slightly more guarded about the evidence they obtained but concluded that the review suggests

> a benefit in reducing the differences in severity of tooth decay (as measured by dmft or DMFT) between classes among five and 12 year-old children. No effect on the overall measure of the proportion of caries free children was detected. However, the quality of evidence is low and based on a small number of studies. The association between water fluoridation, caries and social class needs further clarification

Sugar may be another factor that is linked to social inequalities in oral health. There is evidence that the diet of the less advantaged consists of more processed foods and less fresh foods than the more affluent in society. This is especially the case among the most impoverished families who may live in single rooms where there is no opportunity to prepare food, and as a consequence may have to rely entirely on packaged and take-away foods. Certain types of sweet may also be an inexpensive way of pacifying or rewarding children who are living under difficult circumstances. The literature on smoking among mothers in deprived groups suggests that smoking cigarettes provides a momentary gap in

their otherwise busy or monotonous daily life. The consumption of sweets among children living in deprived circumstances may also fulfil an important role in relieving some of the burden of their living conditions. It also seems plausible that sweets that last longer, such as the boiled sugar variety, may be bought in preference to healthier items from a dental standpoint, such as sweets in the form of bars, which could usually be eaten all at once, thereby reducing sugar exposure frequency.

There are perhaps several plausible ways to take action on sugar both at a 'midstream' and 'downstream' level. In midstream, steps could be considered to produce incentives to manufacturers to limit sugar in processed foods and drinks, or at least to make it clear how much is present. Slightly further downstream there is an acknowledged role for schools in promoting and providing healthy foods, which would be directed at general as well as dental health. Downstream at the level of the individual, steps could be taken to produce effective health promotion material targeted at those from deprived backgrounds to emphasize the role of frequency of sugar intake. Any such intervention would probably require an understanding of the current role of sweet eating among the socially disadvantaged.

The promotion of equitable access to services was identified as a need in the White Paper 'The Health of the Nation'. This considered the need for resource allocation to follow relative need, the availability of proven clinical care, and the removal of barriers to care, particularly for those with poorer health status, and the reduction of variations in the outcome of care across the country. In the General Dental Service steps to try to provide an equitable dental service have included the provision of incentives to register infants from deprived backgrounds for dental care as well as some localized campaigns to increase infant registration in areas where it has been shown to be low.

The interventions discussed so far are predominantly midstream interventions involving communities and groups. There is also a role for interventions at the individual level in helping to reduce health inequalities. It has already been said that the problem with many effective preventive interventions, such as some forms of health promotion, is that they often increase health differences between the affluent and the poor. However, some clinically applied preventive measures can be targeted, such as some forms of individual fluoride-based treatment and the provision of fissure sealants. Both of these will face an initial barrier resulting from children from deprived backgrounds being less likely to attend dental clinics. A further problem will be to classify a 'deprived' individual reliably.

Prevention of oral health inequalities in adulthood

In the United Kingdom, the prevention of social inequalities in health in adults is considered less of a priority than in children. However, they are not entirely separable. The use of preventive health services among adults such as attending for dental check-ups may offer an opportunity for children to attend for dental care also.

In addition to opportunity, there is the issue of transmission of health behaviours between family members; a parent who brushes their teeth every night is probably more likely to encourage their children to do likewise than a parent who brushes irregularly.

The role of patient charges in NHS dentistry as a barrier to the less wealthy does not appear to have been examined in any great detail. Findings from the Adult Dental Health survey (Figure 14.13) have suggested that there is a social class gradient in finding dental care expensive, but this reverses among social class V. This might reflect the role of free dental care that is provided for those on income support, or other indicators of low income, who will tend to be classified as social class V. Access to dental care among the most socially deprived may also be affected by location of dental surgeries. The use of free transportation in poor rural areas has shown that attendance rates at antenatal and child health clinics can be improved by reducing the difficulties that would be involved in the journey to the clinic by other means. Locating drop-in dental surgeries in medical clinics may also be a way of encouraging people who are not registered elsewhere to attend for dental care and may, in particular, help infants to be brought into a dental clinic when they attend for medical care or screening.

A common experience among people when dealing with the National Health Service is a feeling of not knowing what is going on and how this should be dealt with. There is a view that people from professional groups such as lawyers and accountants are better equipped to negotiate their way through the healthcare system thus creating an 'advantage' over those unable to do so. People tend to get on better in conversation with their peers, so dentists are probably more comfortable talking to fellow professionals than anyone else, and this may be a factor in some inequalities in dental care. There is evidence supporting this as a possibility from medical studies. It has been found that people in socially disadvantaged areas prefer to contact practice nurses rather than medical practitioners. There is also evidence that socially disadvantaged people are less likely to be investigated and offered surgery once heart disease has developed and that those who are offered cardiac surgery are less likely to be classified as urgent and have to wait longer than people from affluent backgrounds. It seems unlikely that this is a conscious policy on the part of the medical profession, and may, therefore, be a reflection of factors such as communication although it may also in part reflect attendance by patients at clinics or being excluded by health behaviours such as smoking. Data from the 1998 Adult Dental Health survey (Figure 14.14) suggests there is a social class gradient in being given preventive dental care advice by a dentist. There is a greater than 50 per cent chance that a person from social class I will have received some advice about tooth brushing or gum care from a dentist than someone from social class V. Again this may be influenced by their dental attendance behaviour, but there is also likely to be a communication factor involved as well. People from socially deprived backgrounds also seem more likely to say they feel anxious about attending a dentist, which may be a further reflection of a feeling of lack of control in a clinical setting. There is evidence in medical settings that the choice of agent delivering the intervention may be an important contributing factor to a successful outcome. Studies that have employed people to deliver an intervention drawn either from the same locality or age group or ethnic background have shown that outcome can be enhanced by such measures. Good communication and attentiveness to avoiding unintentional favouritism is something that has to be achieved at the level of individual health practitioners and may be one of the main contributions that they can make to the provision of an equitable health service.

Smoking and alcohol intake are also factors that have a social class gradient. Both affect oral health and can have an even greater effect on general health. The Acheson Committee reported in 1998 that although smoking had decreased overall it had remained stable among people who were the most disadvantaged in society. The committee reviewed evidence about the effects of taxing tobacco as a deterrent and concluded that increasing taxation only seemed to further reduce the disposable income of the least wealthy, many of whom seemed to find their severe hardship itself a deterrent to giving up smoking. For this reason the committee recommended the provision of nicotine replacement patches on prescription, which would at least remove the cost barrier to the most disadvantaged, who can obtain NHS prescriptions free of charge. This recommendation was put into practice in the United Kingdom in 2002.

In addition to affecting the oral mucosa, drinking alcohol is a factor in many assaults and accidents that often lead to teeth being damaged. Deaths from alcohol-related diseases are more than four times higher among unskilled working men than among men from professional groups. There is also a suggestion that problem drinking among the more affluent in society is less harmful to their general health than to that of the poor, as they are protected from some of the deleterious effects of alcohol by their better diet, housing, health care, and other factors. Despite evidence to suggest that trying to price tobacco out of reach of people can reduce the budgets of poor families rather than affect their smoking, the only 'upstream' measure proposed by Acheson Committee was to recommend that fiscal measures should be used to keep the price of alcohol at the same level year on year. Downstream from this the problem of poor people with alcohol problems was seen as a target for intervention as such people often are not able to access services that are available to the general population.

What we know, and what can be done to prevent oral health inequalities

Generally speaking, there is a lack of trials that have looked at the effectiveness of particular dental interventions on social inequalities in oral health. Understandably, most work has concentrated on the common life-threatening medical problems identified by the Department of Health in 1995; coronary heart disease and stroke, cancers, mental illness, HIV/AIDS, and accidents. However, these do tell us a lot about what may or may not work as measures to reduce inequalities in dentistry. On the whole, successful individual interventions are those that accurately target the poor and take some recognition of their needs. Understanding how a behaviour such as smoking fits into the lives of people may be an important first step to designing an effective intervention to reduce or eliminate it. The involvement of people from the same background as those receiving the intervention may also be a key to success. Identifying people on the basis of their social circumstances for intervention also requires good information. Most new deprivation measures are based on information about geographical areas rather than individuals avoiding the need to ask sensitive information from people. However, applying these measures effectively requires accurate geographical information about where people live, quite often in the form of post codes. Gathering such information in the health service accurately is, therefore, crucial to implementing some health improvement schemes and can be aided by health professionals' co-operation in ensuring that address details of patients are gathered completely. There is also a need for properly conducted trials of the ability of oral health interventions to reduce social inequalities in oral health.

There is perhaps no better way to conclude this chapter than to quote the main recommendations of the Acheson enquiry into inequalities in health.

Acheson enquiry recommendations

- that all policies likely to have an impact on health should be evaluated in terms of their impact on health inequalities
- that high priority should be given to families with children
- further steps should be taken to reduce income inequalities and improve the living standards of poor households

Conclusions

- Wherever some form of social stratification is found there are correlated health inequalities.

- The incidence of certain health behaviours differs between social groups (e.g. smoking, heavy drinking, leisure time exercise). However, even when these factors are controlled for (e.g. looking at non-smokers only) the difference in morality rates are still apparent (but reduced) between different groups.

- The effects of deprivation appear to be a personal rather than a community disadvantage. Individuals who are not disadvantaged do not have a higher risk of dying if they live in a deprived area, nor do disadvantaged people who live in advantaged areas gain any benefit from their geographical location.

- Effective health interventions do not always reduce health inequalities between social groups and some may actually increase them. This seems to be behavioural in origin: the socially advantaged may be in a better position to implement healthy lifestyle behaviours than the poor because they are more likely to get health information from health professionals; may have fewer competing life concerns; and

will be in a better position to implement behaviours that have a cost dimension (e.g. healthy diet).

- The only intervention for which systematic reviews show there is limited evidence of effectiveness in reducing social inequalities in oral health (in children) is fluoridation of water supplies (NHS Centre for Reviews and Dissemination, Report 18). However, the quality of evidence was described as low and based on a small number of studies.

Acknowledgements

This research was funded by the Chief Scientist Office of the Department of Health of the Scottish Executive who do not necessarily share the views expressed. Thanks to Margaret Whitehead for supplying Figure 14.2 by Dahlgren, G. & Whitehead, M. (1991). Figures 14.8, 14.11–14.13 were derived directly from the 1998 Adult Dental Health survey data and do not appear in the original survey report.

References

Acheson, D. (1998). *Independent Enquiry into Inequalities in Health*. London: The Stationery Offfice.

Arblaster, L., Entwistle, V., Lambert, M., Forster, M., Sheldon, T., and Watt, I.(1995). *Review of the Research on the Effectiveness of Health Service Interventions to Reduce Variations in Health*. York: NHS Centre for Reviews and Dissemination.

Benzeval, M., Judge, K., and Whitehead, M. (1995). *Tackling Inequalities in Health. An Agenda for Action*. London: King's Fund.

Carr-Hill, R. (1987).The inequalities in health debate: a critical review of the issues. *J. Soc. Policy*, 16, 509–542.

Carroll, D., Davey Smith, G., and Bennett, P. (1996). Some observations on health and socio-economic status. *J. Health Psych.*, 1, 23–39.

Department of Health. (1995). *Variations in Health. What can the Department of Health and the NHS Do?* London: Department of Health.

Jones, C.M., Taylor, G.O., Whittle, J.G., Evans, D., and Trotter, D.P. (1997). Water fluoridation, tooth decay in 5 year olds, and social deprivation measured by the Jarman score: analysis of data from British dental surveys. *Br. Med. J.*, 315, 514–517.

Macintyre, S. (1997). The Black Report and beyond what are the issues? *Soc. Sci. Med.*, 44, 723–745.

Macintyre, S. (2000). Prevention and reduction of health inequalities. *Br. Med. J.*, 320, 1399–1400.

Townsend, P. (1987). Deprivation. *J. Soc. Policy*, 16, 125–146.

Townsend, P., and Davidson, N. (1992) *Inequalities in Health. The Black Report and The Health Divide* (revised edn.) Harmondsworth: Penguin.

15

Oral health promotion and policy

Oral health promotion and policy

Aubrey Sheiham and Richard Watt

Introduction

Oral diseases are important public health problems. They are very prevalent and their impact on both society and the individual are significant. Pain, disability, and handicap from oral diseases are common, and the costs of treatment are a major burden to health care systems (Table 15.1). The causes of dental diseases are known and the conditions are largely preventable. On the basis of those criteria, oral and dental diseases are a public health problem. Furthermore, inequalities in oral health are a problem; disadvantaged and socially excluded population groups suffer higher rates of disease than their more affluent contemporaries. The move towards an evidence-based approach to treatment and prevention has highlighted the limitations of conventional dental health education. Those limitations and the expansion of concepts on health promotion has lead to a wider recognition that there is a need to adopt a more progressive approach to prevention.

In this chapter, oral health promotion will be defined and an outline given of the philosophy underlying the dominant approaches in health promotion, Health For All, and the intersectoral action. The epidemiological basis for strategy is explored and the application of an integrated approach to chronic disease control, the common risk/health approach examined. Case studies using food and periodontal health policies will illustrate the relevance of these approaches to oral health.

Limitations of conventional dental health education

Dental health education aims to promote oral health through educational means, principally the provision of information to improve oral health knowledge and awareness. Through the acquisition of knowledge, a change in behaviour is then considered likely to occur. This rather simplistic and outdated approach has dominated dental health education practice for many years but fails to acknowledge the complexities of human behaviour and the importance of the broader social, economic, and environmental factors determining behaviour change. How effective is the educational approach in promoting oral health?

Several effectiveness reviews have been undertaken to assess the quality and effect of dental health education interventions (Brown, 1994; Schou and Locker, 1994; Kay and Locker, 1996, 1998; Sprod et al., 1996). In broad terms, all the reviews have adopted a similar method: a systematic search of the published and unpublished literature to determine the overall impact of interventions on a range of outcomes. The common findings of these reviews are shown in Table 15.2.

The effectiveness reviews also identified that many interventions were poorly designed, inadequately evaluated and lacked a theoretical basis. It is apparent that a different approach is required to promote oral health and reduce inequalities across the population.

The need for an 'upstream approach'

The present dominant approach to prevention is recognizable in the following allegory. A man was standing by the side of a river

Table 15.1 Criteria for a public health problem

- Prevalence of the condition is high, or if uncommon, the condition should be serious.
- Impact of condition on individual's quality of life (pain, discomfort, functional limitation, social isolation).
- Impact on wider society (costs of treatment, time off school or work).
- Condition preventable and effective treatments available.

Table 15.2 Common findings of effectiveness of dental health education reviews

- Improving individuals' knowledge of oral health can be achieved for short periods, but effects on behaviour are very limited.
- Information alone does not produce long-term behaviour changes.
- Interventions at an individual level are effective at reducing plaque levels only in the short term.
- School based toothbrushing campaigns aimed at improving oral hygiene are largely ineffective.
- Mass media campaigns are ineffective at promoting either knowledge or behaviour change.
- Very few studies have assessed the effects of dental health education on sugars consumption.

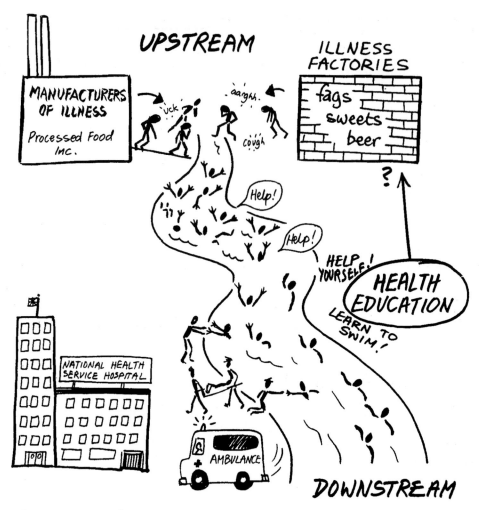

Figure 15.1 Upstream-Downstream approaches

and heard a cry of a drowning person (Figure 15.1). He jumped in to rescue him, pulled him to the bank, and applied artificial respiration. Just as the rescued man was recovering, there were more cries from other drowning people. In jumped the rescuer, brought some back and resuscitated them. The rescuer could not cope on his own so he got some helpers and machines. Still he could not cope. So they worked faster in teams—four-handed and six-handed—with more complex equipment. The numbers of drowning people became so numerous that some could not be rescued before permanent damage occurred. How could he stop them from drowning? Swimming lessons were the solution. These rescuing and training activities kept him so busy that at no time did he stop to consider why people who could not swim were in the river. Who was pushing them in upstream? (McKinlay 1974).

The dentist's concentration on 'downstream' victim-blaming distracts attention from the 'upstream' activities of the confectionery, food and drink companies who are 'pushing people into the water'. Health workers usually intervene only after the damage

has been done. Instead of expending so much effort on downstream and midstream activities, more efforts should be directed at making the river shallower, so that people do not have to learn to swim—making healthier choices the easier choices (Milio 1986)—and controlling the activities of those pushing people into the water—a direct attack on the determinants of health.

Definitions of health promotion

The modern health promotion movement has emerged out of the need for a fundamental change in strategy to achieve and maintain health. It is based on a public health philosophy that should encompass the prevention of disease at a primary level, and secondly, the promotion of health (Milio 1988). These two concepts, when applied to developing environments which promote healthier choices for people in coping with their lives, need to be adopted in a manner that encourages those choices to be the easiest choices (Milio 1986). Health promotion can be considered 'as the combination of educational and environmental supports for actions and conditions of living conducive to health' (Green and Kreuter 1990). Strategies to change 'the range of options available to people and to make health-promoting choices easier and/or to diminish health damaging options by making them more difficult to choose' (Milio 1986). Another definition is 'health promotion is the process of enabling individuals and communities to increase control over the determinants of health and thereby improve their health. Health promotion represents a mediating strategy between people and their environment, combining personal choice and social responsibility for health to create a healthier future' (WHO 1984). It is directed to the underlying determinants as well as the immediate causes of health. The causes of the causes.

Health promotion involves:

- Preventing disease at a primary level
- Making health-promoting choices easier
- Combining personal choice and social responsibility for health

The dominant philosophy, primary health care and health promotion

The Declaration of Alma Ata (WHO 1978), and the subsequent development of the WHO strategy for 'Health for All by the Year 2000' effectively set the agenda for the 'new public health' and health promotion movements. The principles in the Declaration of Alma Ata can be summarized by five principles:

- Equitable Distribution. Governments must endeavour to equitably distribute those variables which influence health.

- Community Participation. Individuals and communities should participate in all decisions which affect their health.

- Focus on Prevention. The focus of health planners and funding must shift from medical/dental care to prevention and health promotion.

- Appropriate Technology. Emphasis should be on the most appropriate technology and personnel to deal with problems.

- A Multi-sectoral Approach. Solutions to ill-health cannot be solved only by the health sector. Social, economic, agriculture, education sectors must co-ordinate policies that affect health.

Establishing healthy public policy is one of the five means for achieving the goal of Health for All by the Year 2000. The others are creating supportive environments, strengthening community action, developing personal skills, and reorienting health services (WHO 1986). The Ottawa Charter also included three process methods—mediation, enablement, and advocacy—through which people could begin to take more control over their health (WHO 1986). Healthy public policy is characterized by an

Table 15.3 The Ottawa Charter (WHO 1986)

Themes and key areas for health promotion action –

- Promoting health through public policy: by focusing attention on the impact on health of public policies from all sectors, and not just the health sector.

- Creating a supportive environment: by assessing the impact on health of the environment and clarifying opportunities to make changes conducive to health.

- Developing personal skills: by moving beyond the transmission of information, to promote understanding, and to support the development of personal, social and political skills which enable individuals to take action to promote health.

- Strengthening community action: by supporting concrete and effective community action in defining priorities, making decisions, planning strategies and implementing them to achieve better health.

- Reorienting health services: by refocusing attention away from the responsibility to provide curative and clinical services towards the goal of health gain.

explicit concern for health and equity in all areas of policy and by accountability for health impact. In health care, equity is based on Aristotle's dictum that there is no greater injustice than to treat unequal cases equally. Equity requires that people who are alike in relevant respects be treated in like fashion, and people who are unlike in relevant respects be treated appropriately in unlike fashion. This corresponds to horizontal equity—like treatment of like individuals, and vertical equity—the unlike treatment of unlike individuals (Culyer 1993).

The term inequity '… refers to differences which are unnecessary and avoidable but, in addition, are also considered unfair and unjust'. (Whitehead 1991). Reducing inequalities in health is established as one of the prime tasks of health promotion (WHO 1984). Equity is an ethical principle and it is unsurprising that the ethical principles underlying health promotion conform to the Declaration of Helsinki and include respect for persons, beneficence, non-maleficence and justice.

The Ottawa Charter included the concept of healthy public policy (Table 15.3). This goes beyond the health care system. It is concerned with the health implications of all policies including economic, employment, agriculture, housing, transport, and environment policies recognizing that improvements in health comes from a multi-sectoral rather than a purely health sector approach. Milio (1987) defined healthy public policy as 'ecological in perspective, multi-sectoral in scope and participatory in strategy'. Healthy public policy stresses the need to analyse and understand the broad beliefs and cultures of the community as well as those of the professionals who act as advocates, and the functioning of local and central government. Understanding the existing policy environment is central to the development of healthy public policy.

General principles of oral health promotion

Oral health promotion has emerged in line with developments in general health promotion. Oral health promotion strategies should be based upon the following guiding principles:

- Base action upon a comprehensive needs assessment using both normative and lay measures of need
- Develop a range of clearly stated and challenging goals
- Preventive rather than curative approaches—promote public health measures to the public and public authorities, e.g. fluoride in water.
- Be based upon contemporary theories of individual and organizational change
- A re-orientation from prescription to supportive health promotion methods—redress the balance of influence and make healthier choices easier. Promote self-esteem and facilitate decision-making skills rather than be prescriptive.
- Combat the influence of those interests which produce and profit from ill health. This involves controls on industry-sponsored educational materials in schools, advertising, and campaigns to reduce barriers to good oral health.
- Public health rather than individually focussed programmes.
- Focus on the social causes of ill health rather than a victim-blaming approach—acknowledging the limited real choices available to any individual.
- Address the underlying determinants of oral health.
- Tackle causes that are common to a number of chronic diseases.
- Supportive rather than authoritarian styles of action.
- A commitment to distribute success equitably
- Ensure actions are evidence based.
- Community participation rather than professionally dominated activities.
- Working in partnership with key groups and agencies.

Selecting a strategy is influenced by these criteria and philosophical, professional, and political perspectives. The epidemiological basis for strategy selection for oral health promotion is the Common Risk Factor Approach and the Whole Population Strategy (Rose 1992).

Health promotion strategy

- Analyse and understand the broad beliefs of the community as well as those of the professionals who act as advocates
- Develop a range of clearly stated and challenging goals
- Ensure actions are evidence based

An integrated common risk/health factor approach

The solutions to the chronic disease problems are solutions shared with other health workers, educators, and the community. The strategies to mitigate the health problems are incorporated in the Ottawa Charter for Health Promotion. They are: community action and support, environmental change, legislation, improving personal skills, and empowering people to become stakeholders in society, and collectively work to change the structures which determine their health. Significant control of dental diseases can mainly be achieved in terms of social policy. The task of oral health workers is to convince policy makers and society to undertake the specific social measures which are required to solve general and oral health problems, and to participate in the implementation of these policies.

The determinants of chronic diseases

Health education policy and interventions have focused on health behaviours and have been relatively inattentive to social contextual factors that are related to health behaviours in general. Lifestyles are commonly considered as important aetiological causes of morbidity and mortality. Others interpret lifestyle as a composite expression of the social and cultural circumstances that condition and constrain behaviour, in addition to the personal decisions the individual may make (Green and Kreuter 1990). But the apparent simple acts are enmeshed in more complex lifetime habits and social circumstances associated with lifestyle (Graham 1990). Living conditions provide the context in which lifestyles are sustained.

Social determinants have rightly taken a more prominent position in recent policy discussions (Marmot and Wilkinson 1999). The principal determinants of health and disease are social and economic conditions, culture, and other environmental factors (Marmot and Wilkinson 1999). Social structure is the true aetiological agent in most chronic diseases. Most behaviours are socially patterned and often cluster with one another. This patterned behavioural response has led Link and Phelan (1995) to consider situations that place individuals 'at risk of risks'. Indeed some epidemiologists promote the notion of the 'social production' of disease (Krieger 1994). The social environment has, therefore, become more significant for health (Sheiham 2000).

Health promotion is directed at the underlying determinants, the causes of the causes, as well as the immediate causes of ill health. The immediate causes of the major dental diseases, caries and periodontal disease are diet, dirt (plaque), and smoking. Oral mucosal lesions, oral cancer, temporomandibular joint dysfunction and pain are related to tobacco, alcohol, and stress and trauma to teeth and jaws to accidents (Fig 15.2). As these causes are common to a number of other chronic diseases such as heart disease, cancer, strokes, accidents, it is rational to use a common risk factor approach (Sheiham and Watt 2000).

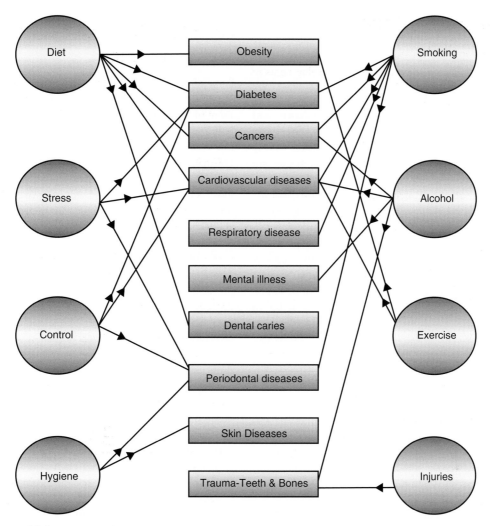

Figure 15.2 Common risk factor approach

A common risk/health factor approach—an integrated approach

The key concept underlying the integrated common risk approach is that promoting general health by controlling a small number of risk factors, may have a major impact on a large number of diseases at a lower cost, greater efficiency, and effectiveness than disease-specific approaches. Savings may be made by coordinating the work done by various specialist groups and organizations. Decision-makers and individuals will be more readily influenced by measures directed at preventing heart diseases, obesity, stroke, cancers, diabetes, as well as dental caries than if dental disease-specific recommendations are made alone.

There are basically two approaches for an equity-oriented health policy: focusing on actions or on specific risk factors to reduce specific diseases and public policies aimed at improving health conditions, in general, and among those at particular risk. The new public health policy is no longer oriented to single diseases. The Common Risk/Health Factor Approach (CRHFA) distinguishes between actions aimed at reducing 'risk factors' and actions promoting 'health factors'. The strategy includes efforts to improve health by reducing risks, promoting health, and strengthening possibilities to cope with 'given' risk factors—creating supportive environments, reducing the negative effects of certain risk factors and facilitating behaviour changes. One of the principles of health promotion is to focus on the whole population rather than on disease-specific at-risk groups. A major benefit of the Common Risk/Health Factor Approach is the focus on improving health conditions in general for the whole population and for groups at high risk. It thereby reduces social inequities.

Concepts of common risk factors must inform public health work and education. A number of chronic diseases such as heart disease, cancer, strokes, accidents, and oral diseases have risk factors in common and many risk factors are relevant to more than one chronic disease. Preventive strategies based upon CRHFA will exert a favourable effect, not only on a single disease but simultaneously on several conditions.

The epidemiological basis for CRHFA

The major risk factors for chronic diseases are smoking; diets high in saturated fats and sugars, and low in fibre, fruit and vegetables; alcohol; accidents; a sedentary lifestyle, stress; and low control and environmental pollution (Sheiham and Watt 2000). Numerous expert committees have concluded that particular diets, namely those high in saturated fatty acids, non-milk extrinsic sugars and low in polyunsaturates, fibre and vitamins A, C, and E are associated with coronary heart disease, stroke, diabetes, cancers, obesity, and dental caries. Increasing scientific evidence from epidemiological, clinical, and other relevant research has been accumulated to show that non-milk extrinsic sugars are a cause of a range of diseases, especially dental caries. Sheiham, claims that *'Dental caries is a sugar-dependent infectious disease'*, a conclusion supported by most contemporary scientific evidence (Rugg-Gunn and Nunn 1999). A reduction in non-milk extrinsic sugars intake is desirable in view of their cariogenicity, as well as other harmful effects on general health. The World Health Organization and COMA recommended reductions in non-milk extrinsic sugars (NMES) to a maximum of 10 per cent of energy intake.

Smoking has been implicated in a large number of diseases. It is estimated that smoking causes about 30 per cent of all cancer diseases and deaths. They also have more periodontal disease and other diseases of the oral mucosa.

High alcohol consumption increases the risk of a wide variety of conditions such as raised blood pressure, liver cirrhosis, cardiovascular disease, and cancers. In addition, many social problems such as family violence, crime, and injuries are linked with heavy alcohol use. Trauma to the head often includes fractures of the jaws and teeth.

Dirt causes inflammation of the skin and mucosa. Dental plaque (dirt) is the main cause of gingival inflammation and periodontitis. Similarly, biofilms of bacteria on the skin, if not washed away, lead to pimples and more serious skin conditions.

Injuries are responsible for many deaths in both developing and developed countries. Accidental injury is the most important cause of death and hospital admission among children and young people in the UK, Europe, and US. The prevalence of dental trauma among children and young people is about 15 per cent.

Clustering of risk factors

Some of the risk factors cluster in groups of people. Changing one of the factors may influence the others. People who smoke are more likely to eat a diet high in fats and sugars and low in fibre, polyunsaturated fatty acids, fruit, and nutrient rich foods containing Vitamins A, C, and E, take less exercise and drink more alcohol than non-smokers (Sheiham and Watt 2000). The clustering of risk factors in individuals and groups, particularly those at the lower social groups suggests that preventive approaches should be directed at clusters of risk factors common to a number of diseases and the social structures which influence individuals' health risks.

Population and High-risk strategies

The economic rationale for preventive measures depends on the prevalence of the disease: when the prevalence is very low, and the diseases not serious, the returns often do not justify the intervention. For example the cost per caries lesion saved increases as the level of decay in a population decreases. At the lower levels of dental caries, now prevailing in most industrialized countries, the traditional preventive methods such as fluoride rinsing, professionally applied fluorides, and intensive chairside dental health education need to be justified because the cost effectiveness is borderline.

Concern for reducing disease in people with severe caries or periodontal disease rests on the assumption that those predisposed to develop many cavities and pockets are distinguishable from those at low risk. That implies some means of identifying those in special need. The high risk strategy aims to identify people who may develop disease in the future by the use either of a predictive marker or of an early feature of the disease which precedes its clinical manifestation so that efforts can be focussed on them (Fig. 15.3). Screening is used to detect those individuals at high risk for close monitoring and special preventive treatment.

One advantage of the high risk strategy is that any preventive intervention which is undertaken is appropriate to the individual concerned, who has a high probability of future disease (Rose

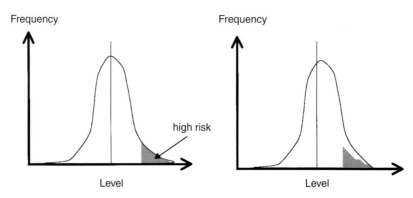

Figure 15.3 High risk approach

1992). A corollary is that those at risk, once identified and told, are likely to be better motivated to participate in the care offered. This assumes that the intervention is sensitive to the behavioural ability of the person, and their social and economic circumstances. A further advantage is that those not at risk do not have to undergo preventive treatment. Finally, the high risk strategy conserves valuable resources by directing services where the need and potential benefits are likely to be greatest. However this does not necessarily imply that the overall ratio of benefits to costs is favourable.

To be useful in predictive case-finding, a test must detect the majority of high risk children and at the same time identify those at low risk. To be more precise, they must have high sensitivity, otherwise many with potential caries will not be identified, as well as a high specificity to prevent excessive dilution of the high risk group with subjects who are, in fact, at comparatively low risk. A practical way of looking at the imperfections in screening tests is to consider sensitivity and specificity in terms of screened patients whose test result is wrong. A review of the literature on the available predictors of caries found that none are of sufficient sensitivity and specificity (Johnson 1991; Sheiham and Joffe 1991). The best indicator of future caries in individuals is past caries experience, but prior disease is not a reliable predictor of future disease. Although the future course of disease is difficult to predict accurately in particular individuals, epidemiological data allow us to see what the future patterns of caries in groups of children could be, if their caries status when they are young is known. This allows prediction not only of what the DMF for 10-year-olds will be when they are 18, but which teeth will become carious and which surfaces will be attacked (McDonald and Sheiham 1992). These predictions allow planning of the numbers and types of dental personnel required in the future, but not identifying which child will need therapy.

In addition to reliability and validity, there are several factors to be considered before undertaking or advising the use of a screening test. The recommended intervention needs to be successful in reducing the incidence and/or severity of the disease. When the aim is the detection of one or more markers rather than disease itself, one must ensure that the overall effect will have more benefits than disadvantages from the point of view of the child being screened. The test itself must be acceptable to the subject in terms of inconvenience, discomfort, and risks of side-effects. Furthermore, it must be simple and capable of rapid application to large numbers of subjects (Burr and Elwood 1985).

To summarize, the high risk strategy for preventing caries and periodontal diseases has several drawbacks, and if relied upon exclusively it cannot be expected to make a major impact on the disease. The current preoccupation with markers of disease prediction is misdirected and is unlikely to produce information of use to control dental diseases.

Whole population strategy

Fortunately another strategy which complements the use of the high risk strategy is the whole population strategy (Fig. 15.4). The concepts of the whole population strategy have been adopted by the World Health Organization (WHO 1984) and incorporated as Principles of Health Promotion:

- Focus on whole population rather than on disease-specific at-risk groups.

- Action should be addressed towards the many factors influencing health in order to ensure that the 'total environment, which is beyond the control of individuals, is conducive to health'.

In many industrialized countries today compared with twenty years ago, dental health in children and young adults is markedly better. This improvement has come about as a result of changed norms of behaviour in the population as a whole, together with an alteration in manufacturing practices and the addition of fluoride to toothpaste. The commonsense view, that modern dentistry can take much of the credit by having identified the causes and methods of prevention, is only a small part of the picture (Nadanovsky and Sheiham 1994). The improvement of health as a result of wider social factors is not confined to caries. Concerning the major epidemic diseases which have declined dramatically during the past hundred years, McKeown examined a number of factors,

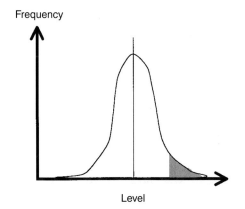
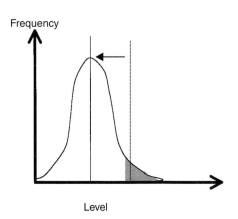

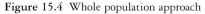

Figure 15.4 Whole population approach

including medical progress, which might have contributed to their reduction (McKeown 1979). The contribution of the medical profession, even immunization, was quite limited.

The implication of these findings is that major improvements in the prevention of disease tend to follow major social changes, whether these are alterations in social norms (dietary patterns, oral cleanliness, contraception), in the availability of key resources (fluoridated toothpaste, quality, and quantity of food) or as a result of engineering (fluoridation of water supplies, clean water, effective waste disposal). There is no reason why a similar approach should not prove equally successful in the future.

Just as the high risk strategy requires a scientific basis, both in technical matters and evaluation, the same is true of the whole population strategy. It depends upon epidemiological, sociological, and other research to identify important determinants of the disease in question, and acting to change their prevalence in the appropriate direction. In the case of caries, the determinants which are open to intervention are sugars consumption and the protective influence of fluoride: the distribution of caries (DMF) depends on the distributions of these exposures. Altering whole exposure distributions may be the most effective way of reducing the prevalence of caries, both in the population as a whole and also specifically among those who are at highest risk. Such a strategy does not exclude the use of a high risk strategy as well, in appropriate circumstances. The scientific basis for the whole population strategy has been outlined by Rose (1992). He draws the distinction between two kinds of aetiological questions: the first seeks the causes of cases: 'Why do some *people* get caries at this time?', and the second seeks the causes of incidence 'Why do some *populations* have much caries while in others it is uncommon?'.

The whole population strategy (WPS) attempts to control the determinants, removing the underlying causes. Therefore, it has great benefits to all sections of the population. This was illustrated by the decline of caries. The WPS approach is behaviourally appropriate. The aim is to alter social norms; when that norm is accepted and institutional changes have occurred, then reinforcement of the behaviour is unnecessary. Examples of such institutional changes are the adaptation of their products on the part of industry (fluoridated toothpaste, low sugar snacks), and government action such as a food and health policy including reduction in sugars. The more effective the basic prevention for the group, the smaller will be the subgroup that will require individualized prevention and treatment.

The whole population strategy can be used flexibly. For example, it can be directed at a designated part of the total population such as a school, district or part of a district—a directed population strategy. This remains different from the high risk strategy in that it does not use screening of individual subjects for risk factors (Sheiham and Joffe 1991).

The whole population strategy, relies heavily on intersectoral planning—involving on the macro level, Ministries of Environment, Food and Rural Affairs, Education, Employment, Foreign Affairs as well as the Health Ministry, and on a micro level,

interdisciplinary planning: getting teachers, primary health workers, community development, and social workers to co-ordinate their efforts. This approach sets the agenda and establishes norms. For example, the idea that excessive consumption of sugars is detrimental to health is a widely accepted belief and many food and drink manufacturers feature 'no sugar added' on their labels as a positive selling feature. Once the norm has been established, efforts should be made to institutionalize them by a reduction in subsidies to produce and promote the product, controls on advertising and on imports, by encouraging the production of low- and no-sugars alternatives, and by changing education materials.

A common risk/health factor approach

- Risk factors include diet, stress, hygiene, smoking, alcohol, exercise, injuries
- Focus on whole populations rather than on disease specific at-risk groups
- Develop a co-ordinated and planned approach

Settings for oral health promotion action

Traditionally dental health education was undertaken within schools targeting schoolchildren. Why was this the case and what are the limitations of this approach? In line with developments in health promotion policy, those working in oral health promotion have increasingly adopted a more holistic approach which involves activity in a range of different settings with a variety of partners. Figure 15.5 presents a range of settings and complementary actions relevant to the promotion of oral health. Working in this way provides an opportunity practically to integrate oral health activity into other areas of policy and practice. It also enables oral health promoters to target influential decision makers to ensure that oral health issues are addressed at a senior level within organizations and agencies.

Intersectoral action—working in partnerships

The central focus of the WHO Health For All 2000 approach is an intersectoral approach (WHO 1981). This approach recognizes that economic, environmental, and social changes should underlie individual behaviour change. Promoting health requires the involvement not only of health professionals, but of all sectors of society, in both public and private spheres.

A wide range of partners have an important part to play in the promotion of oral health (Table 15.4). The challenge facing oral health promoters is highlighting the significance and relevance of oral health to other professionals, agencies, and sectors. The Common Risk/Health Factor Approach provides a theoretical basis for this, as does recognition of the impact of oral health on quality of life.

Act-ivity	Settings					Target Group					
	Community	Education	Primary care	Regional/ National projects	Workplace	Pre-school	Young people	Adults	Older people	Disabled groups	Professionals
Education											
Legislation											
Regulation											
Fiscal											
Organisational change											
Community Development											
Reorientation of health system											

Matrix for the integration of potential settings, target groups, and activities for oral health promotion (Modified from Leeds Health Promotion Service 1995).

Figure 15.5 Settings approach to oral health promotion

Table 15.4 Potential partners in oral health promotion

- Health professionals, for example doctors, health visitors, pharmacists, district nurses
- Education services, for example teachers, school governors, parents
- Local authority staff, for example carers, planning departments, social workers, catering staff within care homes, local politicians
- Voluntary sector, for example Age Concern, Pre-school Learning Alliance, Terrence Higgins Trust, Mind
- Commerce and industry, for example food retailers, food producers, advertising industry, water industry
- Government, local, national, and international

Stages in planning an oral health promotion strategy

To promote oral health and reduce inequalities requires a coordinated and planned approach. Ad hoc interventions are unlikely to be effective and are therefore a waste of public resources. At a local district or national level the planning cycle outlines stages in the planning process (Figure 15.6). Each stage in the process should link together with the next to create a cohesive plan of action.

Stage 1: Assess the needs of the population

It is essential that any strategy should address the needs of the population it is aiming to assist. In the UK a great deal of valuable information is available on the oral health needs of the population. British Association for the Study of Community Dentistry (BASCD) survey results of dental health in 5, 12, and 14 year old children in a district provide some useful indications of oral health needs in the child population. Very limited epidemiological data are available, however, for the adult population at the local level. National oral health surveys of children and adults in the UK have been conducted over the last 30 years, which provide useful data on the changing trends in oral health across the population. Normative assessments of oral health, although very important, provide only a clinical perspective on the needs of the population. Other indicators of need are also required to ensure that a broad view is taken to determine the priorities of the population (Table 15.5).

Stage 2: set goals for change

Clear measurable goals are prerequisites for policy. If you do not know where you want to be, you will not know when you have arrived there or by the best route. Achievable or desirable levels of health provide plausible measures for goal setting.

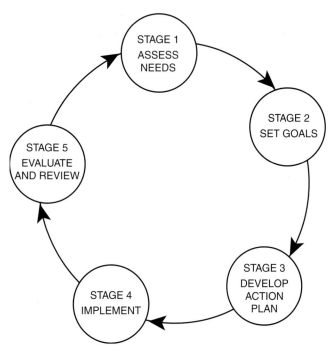

Figure 15.6 Planning cycle

Table 15.5 Information required for an oral health promotion needs assessment

- Clinical overview of patterns of health and disease
- Socio-demographic population profile
- Key data on oral health determinants in population e.g. NMES consumption, smoking rates
- Existing relevant policy initiatives and service provision
- Resources available, e.g. personnel, finances
- Public concerns and demands

An overall oral health goal is to achieve

a natural, functional, acceptable dentition, which enables an individual to eat, speak, and socialize without discomfort, pain, or embarrassment for a lifetime, and which contributes to general well being. In practical terms that is, the retention throughout life of a functional, aesthetic, natural dentition of not less than 20 teeth and not requiring recourse to a prosthesis (WHO 1982).

Goals for acceptable levels of oral health were proposed by a group of Chief Dental Officers from Northern European Countries (Table 15.6). In addition, an acceptable level of oral health would include:

- Satisfactory prosthetic replacement of any missing dental unit which obviously detracts from aesthetics.

Table 15.6 Suggestions for acceptable levels of dental health by age (WHO 1982)

Age	Mean no. of missing teeth	DMF	Periodontal status
12	0	2	0 teeth with pockets >3 mm
15	0	3	0 teeth with pockets >3 mm
18	1	4	0 teeth with pockets >3 mm
35–44	2	12	Fewer than 7 teeth 0 teeth with pockets >4.5 mm
65–74	10	12	20 functional

- Freedom from pain.
- No unacceptable deposits.
- No unacceptable intrinsic anomalies.
- An occlusion, which is functionally and cosmetically acceptable.

Goals for oral health can be expressed in terms of health, disease, health promotion, and training:

- Oral health goals, for example, caries free levels.
- Disease goals such as oral cancer rates.
- Health promotion goals like development of healthy public policies in nutrition,
- Training goals, for example, skills development of workforce

Stage 3: Develop an action and evaluation plan

Based upon the goals already set, an action and evaluation plan is required to outline the scope and detail of the strategy. Based upon the principles outlined above, it is essential that a broad range of complementary actions are included in any oral health promotion strategy. Reliance solely on health education interventions is unlikely to produce any sustained long-term improvements in oral health. The approaches outlined in the Ottawa Charter provide exciting and innovative ways to tackle the underlying determinants of oral diseases in society. An important element in the action planning is the identification of potential partners and allies for change.

The evaluation of oral health promotion has been a neglected area of practice for many years. Assessing the effects of interventions and providing feedback to practitioners and the population should be considered as core elements in any oral health strategy. Quality evaluation requires adequate resources and personnel with the necessary skills and experience (WHO 1998). Health promotion evaluation can highlight changes in a range of outcomes relevant to the actions implemented (Nutbeam 1998). In oral health promotion evaluation a variety of outcome measures can be used to assess changes achieved at different points in the process of implementation (Watt *et al.* 2001).

Stage 4: implement plan

Only when the first stages have been completed should implementation commence. Failure to fully plan out the intervention invariably results in a disappointing outcome.

Stage 5: evaluate and review progress

Evaluating and reviewing the outcomes of the strategy identifies successes and failures, both of which are important to consider and reflect upon.

Public health approaches to caries and periodontal disease prevention

Food and nutrition policy to reduce non-milk extrinsic sugars levels

The main elements of food and nutrition policy are:

- to ensure the adequacy of the national diet in terms of its quantity, quality and variety at affordable prices;
- to ensure authoritative expert advice to Government, food producers and manufacturers, the public, hospitals, nurseries, schools and ;
- to give support to health and other professionals;
- to provide information about individual foods including labeling;
- to monitor trends in disease, health, nutritional status and diet;
- to undertake research to establish a sound scientific basis for policy.

The principal objective is to implement locally devised Food and Health Policies.

> A concerted set of actions based on scientific principles and intended to ensure the safety and the nutritional quality of the food supply and the accessibility of good, affordable, and properly labeled food for all population groups, as well as to encourage and facilitate the healthy use of food. Such policies are more likely to succeed where they reflect a consensus between all the parties concerned with the interest of the population in the foreground, and where there is government involvement and support (WHO 1990).

There are a range of possible roles for government to promote health through sponsored nutrition policies and programmes:

- development and use of cost-efficient mass strategies in nutrition education;
- advocacy for regulation of food standards, nutrient labeling, and advertising;
- formation of intersectoral mechanisms between government departments, NGOs, and the private sector to promote nutritional concerns in policy making, to coordinate efforts/avoid duplication and to coordinate desired changes;

- subsidies for primary food industries to encourage product development consistent with dietary guidelines;
- development of policy and guidelines for dietary practice in government institutions serving food (schools, hospitals, prisons, office canteens, trains);
- 'honest brokerage' of information: opposing misinformation;
- development of and participation in a national research strategy in nutrition; and
- training of health personnel in minimum standards of nutritional knowledge and skill.

It is desirable to:

- discourage importation and manufacture of sugar and sugar-containing products, particularly confectionery, biscuits, baby foods, and soft drinks;
- develop an agriculture policy to discourage growing sugar as a major cash crop;
- remove all NME sugars from infant and baby foods, paediatric medicines, fruit juices, and vitamin preparations;
- reduce the levels of NME sugars in commonly used foods and make available more sugar-free foods;
- reduce the NME sugars content of confections and drinks, and make available sugar-free foods and snacks and drinks;
- develop a catering policy in schools, colleges, large industries, institutions. The policy should ensure the provision of foods low in NME sugars;
- introduce an education policy stressing that NME sugars are nutritionally poor and decrease the nutrient density of foods;
- control advertising and misleading labels on products.

Policies to improve periodontal health

In a recent review of mechanical oral hygiene practices, Frandsen (1986) came to some important conclusions which have implications for public health aspects of periodontal disease. The conclusions are:

- There is no scientific evidence that one specific toothbrush type and design is more superior at removing plaque.
- The roll technique of toothbrushing is the least effective in removing plaque; no single method was superior to other methods.
- The optimal frequency and starting age for scaling and polishing has not been determined. The 6-month interval is unsubstantiated and is too general a recommendation.
- Regular instrumentation and polishing should not be carried out at disease-free sites.
- The role of root planing is questionable.
- Scaling, polishing, root planing, and surgical treatment of shallow periodontal pockets results in permanent loss of attachment.

Strategies for controlling periodontal diseases

Although severe periodontal disease is not widespread, the fact that the costs of treating the disease are high because of the organization of dental care, does qualify it as a dental public problem. In addition, the symptoms of periodontal diseases such as bleeding, halitosis, gingival recession, and tooth loss have an impact on many people. Furthermore, we have sufficient information to control the common forms of the disease (Sheiham 1991).

Four strategies can be considered:

- population strategy for altering behaviours and in particular oral cleaning effectiveness to reduce the dental plaque level of the community.
- secondary prevention strategy to detect and treat people with destructive periodontal disease.
- high-risk strategy for bringing preventive and therapeutic care to individuals at special risk.
- combined population, secondary prevention and high-risk strategy.

The high risk strategy screens people to identify those with unacceptably high plaque scores. Effective periodontal care for the high risk groups is difficult to achieve and maintain and costly in time and resources. A population strategy aims to reduce the plaque level of the whole population; moving the distribution curve to the left. Such a strategy saves more teeth than a high risk one, because, although high risk people lose more teeth per person, there are more low than high risk people. A whole population strategy, by lowering the overall plaque score, reduces the number of high risk people. A secondary prevention strategy aims to treat all persons with signs of early periodontal diseases such as gingivitis and shallow periodontal pockets. Current concepts of periodontal diseases and their treatment referred to earlier, cast serious doubts on the justification for such a strategy.

The population strategy is most likely to benefit the periodontal health of the majority of people because a small reduction overall of plaque per year will reduce the general level of periodontal disease. This should lead to the extraction of fewer teeth than if the bulk of resources is concentrated on a small number of high-risk people or on treating all those with early signs of periodontal diseases.

Case studies—health policies

- Food and nutrition policy to reduce non-milk extrinsic sugar levels
- Population strategy to reduce the dental plaque level of the community
- Secondary prevention strategy to detect and treat people with destructive periodontal disease

Practical examples of oral health promotion using the CRHFA and Ottawa Charter

Food in nurseries

Rather than focusing only upon caries prevention, an alternative approach is the development of a holistic nutrition programme, which aims to improve the overall nutritional status of preschool children. Such an approach will not only reduce non-milk extrinsic sugars consumption and hence improve oral health, but will also improve the overall quality of preschool children's diet, and thereby promote their growth and future development.

The range of potential partners involved in a preschool health promotion nutrition programme is outlined in Figure 15.7, together with the various actions that may be adopted. A wide range of sectors are involved in the food chain all of whom have a potential role. Rather than only focus attention on the consumers of food, this approach recognizes the importance of influencing key groups from food producers, to manufacturers to government departments (Sanderson 1984). Health education forms only one component part of the overall programme, and can be targeted at a range of influential partners and professionals, not only the public. Other complementary actions can address cost and access issues in relation to food.

In Brazil food policies in state nurseries have not only substantially reduced sugars consumption and improved the nutritional quality of the diet, but successfully reduced caries increments over a one year period (Rodrigues *et al.* 1999). The catering staff were allocated less sugar for cooking and baking and natural fruit

	Producer	Processor	Manufacturer	Inter mediaries	Caterers	Consumers	Government	Pressure Groups	Health Service Treaters
EDUCATION	—	—	—	—	—	—	—	—	—
PRICING	—	—	—	—	—		—		
PROVISION	—	—	—	—					
REGULATION	—	—	—	—	—	—	—	—	—

Figure 15.7 The food health policy matrix—a framework for identifying priorities for promotion of healthier eating (Sanderson 1984).

drinks replaced sugary drinks. Similar food policy guidelines have been introduced for nurseries, children in care and residential homes for older people in Britain (Caroline Walker Trust 1995; Caroline Walker Trust 1998).

Health promoting schools

An emerging dental public health problem in many countries is trauma to teeth and jaws, which is both expensive to treat and has a considerable impact on individuals' quality of life. The causes of dentally related trauma in children is accidents at school in relation to fighting, bullying, and sports. The individualized approach to prevention of trauma to front teeth is to treat children with protruding teeth by orthodontics or encourage the use of gum guards. This approach has had a minor effect on preventing trauma.

The WHO Health Promoting Schools programme offers an alternative approach to tackling the problem of dental trauma amongst adolescents (Moyses *et al.* 2002). Such an approach focuses upon the influence of the social and physical environment on health. The concept of the Health Promoting School places emphasis upon developing a range of complementary policies and actions to promote the health and well being of students, staff, and the wider community involved in the school. *A Health Promoting School can be characterized as a school constantly strengthening its capacity as a healthy setting for living, learning, and working.* In relation to accidents and the prevention of dental trauma, a wide range of actions and policies are possible (Table 15.7). All these depend upon collaborative working between staff, students, parents, education authorities, local government and health professionals.

The role of dentists in oral health promotion

Most dental public health officer involvement will be as health advocates. Health advocacy is the actions of health professionals and others with perceived authority in health, to influence the decisions and actions of individuals, communities, and government which influence health. Health advocacy involves educating senior government and community leaders and journalists—decision-makers in general, about specific issues, and setting the agenda to obtain political decisions that improve health of the population. To increase effectiveness, advocates work within the dominant philosophy in public health, namely, building partnerships with the community, other professional groups, and other sectors. They place their skills at the disposal of the community. Being on tap not on top.

Dentists must become team members in advocacy and education working with other organizations, government sectors, and with community organizations. The role of individual practitioners in prevention, is limited. Public health dentists should work as health advocates and co-ordinate local health promotion initiatives by first establishing a local Oral Health Promotion Group (OHPG) to develop an action plan, using goals and strategies as guidelines. They and other health promoters should work with industry to improve key products (such as low sugars and sugar-free snacks and drinks). Other interventions require government action, most notably developing policies on sugar production and promotion, safer environments to enhance social cohesion and reduce violence and accidents.

Dental practitioners should:

- maximize use of available staff, including dental therapists, oral health promoters, and hygienists and other local resources, including community groups,

- agree on local initiatives, aimed, for example, at those at particular risk of chronic diseases or those who may prove particularly susceptible to behaviour change (e.g. adolescents)

- agree on a means for assessing, recording, and monitoring diet in the whole practice population,

- develop means for the delivery of effective counselling to promote healthy nutrition

- agree on targets which will allow these practice-based initiatives to be evaluated

Within the health service oral health promoters should be active in the training of other primary health care workers (including dental) and care workers outside the health services. Support should be given to carers in the youth education and welfare services. This should include the promotion of oral health of individual workers, as they are unlikely to accept responsibility to promote good oral health habits in their clients unless they are supported in their efforts to achieve good oral health for themselves.

Conclusions

The main reasons for the dramatic decline in dental caries in industrialized countries are related more to health promotion

Table 15.7 Prevention of oral injuries through Health Promoting Schools

- Personel and social education aimed at developing life skills—focus upon conflict resolution, dealing with relationship problems and health skills in relation to the misuse of alcohol and drugs.

- School policy on bullying and violence between students to create a supportive social environment within school.

- Physical environment—play areas, sports fields all monitored for safety and security.

- School health policy—resources and training for staff in first aid procedures.

- Alcohol policy—restriction on alcohol consumption within school premises.

- Provision of mouth guards—accessible and affordable sports protection.

- Links with health services—procedures for emergency treatment established, screening programmes staff training and support in health issues.

than to dental services (Nadanovsky and Sheiham 1994). All preventive measures require economic, social, and political strategies to ensure their acceptance, implementation, and effectiveness. A public oral health strategy directed at reducing the consumption of sugars, and promoting water fluoridation and fluoridated toothpaste will reduce the prevalence of dental caries to a level where it will be an insignificant problem. The policies and community health promotion presented here have been widely accepted by international, national, and local groups as well as public and community health practitioners. By adopting a health promotion, common risk/health factor approach and integrating oral health with general health policies, policies to promote oral health should become more effective and efficient. What is more, oral health will cease to be marginalized. Dentists must become team members in advocacy and education with other organizations, government sectors, and with community organizations.

References

Brown, L. (1994). *Research in dental health education and health promotion: a review of the literature. Health Education Quarterly*, 21, 83–102.

Burr, M.L. and Elwood, P.C. (1985). Research and development of health promotion services—screening. In *Oxford Textbook of Public Health*, Vol III (ed. W.W. Holland, R. Detels and G. Knox), pp. 373–84. Oxford University Press, Oxford.

Caroline Walker Trust (1995). Eating well for older people. Practical and nutritional guidelines for food in residential and nursing homes and for community meals. Report of an expert working group. Caroline Walker Trust, London.

Caroline Walker Trust (1998). Nutritional guidelines for under 5's in child care: Report of an expert working group. Caroline Walker Trust, London.

Culyer, A.J. (1993). *Equity and Health Care Policy. A Discussion Paper*. Research and Policy Group, Premier's Council on Health, Well-being and Social Justice, Ontario. (Mimeo).

Frandsen, A. (1986). Mechanical oral hygiene practises. In *Dental Plaque Control Measures and Oral Hygiene Practices*. (H. Loe, and D.V. Kleinman eds.) pp. 93–116. IRL Press, Oxford.

Graham, H. (1990). Behaving well: women's health Behaviour in context. In *Women's Health Counts* (H. Roberts ed.), Routledge, London.

Green, L.W. and Kreuter, M. (1990). Health promotion as a public health strategy for the 1990s. *Annual Review of Public Health*, 11, 319–34.

Johnson, N. (1991). *Risk Markers for Oral Diseases. Dental Caries: Markers of High and Low Risk Groups and Individuals*. Cambridge University Press, Cambridge.

Kay, L. and Locker, D. (1996). Is dental health education effective? A systematic review of current evidence. *Community Dentistry and Oral Epidemiology*, 24, 231–35.

Kay, L. and Locker, D. (1998). *A Systematic Review of the Effectiveness of Health Promotion Aimed at Promoting Oral Health*. Health Education Authority, London.

Krieger, N. (1994). Epidemiology and the web of causation: has anyone seen the spider? *Social Sciences and Medicine*, 39, 887–903.

Link, B.G. and Phelan, J. (1995). Social conditions as fundamental causes of disease. *J. Health & Behavior*, (Extra Issue), 80–94.

Marmot, M. and Wilkinson, R. (1999). *Social Determinants of Health*. Oxford University Press, Oxford.

McDonald, S.P. and Sheiham, A. (1992). The distribution of caries on different tooth surfaces at varying levels of caries—a compilation of data from 18 previous studies. *Community Dental Health*, 9, 39–48.

McKeown, T. (1979). *The Role of Medicine*. Basil Blackwell, Oxford.

McKinlay, J.B. (1974). A case for refoccussing upstream—the political economy of illness. Proceedings of the American Heart Association. Conference on applying behavioral sciences to cardiovascular risk, pp. 7–17, American Heart Association, Seattle.

Milio, N. (1986). *Promoting Health Through Public Policy*. Canadian Public Health Association, Ottawa.

Milio, N. (1987). *Healthy Public Policy: Issues and Scenarios*. Symposium on Healthy Public Policy, Yale University.

Milio, N. (1988). Making healthy public policy. *Health Promotion*, 2, 263–74.

Moysés, S.T., Moysés, S.J., Watt, R.G. and Sheiham, A. (in press). The impact of health promotion schools policies on oral health of 12 year olds. *Health Promotion International*

Nadanovsky, P. and Sheiham, A. (1994). The relative contribution of dental services to the changes and geographical variations in caries status of 5- and 12-year-old children in England and Wales in the 1980s. *Community Dental Health*, 11, 215–223.

Nutbeam, D. (1998). Evaluating health promotion—progress, problems and solutions. *Health Promotion International*, 13, 27–44.

Rodrigues, C.S., Watt, R.G., and Sheiham, A. (1999). Effects of dietary guidelines on sugar intake and dental caries in 3-year olds attending nurseries in Brazil. *Health Promotion International*, 14, 329–35.

Rose, G. (1992). *The Strategy of Preventive Medicine*. Oxford University Press, Oxford.

Rugg-Gunn, A. and Nunn, J. (1999). *Nutrition, Diet and Oral Health*. Oxford University Press, Oxford.

Sanderson, M. E. (1984) Strategies for implementing NACNE recommendations. *Lancet*, **10**, 1352–6.

Sheiham, A. (1991). Public health aspects of periodontal diseases in Europe. *Journal of Clinical Periodontology*, **18**, 362–9.

Sheiham, A. (2000). Improving oral health for all: focussing on determinants and conditions. *Health Education Journal*, **59**, 351–63.

Sheiham, A. and Joffe, M. (1991). Public dental health strategies for identifying and controlling dental caries in high and low risk populations. In: *Risk Markers for Oral Diseases. Dental Caries: Markers of High and Low Risk Groups and Individuals* Vol. 1. (ed. N.W. Johnson), pp. 445–8. Cambridge University Press, Cambridge.

Sheiham, A. and Watt, R.G. (2000). The common risk factor approach: a rational approach for promoting oral health. *Community Dentistry and Oral Epidemiology*, **28**, 399–406.

Schou, L. and Locker, D. (1994). *Oral health: A Review of the Effectiveness of Health Education and Health Promotion*. Dutch Centre for Health Promotion and Health Education, Amsterdam.

Sprod, A., Anderson, R., and Treasure, E. (1996). *Effective oral health promotion. Literature Review*. Health Promotion Wales, Cardiff.

Watt, R.G., Fuller, S.S., Harnett, R., Treasure, E.T., and Stillman-Lowe, C. (2001). Oral health promotion evaluation—time for development. *Community Dentistry and Oral Epidemiology*, **29**, 161–6.

Whitehead, M. (1991). The concepts and principles of equity and health. *Health Promotion*, **6**, 217–28.

World Health Organization (1978). Alma-Ata 1978: Primary Health Care. Report of the International Conference on Primary Health Care, Alma-Ata, USSR, September 1978. World Health Organization, Geneva.

World Health Organization (1981). *Global Strategy for Health for All by the year 2000*, WHO, Health for All Series No. 3, World Health Organization, Geneva.

World Health Organization (1982). *A Review of Current Recommendations for the Organization and Administration of Community Oral Health Services in Northern and Western Europe*. Report of a WHO Workshop. World Health Organization Regional Office for Europe, Copenhagen.

World Health Organization (1984). *Health Promotion. A Discussion Document on the Concept and Principles*. World Health Organization Regional Office for Europe, Copenhagen.

World Health Organization (1986). *The Ottawa Charter for Health Promotion. Health Promotion 1*, pp. iii–v. World Health Organization, Geneva.

World Health Organization (1990). *Food and Nutrition Policy for Europe*. Report of a WHO Conference, Budapest 1990, p. 12. EUR/ICP/NUT 133. World Health Organization Regional Office for Europe, Copenhagen.

World Health Organization (1991). *Diet, nutrition, and the prevention of chronic diseases*. Technical Report. Series 797, World Health Organization, Geneva.

World Health Organization (1998). *Health Promotion Evaluation: Recommendations to Policy Makers*. Copenhagen: World Health Organization, Geneva.

16

Developing the concept of prevention—evidence-based dentistry

Developing the concept of prevention—evidence-based dentistry

John Murray

Introduction

Evidence that the oral health of a community is improving can be shown by properly coordinated epidemiological studies. Evidence that a particular treatment is an improvement on previously accepted treatments or protocols is best shown by systematic reviews, prospective clinical studies, ideally by randomized control trials.

Secular decline in caries in children

The suggestion that the dental caries rates in English children were declining was cautiously put forward by Palmer in 1980. The theme of a decline in dental caries took on an international flavour when a conference was held in Boston in 1982. Speakers from Denmark, Ireland, the Netherlands, New Zealand, Norway, Scotland, Sweden, and the United States all confirmed that a downward trend in dental caries in children and young adults had occurred in the 1970s (Glass 1982, Table 16.1).

Data from the Netherlands was important, because it showed that the decline in caries had occurred in both primary and permanent dentitions (Figs 16.1 and 16.2). Perhaps the most important diagram illustrating the downward trend was compiled from the WHO Global Oral Data Bank (Fig. 16.3), giving DMFT values in 12-year-old children using the period 1967–83, from nine 'westernized' or developed countries. This decline in caries in permanent teeth in children and adolescents should lead to a greater retention of teeth in adult life.

Trends in edentulousness

The standard of dental health in a country depends in part on the attitude of the population to dental care, and the resources available for dental treatment. There is also a historical perspective in that treatment available to a population in the past often makes itself felt in the statistics of the present. For example, the 'management' of periodontal disease during the 1930s to 1950s in the UK, by the extraction of teeth and the provision of dentures, has

Table 16.1 Declining dental caries in various countries (references in Glass 1982)

Author	Country	Age of subjects (years)	Year of examination	Mean DMFT
Fejerskov *et al.*	Denmark	20	1972	16.6
Fejerskov *et al.*	Denmark	20	1982	11.8
O'Mullane	Eire	8–9	1961	8.0
O'Mullane	Eire	8–9	1979	4.4
Brown	New Zealand	12–13	1950	7.9
Brown	New Zealand	12–13	1982	4.1
Von der Fehr	Norway	15	1970	32.0*
Von der Fehr	Norway	15	1979	15.0*
Downer	Scotland	10	1970	5.0
Downer	Scotland	10	1980	3.6
Carlos	USA	6–11	1971–74	1.7
Carlos	USA	6–11	1979–80	1.1
Carlos	USA	6–11	1971–74	6.2
Carlos	USA	6–11	1979–80	4.6

*DMFS values.

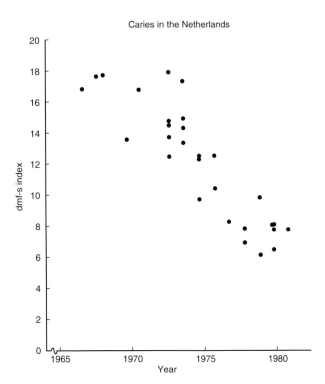

Figure 16.1 dmfs values for 6-year-old children from the Netherlands. (Kalsbeek 1982.)

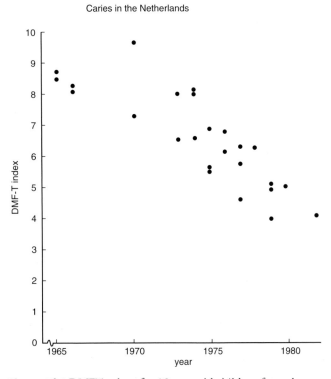

Figure 16.2 DMFT values for 12-year-old children from the Netherlands. (Kalsbeek 1982.)

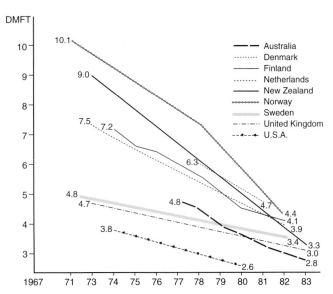

Figure 16.3 Trends in dental caries 1967–83 DMFT as 12 years. (Source: Who Global Oral Data Bank: Renson et al. 1986.)

Table 16.2 Prevalance of edentulousness in various European countries (WHO 1986).

Country	Per cent edentulous	
	35–44 yrs	65+ yrs
Austria	–	30
Denmark	8.0	60
Finland	15.0	65
GDR	0.5	58
Hungary	–	18
Ireland	12.0	72
Malta	–	50
Morocca	2.8	–
Netherlands	18.0	70
Poland	13.5	–
Portugal	2.0	–
Sweden	1.0	20
Switzerland	–	25
United Kingdom	13.0	79

resulted in a high prevalence of edentulousness. The finding in the first national survey in England and Wales carried out in 1968 that 37 per cent of adults over the age of 16 years had no natural teeth, certainly focused attention on the dental needs of adults (Gray *et al*. 1970). Even if the pattern of dental treatment changed immediately, from extraction towards restoration and prevention, those already rendered edentulous will feature in the statistics until they die. A summary of edentulousness in various European countries (WHO 1986) shows the UK almost at the bottom of the list in terms of edentulousness at two age groups (Table 16.2). Edentulousness has continued to decline in the UK. The proportion of

Table 16.3 Predictions of total tooth loss in the United Kingdom (Kelly *et al.* 2002)

Age	Percentage edentate in 1998	Predicted future levels for 2008	2018	2028
16–24	0	0	0	0
25–34	0.5	0	0	0
35–44	1	1	1	1
45–54	6	2	2	2
55–64	20	9	5	5
65–74	36	23	12	8
75–84	53	39	26	15
85 and over	81	55	44	31
All	13	8	5	4

adults aged 16 and over in this category fell to 29 per cent in 1978, 21 per cent in 1988, and 13 per cent in 1998.

The 1998 UK Adult Dental Health Survey gave a prediction of future levels of total tooth loss up to 2028, indicating a continuing marked decline in edentulousness even over the age of 85 years (Table 16.3). However, for very elderly people (85 and over) it is obvious that complete dentures will still be needed; 81 per cent of this age group were edentulous in 1998; this proportion, at current projections, is due to fall to 31 per cent by 2028.

Trends in the dentate adult population

The 1998 Adult Dental Health Survey provided important information on the status of dentate adults. The overall picture for dentate adults of all ages conceals large differences in the disease and treatment experience of each age cohort. Among young people the level of disease experience is low, while in the middle age groups there is a greater reliance on restorative treatment. In the oldest age group (those aged 55 or more) missing teeth form a large part of the overall tooth condition and make a significant impact on the overall mouth status (Kelly *et al.* 2000) (Fig. 16.4). The challenge for the future, in terms of prevention, is to maintain the number of sound untreated teeth in the 16–24-year-old cohort, through to age 55 years and beyond.

Trends in oral health

- Decline in caries in children observed from the late 1970's
- Benefits observed in both dentitions
- Edentulousness in Britain was high in the 1970s but is improving dramatically.
- 30 per cent of those over 85 years will need complete dentures, even in 2028
- Discernable improvements in the pattern of restoration and tooth loss in the dentate population

Impact of evidence-based dentistry on clinical practice

In addition to primary prevention of disease, the impact of a preventive approach can also be found in the efforts made to identify best practice, avoid unnecessary treatment, provide the most appropriate care, and reduce the need for further intervention.

Impacted wisdom teeth

The prophylactic removal of impacted wisdom teeth, has been the subject of considerable debate recently. Firm views for and against the practice of removing impacted wisdom teeth have been expressed; a systematic review came to the following conclusions: (NHS Centre for reviews and dissemination 1998):

- Third molar surgery rates vary widely across the UK.
- Around 35% of third molars removed for prophylactic purposes are disease free.
- Surgical removal of third molars can only be justified when clear long-term benefit to the patient is expected.
- It is not possible to predict reliably whether impacted third molars will develop pathological change if they are not removed.
- There are no randomiszed control studies to compare the long term outcome of early removal with retention of pathology-free third molars.
- In the absence of good evidence to support prophylactic removal, there appears to be little justification for the routine removal of pathology-free impacted third molars.
- To ensure appropriate treatment referrals, waiting lists for the surgical removal of third molars should be monitored through a process of audit.

In a recent study to identify the least costly, most effective and most cost-effective management strategy for a symptomatic disease-free mandibular third molar, it was concluded that retention of these teeth is less costly to the NHS, more effective for the patient, and more cost effective to both parties than removal. However, should the likelihood of developing repeat episodes of pericoronitis, periodontal disease, and caries increase substantially, then removal becomes the more cost-effective strategy (Edwards *et al.* 1999).

The 'Key Message' in the compendium 'Clinical Evidence' was 'We found limited evidence suggesting that the harm of removing asymptomatic impacted wisdom teeth outweigh the benefits' (Clinical Evidence 2001).

Dhariwal, Goodey, and Shepherd (2002) provided some important data in their review of trends in Oral Surgery in England and Wales 1991–2000. The frequencies of oral surgical procedures was derived from the Dental Practice Board Digest of Statistics. The number of impacted third molar extractions in the General Dental Service increased steadily until 1997, after which there was a 32 per cent decrease to 2000 (Fig. 16.5) coinciding with the

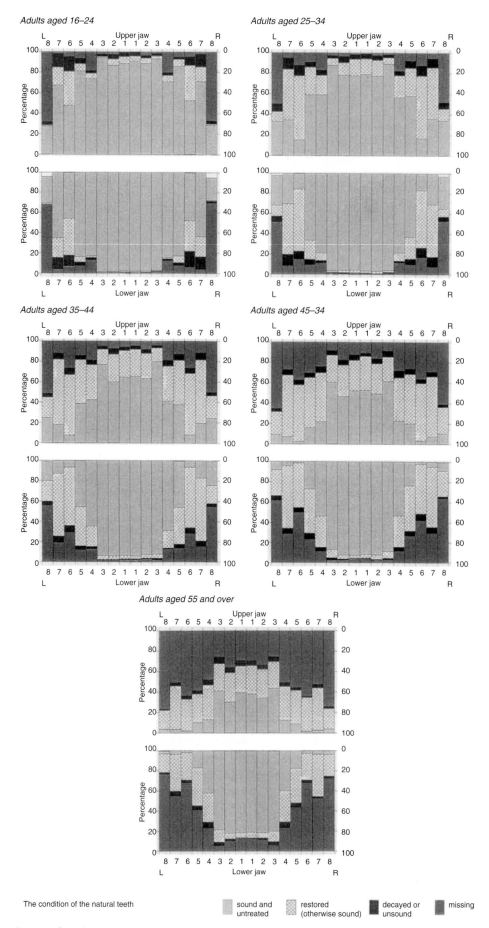

Figure 16.4 Distribution of tooth conditions around the mouth in dentate patients in the UK 1998. (Kelly *et al.* 2000.)

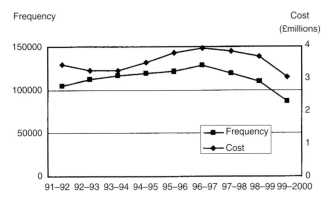

Figure 16.5 Frequency and cost of impacted third molars extractions in GDS 1991–1999. (Dhariwal, Goodey and Shepherd 2002.)

shift in emphasis to a more conservative approach to the management of impacted wisdom teeth.

Protecting the lingual nerve during lower third molar removal

Robinson and Smith (1996) reported that surgery with lingual flap retraction resulted in lingual sensory disturbance in 6.9 per cent of cases, whereas surgery without lingual flap retraction resulted in lingual sensory disturbance in 0.8 per cent of cases. They concluded that, for the majority of cases involving lower third molar removal, lingual retraction should be avoided. This conclusion was supported by Gargallo-Albiol *et al.* (2000).

Periodontal surgery vs. non-surgical approach

In periodontics, there has been considerable expansion over the last 20 years of the evidence base for non-surgical management as the principal intervention for the treatment of periodontal diseases. The initial evidence emerged from pivotal clinical studies reported in the 1980s. For example, non-surgical treatment, scaling, and root planning, was found to be comparable, with respect to long-term clinical outcomes, to three different surgical procedures using a split mouth design (Hill *et al.* 1981). At the same time, a series of reports by Badersten's group confirmed the long-term effectiveness of scaling and root planning, and demonstrated clearly that this treatment is effective, even in very deep pockets (8–12mm) for which periodontal surgery would previously have been thought to be both essential and inevitable (Badersten *et al.* 1984).

The biological basis for periodontal healing following treatment is also now better understood. It is widely accepted that periodontally affected tissues, including the ulcerated pocket epithelium, retain the inherent capacity for regeneration. The indications for some surgical procedures such as soft tissue or pocket curettage, pocket elimination, and bone resection are no longer apparent. The objective of scaling and root planning is to achieve a root surface that is free of plaque and calculus deposits,

as well as bacterial endotoxins and which is, therefore, biologically compatible with the formation of a long junctional epithelium. Perhaps a better description and a more contemporary term for this process is root surface debridement.

One of the traditional disadvantages with subgingival instrumentation has been the restricted access to deep pockets, furcations, and other anatomically complex sites. To some extent, this problem has been overcome by the introduction of new generation instruments, both manual and power-driven, which have improved the efficiency of root instrumentation. Furthermore, residual pathogens that might remain following root planning, for example in the pocket epithelium or the adjacent connective tissues, can be targeted more specifically using locally delivered, slow-release antimicrobials that have been introduced during the 1990s. This means that the aims of root surface debridement can now be achieved more effectively and consistently than has hitherto been possible and the need for periodontal surgery has been reduced considerably.

Endodontics—Retreatment vs. root-end surgery

Root canal treatment usually fails because of persistent root canal infection. This can be managed non-surgically by cleaning and resealing the pulp space, or surgically to remove the root-end (apicectomy) and periapical lesion before filling the root entrance to seal in its contents.

Many studies have evaluated surgical and non-surgical retreatment individually, with highly variable and conflicting results (reviewed by Friedman 1998). Few have directly compared surgical and non-surgical outcomes, but neither the retrospective study of Allen (1989), nor the prospective, randomized investigation of Kvist and Reit (1999) showed any systematic difference. Decision-making is, therefore, based on individual case-related factors, which usually favour the less invasive non-surgical approach (European Society of Endodontology 1994).

Data from the Dental Practice Board Digest of Statistics (Dhariwal, Goodey, and Shepherd 2002) show that the annual number of apicectomies fell by 56 per cent between 1991–92 and 1999–2000 (Fig. 16.6).

Recent and rapid technological advances in non-surgical and surgical endodontics (operating microscopes, NiTi rotary instrumentation, thermoplastic obturation, ultrasonic retropreparation, new retrofilling materials) may reinforce or change this view, but evidence on their clinical effectiveness is not yet available.

Notable changes in clinical practice, moving towards a more conservative approach to

- removal of impacted wisdom teeth
- need for periodontal surgery
- non-surgical endodontic treatment

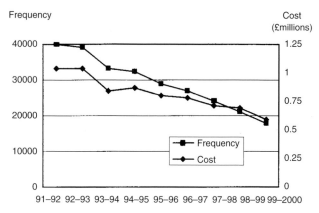

Figure 16.6 Number and costs of apicectomies in the GDS in England and Wales 1991–1999

Treatment of aphthous ulcers

The aims of treatment of aphthous ulcers (see Chapter 11) are to reduce pain as well as the frequency and duration of ulceration, with minimal adverse effects. Suggested treatments include topical corticosteroids, chlorhexidine, and hexidine. Nine small randomized control trials found no consistent effect of topical corticosteroids on the incidence of new ulcers, compared with control preparations. They found weak evidence that topical corticosteroids may reduce duration of ulcers and hasten pain relief, without causing notable local or systemic adverse effects. Randomized control trials (RCTs) have found that chlorhexidine gluconate mouth rinses may reduce the duration and severity of each episode of ulceration, but do not affect the incidence of recurrent ulceration. There is no evidence of benefit from hexidine mouthwash or from a proprietary antiseptic mouthwash compared with control mouthwashes (Clinical Evidence 2001).

Oral mucositis in patients receiving chemotherapy

Oral mucositis is a well-known complication of chemotherapy (see Chapter 11). Clarkson, Worthington and Eden (2001) evaluated the effectiveness of oral and topical prophylactic agents for oral mucositis and oral candidiasis in patients with cancer (excluding head and neck cancer) compared with placebo or no control. Only randomized and quasi-randomized controlled trials were eligible for inclusion in their review. Only ice chips showed any benefit in preventing mucositis. None of the other seven agents examined (chlorhexidine, prostaglandin, glutamine, sucralfate, molgramostim, camomile, and allupurinol mouthwash) showed any benefit.

Infective endocarditis, dentistry, and antibiotic prophylaxis

In a recent article Seymour *et al*. (2000) suggested that it was time for a re-think on antimicrobial prophylaxis in dentistry. The authors point out that dental procedures, especially those that result in a bacteraemia, are frequently blamed for infective endocarditis (IE), hence the need for antibiotic prophylaxis to cover such procedure in at risk patients. This has been the clinical doctrine and teaching for the past 50 years. Recent evidence from the USA and the Netherlands challenges the practice of prescribing antibiotics before dental procedures to prevent endocarditis. In addition there is increasing concern over the unnecessary use of antibiotics. They summarized the situation as follows:

> Four recent studies of endocarditis patients either fail to show a dental connection with infective endocarditis, or can only show a small one, although the study designs are low in the hierarchy of validity and can be criticised. Other contributors to the debate add that the dangers of chemoprophylaxis outweigh the dangers of endocarditis and that chemoprophylaxis is poorly identified even when at risk patients are identified. Indeed there is evidence to suggest that spontaneous bacteraemia (rather than dental treatment) are most likely to be the cause of IE in at-risk individuals. If this is the case, then the use of antibiotic prophylaxis needs to be reconsidered and a greater emphasis placed on improving oral health in these patients.

Antibiotic cover for patients with joint prostheses

Antibiotic prophylaxis for patients with prosthetic joints still remains a contentious issue, despite reports and guidelines from the British Society for Antimicrobial Chemotherapy, the American Dental Association, the American Academy of Orthopaedic Surgeons, the British Orthopaedic Association, and the British Dental Association. Seymour *et al*. (2002) comment that very few orthopaedic surgeons request dental advice before joint replacement, but many insist on antibiotic cover before dental treatment. They believe that 'patients would be better served all round, and hence at a lesser risk of joint infection, if they attended to their oral health before surgery, as opposed to relying upon the dubious practice of antibiotic prophylaxis'.

Organization of services—clinical governance

Virtually every branch of dentistry can point to changes either in clinical practice, in order to prevent untoward incidents, to developments in clinical guidelines, aimed at focusing action on those most likely to benefit, or to improving the organization of services.

At a corporate level all organizations, whether dental practices, dental schools or hospitals must embrace clinical governance: 'a framework through which organisations are accountable for continuously improving the quality of their services and safeguarding high standards of care by creating an environment in which excellence in clinical care will flourish'. Figure 16.7 shows

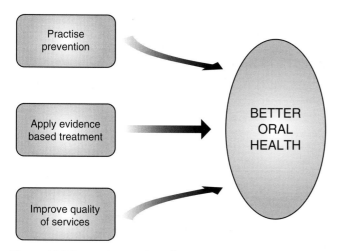

Figure 16.7 Prevention, evidence based treatment, and clinical governance.

in diagrammatic form how prevention, evidence-based treatment, and clinical governance can work together to improve oral health.

The six monthly recall examination

The Department of Health asked the West Midlands Technology Assessment Group to carry out a 'rapid systematic review' of the Clinical Effectiveness and Cost Effectiveness of Routine Dental Checks. From a pool of over 2500 citations and abstracts, the results of 29 studies were considered in detail. For the investigation of the relationship between dental check-up frequency and measures of caries, there was a preponderance of studies reporting an increase in caries and a decrease in the number of teeth, and a decrease in fillings with decreasing dental check-up frequencies in permanent teeth.

Considering periodontal disease, with the exception of one single study reporting a significant increase in attachment level with increasing dental check-up frequency, there was no consistency in the detection of the effect of different dental check frequencies on the permanent dentition and bleeding, probing depth, presence of plaque or calculus, gingivitis; and periodontal health.

Two studies involving oral cancer demonstrated a significant increase in tumour size and advancement of the stage at diagnosis with a decrease in dental check-up frequency for checks at 12-month intervals.

The study concluded that there is little existing evidence to support or refute the practice of encouraging 6-monthly dental checks in adults and children (Taylor personal communication). The analysis demonstrated that cost-effectiveness varies across risk groups, and therefore, consideration should be given to whether a population re-call policy or a re-call policy based on risk would be more acceptable. There is a need for further primary research addressing the role of the dental check and its effectiveness in different oral diseases.

Services for children born with cleft lip/palate

Studies by the Royal College of Surgeons Audit Committee and the Clinical Standards Advisory Group showed that the results from most centres in Britain compared unfavourably with long-term results from the best units in Europe. Over 70 surgeons were involved from 57 centres in the United Kingdom. As there are about 1000 babies born with this condition every year, most surgeons were 'low-volume operators'. The CSAG report, accepted by the Government in 1998, suggested that services should be concentrated into a small number of expert centres (between 8–15 centres for the whole of the UK), fully staffed and equipped with appropriate facilities. The concentration of services does not in itself guarantee improved outcomes, but does allow a smaller number of surgeons to become 'high-volume operators'. The outcomes from each centre must be audited rigorously, both within the UK and compared with the best in Europe, to ensure an improvement in standards. Thus, not only does the expertise of the individual specialists involved (surgeons, orthodontists, paediatric dentists, speech and language therapists etc.) need to develop, but the organization of services provided by each centre, must continually improve.

Changes in clinical practice include

- Need for antimicrobial prophylaxis
- New guidelines on six monthly examination

Conclusions

The issues raised in the previous two sections reflect my personal views concerning the changing practice of dentistry since the first edition of this book was published twenty years ago. The list is by no means comprehensive: the reader may well point to other aspects which might have been included.

A more reflective or evidence-based approach to dental disease and its management can now be discerned. Further developments, both individual and corporate, are required if the practice of dentistry, and the oral health of the population, is going to continue to improve. At the individual professional level, a personal commitment to continuing professional development is required, and will be regulated in the UK by the General Dental Council. At a corporate level all organizations must continuously improve their services.

Finally, and of greatest importance, the public at large must appreciate the vital role they have to play in maintaining their own oral health. It is hoped that this book helps to stimulate and guide changes in all sectors of the oral health community, so that further improvements in oral health are achieved.

References

Allen, R.K., Newton, C.W., and Brown, C.E. (1989). A statistical analysis of surgical and nonsurgical endodontic retreatment cases. *Journal of Endodontics*, **15**, 261–6.

Badersten, A., Nilveus, R., and Egelberg, J. (1984). Effect of nonsurgical periodontal therapy. II. Severely advanced periodontitis. *Journal of Clinical Periodontology*, 11, 63–76.

Clarkson, J.E., Worthington, H.V., and Eden, O.B. (2001). Interventions for preventing oral mucositis or oral candidiasis for patients with cancer receiving chemotherapy (excluding head and neck cancer). Update Software Ltd, The Cochrane Library, 3.

Clinical Evidence (2001). A compendium of the best available evidence for effective health care. BMJ Publishing Group, London.

Dhariwal, D.K., Goodey, R., and Shepherd, J.P. (2002). Trends in oral surgery in England and Wales 1991–2000. *Br. Dent. J.*, 192, 639–45.

Edwards, M.J., Brickley, M.R., Goodey, R.D., and Shepherd, J.P. The cost, effectiveness and cost effectiveness of removal and retention of asymptomatic, disease free third molars. *Br. Dent. J.*, 187, 375.

European Society of Endodontology (1994). Consensus report of the European Society of Endodontology on quality guidelines for endodontic treatment. *International Endodontic Journal*, 27, 115–24.

Friedman, S. (1998). Treatment outcome and prognosis of endodontic therapy. Chapter 15 In: D., Orstavik T.R., Pitt Ford (eds) *Essential Endodontology: Prevention and Treatment of Apical Periodontitis*. Oxford, Blackwell Science: 367–401.

Gargallo-Albiol, J., Buenechea, R., and Gay-Escoda, C. (2000). Lingual nerve protection during surgical removal of lower third molar. A prospective randomised study. *Int. J. Oral. Maxillofac. Surg.*, 29, 268–71.

Glass, R.I. (ed) (1982). The first international conference on the declining prevalence of dental caries. *J. Dent. Res.*, 61, (Special Issue), 1301–83.

Gray, P.G., Todd, J.E., Slack, G.I., and Bulman, J.S. (1970). *Adult Dental Health in England and Wales in 1968*. HMSO, London.

Hill, R.W., Raamfjord, S.P., Morrison, E.C., Appleberry, E.A., Caffesse, R.G., Kerry, G.J., and Nissle, R.R. (1981). Four types of periodontal treatment compared over 2 years. *Journal of Periodontology*, 52, 655–62.

Kalsbeek, H. (1982). Evidence of decrease in prevalence of dental caries in the Netherlands: an evaluation of epidemiological caries survey on 4–6 and 11–15 year old children between 1965 and 1980. *J. Dent. Res.*, 61 (Special Issue), 1321–6.

Kelly, M., Steele, J.G., Nuttall, N., Bradnock, G., Morris, J., Nunn, J.H., Pine, C., Pitts, N., Treasure, E., and White, D., (2000). *Adult Dental Health Survey. Oral Health in the United Kingdom 1998*, Government Statistical Service, HMSO.

Kvist, T., and Reit, C. (1999). Results of endodontic retreatment: a randomised clinical study comparing surgical and nonsurgical procedures. *Journal of Endodontics*, 12, 814–7.

The management of patients with impacted third molar (wisdom) teeth. NHS Centre for Reviews and Disseminations (1998).

Palmer, J.D. (1980). Dental health in children—an improving picture? *Br. Dent. J.*, 149, 48–50.

Robinson, P.P., and Smith, K.G. (1996). Lingual nerve damage during lower third molar removal: a comparison of two surgical techniques. *Br. Dent. J.*, 180, 456–461.

Seymour, R.A., Lowry, R., Whitworth, J.M., and Martin, M.V. (2000). Infective endocarditis, dentistry and antibiotic prophylaxis; time for a rethink? *Br. Dent. J.*, 189, 610–6.

Seymour, R.A., Whitworth, J.M., and Martin, M. (2002). Antibiotic cover for patients with joint prostheses—Still a dilemma for dental practitioners. Personal Communication.

World Health Organization (1986). *Country Profiles on Oral Health in Europe 1986*. WHO, Geneva.

Index